Pediatrics, Child and Adolescent Health

Pediatrics, Child and Adolescent Health is a book series with publications from a multidisciplinary group of researchers, practitioners and clinicians for an international professional forum interested in the broad spectrum of pediatric medicine, child health, adolescent health and human development.

Joav Merrick, MD, MMedSci, DMSc, born and educated in Denmark is Professor of Pediatrics affiliated with the Division of Pediatrics, Hadassah Hebrew University Medical Center, Mt Scopus Campus, Jerusalem, Israel, Kentucky Children's Hospital, University of Kentucky, Lexington, United States and Professor of Public Health at the Center for Healthy Development, School of Public Health, Georgia State University, Atlanta, United States, the former medical director of the Disability Administration, Ministry of Social Affairs and Social Services, Jerusalem and the founder and director of the National Institute of Child Health and Human Development in Israel. Email: jmerrick@zahav.net.il

nova
Medicine & Health
New York

Pediatrics, Child and Adolescent Health

Adventure Education and Positive Youth Development in Aotearoa, New Zealand
Damian Scarf (Editor)
2022. ISBN: 978-1-68507-753-2 (Softcover)
2022. ISBN: 978-1-68507-848-5 (eBook)

Chronic Disease and Disability: The Pediatric Kidney, Second Edition
Donald E. Greydanus, MD, Dr HC (Athens), FAAP, FIAP (HON) (Editor)
Vimal Master Sankar Raj, MD (Editor)
John D. Rowlett, MD (Editor)
Cheryl Dickson, MD (Editor)
Joav Merrick, MD, MMedSci, DMSc (Editor)
2022. ISBN: 978-1-68507-716-7 (Hardcover)
2022. ISBN: 978-1-68507-850-8 (eBook)

Why Do Children Die? Selective Perspectives on Thanatology in Pediatrics
Donald E. Greydanus, MD, Dr HC (Athens), FAAP, FIAP (HON) (Editor)
Dustin C. Rowland, MS (Editor)
Joav Merrick, MD, MMedSci, DMSc (Editor)
2022. ISBN: 978-1-68507-461-6 (Hardcover)
2021. ISBN: 978-1-68507-597-2 (eBook)

Preventing Child Abuse: Critical Roles and Multiple Perspectives
Vincent J Palusci, MD, MS (Editor)
Frank E. Vandervort, JD (Editor)
Donald E Greydanus, MD, Dr HC (Athens), FAAP, FIAP (HON) (Editor)
Joav Merrick, MD, MMedSci, DMSc (Editor)
2021. ISBN: 978-1-53619-268-1 (Hardcover)
2022. ISBN: 978-1-53619-696-2 (eBook)

Adolescence: International Aspects of Psychological Stress
Supa Pengpid, MPH, DrPH, MBA (Editor)
Karl Peltzer, MA Clin Psych, PhD (Editor)
Joav Merrick, MD, MMedSci, DMSc (Editor)
2021. ISBN: 978-1-53619-341-1 (Hardcover)
2021. ISBN: 978-1-53619-652-8 (eBook)

More information about this series can be found at
https://novapublishers.com/product-category/series/pediatrics-child-and-adolescent-health/

Donald E. Greydanus, Dilip R. Patel,
Ahsan Nazeer, Roger W. Apple and Joav Merrick
Editors

Behavioral Pediatrics II

Neuropsychiatry, Sexuality and Eating Disorders. Fifth Edition

nova
Medicine & Health
New York

https://doi.org/10.52305/WGEQ3285

Library of Congress Cataloging-in-Publication Data

ISBN: 979-8-88697-019-7

Published by Nova Science Publishers, Inc. † New York

Dedication for this 5th Edition

Helen D Pratt, PhD (1948-2020)

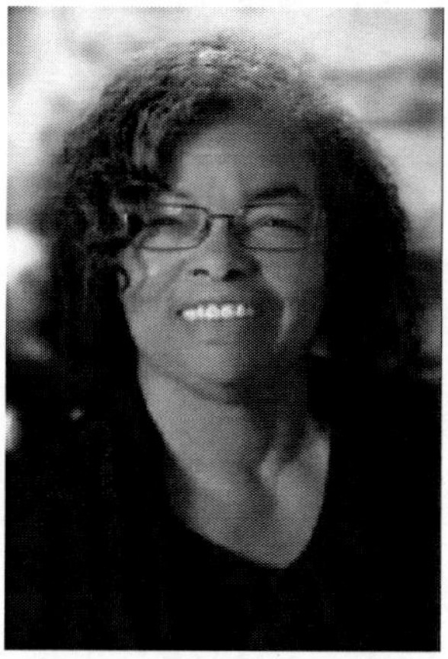

Photography courtesy of Bo Pratt photography

In 1991, Helen D Pratt, PhD became the founding faculty member and Director of Behavioral Pediatrics at Western Michigan University, Homer Stryker MD School of Medicine, formerly known as Michigan State University/Kalamazoo Center for Medical Studies. She remained in that role for nearly 25 years. In addition to her work as a clinician, Dr Pratt was a prolific writer, scholar, presenter and mentor. During her career, she published over 200 journal articles and book chapters. She presented her work at prestigious national and international professional conferences including the American Psychological Association. She was an inspiration to the countless psychology students, medical students and medical residents whom she mentored. She retired from Western Michigan University as Professor Emerita of Pediatric and Adolescent Medicine in 2015.

Starting college at age 30 years, Dr Pratt knew she had less time to pursue her career than traditional students. She was a dedicated, outstanding student who earned her undergraduate degree from the Lee-Honors College at Western Michigan University. She earned her master's and doctoral degrees in clinical psychology from Western Michigan University. Dr Pratt was proud of her accomplishments, valued professionalism, and pursued excellence, while encouraging others to do the same.

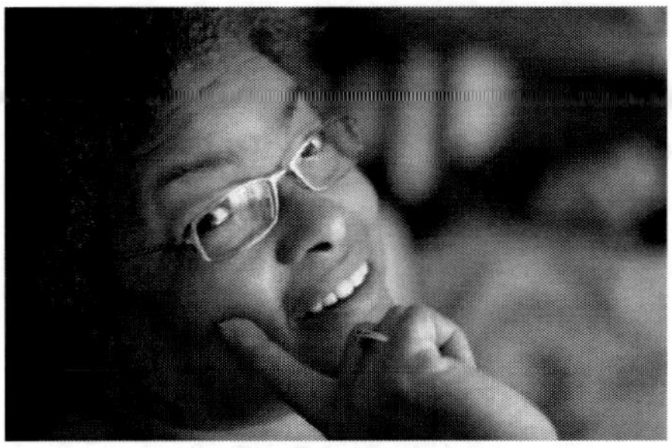

Photography courtesy of Bo Pratt photography

During the development of this book, I had the honor of speaking with her husband, Robert Pratt Jr, MA, and her daughter, Dr Brandy Brown. They told me that making the world a better place was a goal throughout Helen's life. Both her professional and personal life reflected her commitment to improving the world, one person at a time. In addition to supporting and guiding student mentees, Dr Pratt and her husband Bob fostered over fifty foster children; hosted seven international students; and guided, mentored, loved, and supported their own five children. Dr Pratt was especially proud of one of their exchange students from Ghana, Kwabena Oware Adu-Gyamfi. He was encouraged by Dr Pratt to pursue a medical degree when he returned home. He followed her advice, completed medical school, and returned to Michigan to become an outstanding resident at Western Michigan University, Homer Stryker MD School of Medicine.

In addition to her many accomplishments, her husband, Bob, spoke of several of her personal qualities: her wonderful smile, her laugh and her amazing ability to make all people feel comfortable and at ease. Daughter Brandy added that everyone could connect with her.

As I reflect on the legacy of Dr Pratt, it is these personal qualities that I remember most. Her ability to care for people was amazing. It allowed learners, like myself, to hear and accept critical feedback, and integrate that feedback into practice to become better psychologists.

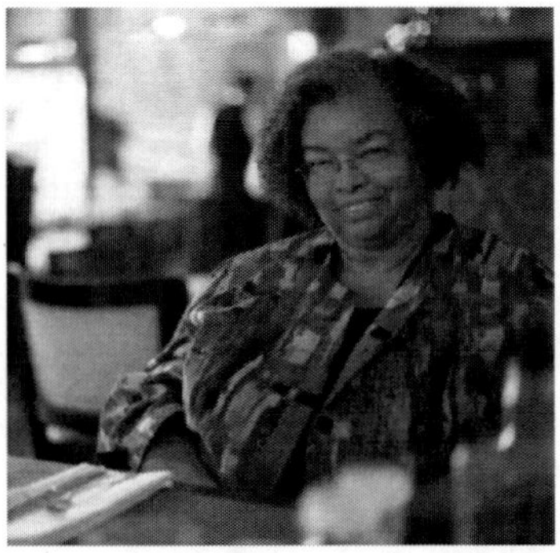

Photography courtesy of Bo Pratt photography

Thank you, Dr Pratt, from all of us whose lives you have touched. Your spirit lives on in how we teach and mentor young physicians, psychologists, family and friends.

Sincerely,

Roger W Apple, PhD

Contents

Forewords

First edition

Greydanus DE, Wolraich M, eds. Behavioral pediatrics, 1st edition. New York: Springer, 1992.

The origins of the term "behavioral pediatrics" are not clear, but we used it in the early 1970s at the University of Rochester to distinguish a program based in pediatrics from those based in child psychiatry. Most behavioral pediatrics programs involved child psychologists working with pediatricians. In the late 1970s the William T Grant Foundation funded 11 Behavioral Pediatrics Programs in the United States aimed at educating pediatric residents about behavioral problems in children. These programs were modeled on a program begun earlier by Dr. Stanford Friedman at the University of Maryland. A key element of all was that they were based in pediatric departments rather than in child psychiatry. This created some confusion and concern, especially among child psychiatrists. I see little reason for conflict, since, although there is some overlap, the two fields deal with different aspects of child behavior, and the very large need cannot be met by child psychiatry alone.

At the end of the Foundation's six years of support of these 11 programs, more than 35 pediatric training programs in the United States had divisions of behavioral pediatrics, and the field seemed well on its way to maturity. This was followed by the organization of the Behavioral Pediatric Society, and in the late 1980s, by the adoption of the Journal of Developmental and Behavioral Pediatrics as the official journal of the Society. All that is left to create a new specialty is a textbook and subspecialty boards. With this textbook, the first of these steps is achieved and the second, subspecialty boards, is now being proposed.

Some will object to a separate subspecialty of behavioral pediatrics. I take pride in being an academic general pediatrician, and I believe that this field includes adolescent medicine and behavioral pediatrics, as well as the area represented by the grandfather of these breakaway societies—the Ambulatory Pediatric Association. While I have had concerns about the separation of behavioral pediatrics from general pediatrics, and from the other pediatric research societies, I do have some difficulty in consistency, since I was one of the original "breakaway pediatricians" who formed the Ambulatory Pediatric Association. Behavioral pediatrics has come of age, and it deserves to be recognized as a separate subspecialty. The task is to integrate its knowledge and skills into the fabric of all pediatric training programs.

This book gives comprehensive coverage of the current status of the field of behavioral pediatrics. It deals very well with the general principles, the skills needed for assessment, and the management of the majority of clinical syndromes. It is authored, appropriately, by a group of authors from many disciplines, including pediatrics and psychology, and it touches on the psychologic aspects of chronic physical disease as well as family problems, including divorce, which puts children at risk. This coverage is very much in the tradition of most medical texts—oriented to the individual and family, and causes and treatments of the problems. There is relatively little in this or any other textbook of pediatrics on the social, cultural, and environmental origins of problem behaviors, or on social policies that may be necessary to prevent or effectively manage many of these problem behaviors of children and youth: better jobs for their parents and a hopeful future for themselves, better education, reduction of discrimination, and social violence. And, at the level of therapy, group approaches, peer counseling, community support groups, and community empowerment are interventions, I believe, the behavioral pediatrician will use more in the future, as well as the individual and family approach so well outlined in this book.

Since this text contains excellent chapters on schizophrenia and depression, which are usually considered the domain of child psychiatry, the question remains, how does behavioral pediatrics differ from child psychiatry? I offer my own idiosyncratic definition: "behavioral pediatrics is what the pediatrician does to diagnose, to treat, and most important, to prevent mental illness and problems behaviors in children." The field obviously overlaps with child psychiatry, but is still distinct. Some problems, such as teen pregnancy, failure to thrive, behavioral aspects of sports medicine, and sexually transmitted diseases, are rarely dealt with by child psychiatrists, and are clearly in the province of the behavioral pediatrician. On the other hand, schizophrenia, autism, and severe depression, while they may—and should—be picked up by the pediatrician, must usually be treated by the child psychiatrist. Given that behavioral pediatrics is a multidisciplinary field and has some overlap with child psychiatry and other disciplines, productive relations between these disciplines still need to be worked out in many institutions.

The challenge to the field of behavioral pediatrics is to learn to work effectively as a team, to develop advocacy skills to promote social policies that deal with the sociocultural causes of problem behaviors, and at the same time, develop the skills to relate to individual patients and their families and to diagnose and manage effectively those problems for which the pediatrician can become competent. This is a big order, but one that this book goes a long way toward helping to achieve. Unless pediatricians learn to deal effectively with these major problems, they will be unable to deal with most pressing and common problem faced by the children and their families today. With a textbook of its own, behavioral pediatrics has come of age.

Robert J Haggerty, MD
President, William T Grant Foundation, Clinical Professor of Pediatrics, New York Hospital/Cornell Medical Center, New York, United States of America

Second edition

Greydanus DE, Pratt HD, Patel DR, eds. Behavioral pediatrics, 2nd edition. New York: iUniverse Publishing, 2006.

When all's said and done, when the doors of the clinic or office close, the pediatrician, family doctor or nurse practitioner will drive home to a late dinner all the time thinking about the social and behavioral challenges presented by his or her young patients that day. The "medical" decision-making, diagnosis and treatment of the principal problems will, on the whole, have been made easy in comparison to the social and behavioral problems presented by the patients. For most practitioners, behavioral training (the psychosocial in the biopsychosocial) occurred years ago. The practitioner may not be conversant with contemporary diagnosis, treatment and psychological perspectives. So fortunately, within the pages of this volume, you will find expert articulation of the behavioral and social dimensions of your challenging cases as well as an excellent presentation of child and adolescent psychological and psychiatric diagnosis and treatment.

There are a number of features of this carefully edited volume that I recommend to you, the reader. The disciplinary "silos" of specialty and subspecialty are breached in a healthy way; the reader is presented with comprehensive coverage of behavior both normal and pathological in children and adolescents in clear prose writing by experts in many disciplines. The writing avoids specialty jargon while clarifying key concepts. This book is an asset not only for those seeking a deeper understanding but those interested in becoming more engaged in diagnosis and treatment of their behavioral disordered young patients. Increasing involvement by primary care clinicians in such treatment is essential in my view if we expect that access to treatment for these relatively common conditions will be available.

More important than the treatment is prevention. Primary prevention remains a "holy grail" awaiting more scientific discovery at least for the serious mental disorders but much is known about secondary prevention (reducing episodes of illness and morbidity) and tertiary prevention (reducing social disability). Prevention in many area of behavioral health can be linked to healthy family behaviors; for example, it is clear that drug use and dependence (including smoking) in adolescents is less common in families that closely monitor their children's activities. The same can be said for other risky behaviors with damaging consequences to health and well-being.

Family doctors, pediatricians, nurses and other primary care providers function as sentinels in the community for much that is happening in our culture and function, to use a current phrase, as "first responders." This volume can be a key resource for "first responders." The role of human behavior in illness and the human behavioral illnesses is so widely prevalent that, as a psychiatrist and a dean, it won't surprise the reader to know that I hope and even expect a high level of behavioral sophistication in those who care for children and adolescents.

Robert Haggerty in his Foreword to the first edition provided a brief history of behavioral pediatrics and attempts a definition of behavioral pediatrics that might distinguish child psychiatry from behavioral pediatrics. Since the first edition of this book, the American Board of Pediatrics (ABP) has recognized the subspecialty of Developmental and Behavioral Pediatrics. The American Board of Medical Specialties in the last several years supported the ABP's application for recognition and the provision of a subspecialty certificate. Behavioral pediatrics is here to stay. But the key question is not how child psychiatry and behavioral pediatrics are similar or different but "are patients better served" to have both. I have no doubt that they are! Dr Haggerty also emphasized the need for us to function in teams—certainly a challenge we have in medical schools—to create curricula that teach provision of care in cross-professional teams. This well-crafted volume covers behavioral pediatrics content and provides a context for effective team delivery of high quality behavioral care to children and adolescents.

Glenn C Davis, MD
Former Dean, College of Human Medicine, Michigan State University, East Lansing, Michigan, United States of America

Third edition

Greydanus DE, Pratt HD, Patel DR, eds. Behavioral pediatrics, Third edition. New York: Nova Biomedical, 2009.

Pediatrics (from two Greek words for child [*pais*] and healer [*iatros*]) is the field of medicine concerned with infants, children and adolescents, their growth and development along with their prospect to achieve full potentials as adults.

Abraham Jacobi (1830-1919), the father of American pediatrics and also the area of social pediatrics, is the name that comes up first to mind when you think about pediatrics. This German Jewish physician graduated from the University of Bonn in 1851, but when he traveled to Berlin to take his state medical exams, he was arrested and held in prison for nearly two years on a charge of promoting political and social reform in the German revolution of 1848. He left Germany and arrived in New York in 1853, where he practiced general medicine, surgery and obstetrics, but his early contributions to the New York Medical Journal helped establish the field of pediatrics. In 1857, Jacobi lectured on childhood diseases of the larynx at the College of Physicians and Surgeons, his first formal pediatric lecture, and in 1860, he accepted a position as professor of infantile pathology and therapeutics at New York Medical College. This appointment signaled a turning point as it was the first pediatric medical position and launched pediatrics as an academic discipline in the United States and during his lifetime all major medical centers in the United States established pediatric departments. He also established the bedside clinical teaching method, a landmark in medical education. In 1865 he accepted the position of clinical professor of diseases of children at New York Medical College and in 1870 the College of Physicians and Surgeons (Columbia University) appointed him professor of clinical pediatrics. He worked at almost every hospital in New York, but he concentrated on the Jews Hospital (later Mount Sinai Hospital), where he set up the first outpatient pediatric clinic in 1874. By 1878, the Jews Hospital had the first department of pediatrics in a United States general hospital.

But the fact is that already much earlier in time pediatrics had been the focus of several Persian physicians. In the 10th century, the famous Persian physician Rhazes (Muhammad ibn Zakariya Razi, 865-925) wrote the first book that we know about (diseases of children, one of his 184 publications) to deal with pediatrics as an independent field of medicine. His teacher Ali ibn Sahl Rabban al-Tabari (838-870), a modern convert of Jewish decent, who produced the first encyclopedia of medicine, was also a pioneer in the field of child development which was discussed in depth in his book, "Firdous al-Hikmah" (Paradise of wisdom). The first work on pediatrics in the Western world was the Book of Children, published in 1545 by Thomas Phaer (1510-1560). The first Hospital for Sick Children in Great Ormond Street in London that we know was founded in 1852 and still today considered one the best pediatric centers in the world.

So where and when does the field of behavioral pediatrics come into the picture? Some will go back to Charles Darwin (1809-1882), who in 1877 published his observations on his first child (A biographical sketch of an infant; Mind 1877; 2:285-94) as a study of human behavioral development. This and his other work inspired and influenced other scholars, which again resulted in major progress in cognition, personality, intelligence testing, learning, psychoanalysis and animal research on human development. In Europe and in Scandinavia, where I grew up and was trained, we would call this special field or area of interest for social pediatrics or even some would say that is it not a discipline, but rather a state of mind. In the

1980s this area in Europe (influenced a lot by the British discipline of community pediatrics) has developed into a field now called child public health involved with the organized efforts of society to develop public health policies to promote child and young people's health, to prevent disease in children and young people, and to foster equity for children and young people within a framework of sustainable development.

In the United States, the Society for Developmental and Behavioral Pediatrics was founded in 1982 in order to improve the health care of infants, children, and adolescents by promoting research and teaching in developmental and behavioral pediatrics. This society of pediatricians and other professionals have worked to encourage research in developmental and behavioral pediatrics with an emphasis on psychosocial issues arising in the context of questions and respond to issues that affect research, teaching, or program development in developmental and behavioral pediatrics and to promote an understanding of and particular interest in the social, educational and cultural influences on children. The work of this society and others resulted in the American Board of Pediatrics in 2002 to accept a subspecialty training in developmental and behavioral pediatrics.

The Journal of Developmental and Behavioral Pediatrics devoted to the developmental and psychosocial aspects of pediatric health care in now in 2009 in its 30th year of publication and this present textbook is now in its third edition.

The present book is a welcome addition to the field of behavioral pediatrics and it will be the textbook that will follow pediatricians interested in this field, in a career and subspecialty in behavioral pediatrics.

Professor Joav Merrick, MD, MMedSci, DMSc
Director, National Institute of Child Health and Human Development, Jerusalem Israel, Medical Director, Office of the Medical Director, Division for Mental Retardation, Ministry of Social Affairs, Jerusalem, Israel and Professor of Pediatrics, Kentucky Children's Hospital, University of Kentucky, Lexington, Kentucky, United States of America

Fourth edition

Greydanus DE, Patel DR, Pratt HD, Calles Jr JL, Nazeer A, Merrick J, eds. Behavioral pediatrics, 4th edition. New York: Nova Science, 2015.

Childhood and adolescence are periods critical for developing life-long good physical and mental health. According to Aristotle in the distant past and to the World Health Organization (WHO) nowadays, there is "no health without mental health," as both are inexorably intertwined. Indeed, poor physical and mental health in childhood and adolescence influence adversely both general health and social and economic outcomes across the lifespan.

The overall prevalence of mental disorders is quite high in the world population at all ages; it is estimated that 10-20% of young people worldwide experience mental health symptoms and express associated behavioral problems in childhood and adolescence. On the other hand, there is increasing recognition of the importance of mental health for the success of global development strategies, and, in particular, the achievement of the United Nations Millennium Development Goals, which include eradication of poverty, education for all, improvement of child and maternal health and combating sexually transmitted infections and other diseases.

Despite the above considerations, mental health promotion for children and adolescents remains a neglected public health issue worldwide.

Recently, the existing mental health "gap" has stimulated synergy in action plans and strategies endorsed by global organizations. The United Nations Educational, Scientific and Cultural Organization (UNESCO) Operational Strategy on Youth 2014-2021 aims to ensure youth access to skills and competencies development for their transition to adulthood. The WHO's Comprehensive Mental Health Action Plan 2013-2020 recognizes the essential role of mental health in achieving universal health and stresses the importance of prevention. In this action plan, the term "mental disorders" is used to denote a range of mental and behavioral disorders that include depression, bipolar disorder, anxiety disorders, schizophrenia, substance use disorders, intellectual disabilities, and developmental and behavioral disorders with onset usually occurring in childhood and adolescence, including attention deficit and hyperactivity disorder and autism. In this action plan, emphasis is placed on the provision of comprehensive, integrated mental health care services in community-based settings.

Many "mental health specialists," including psychiatrists, psychologists, family therapists, social workers, specially trained counselors, nurses, neuroscientists, developmental-behavioral pediatricians and adolescent medicine specialists, engage in the assessment and care of children and adolescents with mental health concerns. However, many primary care clinicians, including general pediatricians, are hesitant to engage in mental health screening, assessment, diagnosis, and treatment. The American Academy of Pediatrics in a Policy Statement in 2009 proposed the requisite competencies of pediatric primary care clinicians that enable them to provide mental health services in primary care settings.

We have only recently recognized that the boundaries between medical specialties are much more porous than originally perceived. Many clinicians are unfamiliar with contemporary evaluation, diagnosis, counselling and treatment of the wide range of developmental and behavioral difficulties faced by children, adolescents, and their families. "Behavioral pediatrics, 4th Edition," provides strong foundations for Developmental-Behavioral Pediatrics, moving away from the purely medical specialty-subspecialty model. The book has evolved through three major editions that have described the essential features of the full range of behavioral child and adolescent disorders. The current 4th edition builds on the goal of its predecessors to provide a deeper understanding of child and adolescent development and behavior and to shed light on deviations from the normal pattern. This carefully edited volume has been developed by a group of experts in Developmental-Behavioral Pediatrics, representing special expertise in their respective subareas. It begins with introducing concepts of normal vs. abnormal behavior and describing behavioral and psychological assessment, follows with description of disorders that more commonly manifest in early life and adolescence, and ends with chapters relevant to neglect and abuse, sexual offenders and concepts of family therapy and pharmacotherapy. The hot topics of assessment in primary care, child and adolescent behavior in chronic illness, and sexuality, are also addressed. A similar structure approach has been taken, where possible, within each chapter, to facilitate the comprehensive understanding of information and to improve its clinical utility to both specialists and non-specialists.

Mental health matters enormously and there is a long way ahead of us to achieve it universally. Childhood and adolescence are critical windows of plasticity from the developmental and behavioral perspectives, and prevention and intervention at these early times are critical. "Behavioral Pediatrics, 4th Edition", represents a timely, up-to-date, state-of-the-art academic effort ultimately aiming to improve the health outcomes of our children and adolescents.

George P Chrousos, MD, FAAP, MACE, MACP
Professor and Chairman, First Department of Pediatrics, Chairholder, UNESCO Chair in Adolescent Health Care, Athens University Medical School, Athens, Greece

Current fifth edition

This fifth edition of "Behavioral pediatrics" covers a wide range of pediatric behavioral conditions that may disrupt the optimal development of infants, children, adolescents and young adults. Approximately 20% of children and adolescents have behavioral/emotional problems. Donald E Greydanus, MD, the senior editor of this and earlier volumes, is a highly skilled academic pediatrician who has many years of experience caring for children and adolescents who have behavioral challenges as well as of training the next generation of child health providers to care for these children. Sadly, children's behavioral conditions are becoming more frequent among children and families over time as our society experiences unprecedented challenges resulting from general cultural unrest and the COVID pandemic that leave the developing child and family struggling during critical periods of children's development. These struggles may affect children's and families' health for years to come.

Behavioral pediatrics is a term coined in the mid-to-late 1960s and early 1970s by Drs Robert J Haggerty and Stanford B Friedman then of the Department of Pediatrics at the University of Rochester (New York). Dr. Friedman provided a broad definition of behavioral pediatrics as "an area within pediatrics which focuses on the psychological, social, and learning problems of children and adolescents" (1). The importance of behavioral problems was also recognized by pediatricians and child psychiatrists at Yale, Johns Hopkins, Boston Children's Hospital, the University of Indiana, and the University of California (UCSF).

Rush Rhees, former President of the University of Rochester, wrote in an introduction to a text on tonsillectomies in 1932: "No age has benefited more from scientific discoveries in medicine than that of childhood" (2). The impact of good nutrition, safe water, pasteurized milk, immunizations, and antibiotics all dramatically improved children's health and set the stage for the focus on the new morbidity of behavioral problems. That is, children's improving biologic health allowed greater attention to incorporating the definition of and treatment of behavioral and psychological problems into the practice of pediatrics. The "new pediatrics" was based partially on the biopsychosocial model of medicine created by George Engel in Rochester (3) with whose work Drs Haggerty and Friedman were aware resulting from their training in Rochester when Dr Engel was defining this model.

Today across the world, children's and adolescents' behavioral conditions are accelerating largely as a result of the unexpected COVID-19 pandemic leaving persons of all ages struggling to maintain and in some instances, retain any sense of equilibrium. Family life at its core is being disrupted, as the economy is uncertain and drew to a halt during the first peak of the pandemic. The economic consequences of complete shutdown of small and major businesses/industries left many wondering from where their very sustenance was coming. Working parents assumed the role of at-home untrained educators of their children with minimal direction from educators as disruption of all aspects of life occurred. The lack of predictability within families, schools, and communities has resulted in alarming anxiety, confusion, and depression among all age groups. The morbidity and mortality resulting from recurrences of COVID sweeping over the world resulted in greater uncertainty and anxiety. The critical importance of behavioral pediatrics now cannot be overemphasized.

This new volume is an important contribution to defining behavioral pediatrics further and providing child health care providers and educators of professionals new insights into the evolving conditions from which our children and their families suffer.

This book is a compendium of topics critical to health care providers' knowledge of optimal physical and emotional health of children, adolescents, and families as well as behavioral conditions resulting from disruptions in the pattern of normal growth and development. The initial section "sets the stage" with a review of normal child and adolescent development, behavioral assessment and follow-up care in the primary care providers' offices, and emerging strategies such as mindfulness to help resolve the children's symptoms. The next section clarifies the developmental disorders, disruptive disorders, and mood disorders and is an introduction to the sections that follow discussing conditions reflected in children's anxiety, depression, and mood disorders. Stress, anxiety, depression and mood disorders often are antecedents to destructive behaviors such as substance use/abuse, attention deficit disorder, suicidal behavior, eating disorders, and other conditions. Recognition of these antecedents is important with the hope of preventing further morbidity. The challenges of chronic illness are well-covered by discussing conditions such as cystic fibrosis and renal disease as models of chronic illness.

In the future, the negative effects psychologically of the COVID pandemic on developing children and adolescents, and their parents should make clearer the biologic and psychosocial manifestations of the conditions covered so clearly in this book. Additionally, we will begin to understand the short- and long-term effects of the immense stress on every age group and the toll resulting on the emotional health of all nations' children and families from a worldwide pandemic. Hopefully rather than destroying a generation of the world's children, we will learn how to strengthen children's and families' resilience.

This book illustrates the great of the field of behavioral pediatrics over six decades. With the addition to the literature of this updated volume, we expect that more primary care pediatric providers will provide improved screening and short-term intervention or referral to children burdened with behavioral conditions to assure that each child is a strong child. I congratulate Dr. Greydanus and his colleagues for this highly important and relevant addition to the literature on behavioral pediatrics.

Elizabeth R. McAnarney, MD
Distinguished University Professor, Chair Emerita, Department of Pediatrics, University of Rochester, Rochester, New York, United States of America

References

[1] Friedman SB, ed. Introduction: Symposium of behavioral pediatrics. Pediatr Clin North Am 1975; 22:55.
[2] Rhees, R. Foreword. In: Kaiser AD, ed. In or out: A critical study of the end results of tonsillectomy. Philadelphia, PA: JB Lippincott, 1932:v.
[3] Engel GL. The need for a new medical model: A challenge for biomedicine. Science 1975;196:129.

Preface

Professionals in psychiatry and psychology work closely with pediatric clinicians in a variety of professional relationships, including co-located and non-co-located mental health settings. Pediatricians provide a wide variety of care to children and adolescents with complex disorders—depending on their training as well as interests—and this book seeks to provide perspectives in behavioral pediatrics, neuropsychiatric conditions, issues of sexuality and and the complex field of eating disorders.

In *the first section*, various neuropsychiatric conditions are considered; after a discussion of concepts of psychosomatic conditions, topics covered are pediatric sleep disorders, tic disorders, enuresis and encopresis.

Section two selects aspects of pediatric sexuality with discussions on an overview of child/teen sexuality, child/teen gender identity and sexually transmitted diseases/infections (**1-3**). In *section three*, the editors provide perspectives on eating disorders: psychiatric perspectives in pediatric obesity, motivational interviewing and childhood obesity, pediatric obesity psychopharmacology, malnutrition, anorexia nervosa in adolescence, and gynecologic/behavioral features of eating disorders (**4, 5**).

Donald E. Greydanus, MD, Doctor Honoris Causa (Athens, Greece)
Professor and Founding Chair, Department of Pediatric and Adolescent Medicine
Western Michigan University, Homer Stryker MD School of Medicine, Kalamazoo, Michigan, United States of America
Email: donald.greydanus@med.wmich.edu

Dilip R. Patel, MD, MBA, MPH
Professor and Chair, Department of Pediatric and Adolescent Medicine, Western Michigan University, Homer Stryker MD School of Medicine, Kalamazoo, Michigan, United States of America
Email: Dilip.patel@med.wmich.edu

Ahsan Nazeer, MD
Associate Professor and Division Chief, Child and Adolescent Mental Health Services (CAMHS), Sidra Medicine, Doha, Qatar
Email: anazeer@sidra.org

Roger W. Apple, PhD
Associate Professor, Chief, Division of Pediatric Psychology, Director, Autism Center, Department of Pediatric and Adolescent Medicine, Western Michigan University, Homer Stryker MD School of Medicine, Kalamazoo, Michigan, United States of America
Email: Roger.apple@med.wmich.edu

Joav Merrick, MD, MMedSci, DMSc
National Institute of Child Health and Human Development, Jerusalem, Israel, Department of Pediatrics, Mt Scopus Campus, Hadassah Hebrew University Medical Center. Jerusalem, Israel, Kentucky Children's Hospital, University of Kentucky, Lexington, Kentucky, United States, Center for Healthy Development, School of Public Health, Georgia State University, Atlanta, United States of America
Email: jmerrick@zahav.net.il

References

[1] Omar HA, Greydanus DE, Patel DR, Merrick J, eds. Pediatric and adolescent sexuality and gynecology. Principles for the primary care clinician, Second edition. New York: Nova Medicine Health, 2021.
[2] Sison AC, Greydanus DE. Deconstructing adolescent same-sex attraction and sexual behavior in the twenty-first century: perspectives for the clinician. Prim Care 2007;34(2):293-304.
[3] Agana MG, Greydanus DE, Indyk JA, Calles JL Jr, Kushner J, Leibowitz S, et al. Caring for the transgender adolescent and young adult: Current concepts of an evolving process in the 21st century. Dis Mon 2019;65(9):303-56.
[4] Klein DA, Sylvester JE, Schvey NA. Eating disorders in primary care: Diagnosis and management. Am Fam Physician 2021;103(1):22-32. Erratum in: Am Fam Physician. 2021;103(5):263.
[5] Greydanus DE, Agana M, Kamboj MK, Shebrain S, Soares N, Eke R, et al. Pediatric obesity: Current concepts. Dis Mon 2018;64(4):98-156.

Section one: Special neuropsychiatric conditions (editor: Donald E Greydanus)

Chapter 1

Concepts of psychosomatic conditions

Roger W. Apple[1,*], PhD, Madhav Patel[2], BS and Keshav Patel[3], MS

[1]Department of Pediatric and Adolescent Medicine, Western Michigan University Homer Stryker MD School of Medicine, Kalamazoo, Michigan, United States of America
[2]Georgetown University School of Medicine, Washington DC, United States of America
[3]Western Michigan University Homer Stryker MD School of Medicine, Kalamazoo, Michigan, United States of America

Abstract

Psychosomatic conditions are generally discussed in broad and general terms that are difficult to conceptualize and have neither specific identified etiological factors nor consensus for treatment. This chapter was written as a broad overview of psychosomatic conditions in order to provide clarity to the topic. Several databases were searched including Medline and PsychInfo and reference lists from relevant publications. Literature was sought out for psychosomatic conditions, somatoform disorders, and medical illnesses with psychosomatic components. A general description of psychosomatic conditions and overarching themes were identified which include: lack of a universal definition, poor compatibility between psychological diagnoses and diagnoses outside of psychology, unclear etiology, psychosomatic factors occur in many illnesses, holistic perspective is preferred, poor patient insight regarding symptoms, strong family influence, and pediatric-liaison teams are strongly encouraged in diagnosis and treatment. Treatment is often highly individualized utilizing cognitive behavioral therapy, pharmacotherapy and pediatric-liaison teams with a bio-psychosocial focus.

Introduction

Understanding psychosomatic conditions is important as they represent a large proportion of primary care patients (1, 2). Psychosomatic conditions refer to illnesses that impact both the

* ***Correspondence:*** Roger W Apple, PhD, Director, WMed Pediatric Autism Center, Associate Professor, Department of Pediatric and Adolescent Medicine, Western Michigan University, Homer Stryker M.D. School of Medicine, 1000 Oakland Drive, Kalamazoo MI 49008-1284 United States.
Email: roger.apple@med.wmich.edu.

In: Behavioral Pediatrics II
Editors: Donald E. Greydanus, Dilip R. Patel, Ahsan Nazeer et al.
ISBN: 979-8-88697-019-7

mind and body. There is a significant amount of difficulty in classifying what exactly qualifies as a psychosomatic condition. There are many illnesses which present as primarily medical conditions that can be impacted by psychological factors (i.e., diabetes mellitus, cancer); conditions that present as a more equal combination of psychological and medical symptoms (i.e., hypertension, fibromyalgia); and conditions that appear primarily influenced by psychological factors causing medical symptoms (i.e., conversion disorders). Effective intervention for psychosomatic conditions often requires treatment by both mental health and medical professionals. This discussion seeks to minimize the confusion by clarifying terminology, providing a general overview as well as description of psychosomatic conditions in addition to its epidemiology, clinical features, diagnosis and treatment.

The concept of psychosomatic medicine is at a crisis point with research failing to provide an accepted explanation of psychosomatic conditions (3). There has not been one single scientific theory that has been able to provide a complete description of psychosomatic conditions; because of this crisis, an integrative approach is supported regarding understanding the phenomena of psychosomatic conditions that moves away from the mind-body dichotomy. Agreement on diagnostic accuracy and the shared conceptual model is needed among mental health and medical professionals with an increased focus on positive criteria as opposed to merely the exclusion of organic disease (4).

Our search

Several databases were searched including Medline and PsychInfo with reference lists from relevant publications (1). Literature was sought out for psychosomatic conditions, somatoform disorders (disorders yielding medical symptoms that are primarily due to psychological factors), and medical illnesses with psychosomatic components. Specific information was sought out for epidemiology, clinical features, diagnosis and treatment. Reviewing such a broad literature base was done to provide a greater depth and breadth of information as well as look for overarching themes and concepts that could help clarify the most salient factors regarding this somewhat ambiguous topic of psychosomatic conditions. One of the most frequently cited and illustrated topics throughout the literature was the ambiguity of terminology. Not only was it the specific terminology that was ambiguous but also the entire concept of what constitutes psychosomatic conditions which will be discussed in the definition section of this review.

Our findings

This treatise provides a general description of psychosomatic conditions and the overarching themes that help clarify this ambiguous topic. Some common overarching themes identified in this work include:

- Lack of a universal definition;
- Poor compatibility between psychological diagnoses and diagnoses outside of psychology;
- Etiology is not clear;

- Most illnesses have psychosomatic influences;
- Holistic perspective is preferred over linear causality models;
- Patients often experience poor insight regarding the connection between psychological and medical symptoms;
- Very strong family influence;
- Pediatric-liaison teams are strongly encouraged in diagnosis and treatment.

Even with such ambiguity, psychosomatic conditions are extremely common in children and adolescents; unfortunately, less than half of these patients receive treatment. Psychosomatic conditions are rarely diagnosed before age 5 and common symptoms often involve family dysfunction and concerns impacted by socio-demographic factors. Physical symptoms include headache, low energy, sore muscles, loss of appetite, back pain, vague aches and pains, dizziness and fainting, anorexia nervosa, and gastrointestinal symptoms (5-8). Due to the complexity and ambiguity of psychosomatic conditions, the diagnosis and treatment is often highly individualized utilizing cognitive behavioral therapy, pharmacotherapy and pediatric-liaison teams with a bio-psychosocial focus.

Definition

Most often the terms *psychosomatic disorders* and *somatoform disorders* are used interchangeably to describe psychosomatic conditions as a constellation of symptoms both psychological and medical that result in somatic symptoms that cannot be explained by organic conditions (5, 7). In more recent times, the term *psychosomatic* has gained criticism due to its lack of explicit reference to social and interpersonal factors that are strongly intertwined with the mind-body relationship (9). Most patients with psychosomatic symptoms seek a medical explanation for their symptoms.

Unfortunately, there is no consensus on a universal definition of what defines the extremely broad and often vague conceptualizations that characterize psychosomatic conditions. In fact, there is little consensus on what qualifies as a psychosomatic disorder. In a review of articles and empirical studies, each source provided their own unique definition in relation to their topic. Defining the general term of *psychosomatic disorders* is particularly challenging because it does not refer to a category of diagnoses, but rather, a subspecialty which had previously been termed *consultation psychiatry* (10-12) and subsequently as *psychosomatic medicine*. *Psychosomatic medicine* was approved as a subspecialty of psychiatry by the American Board of Medical Specialties in 2003 (13).

This name was supported at the time because it had historical value, would likely be approved by regulatory organizations since it did not overlap with other subspecialties, and is utilized in the names of journals in the field including *Psychosomatics,* the *Journal of Psychosomatic Research,* and the *Journal of Psychosomatic Medicine* (14). However, several psychiatrists criticized the name, as it conveys a singular focus on somatoform disorders caused uni-directionally by psychological etiologies. This limited implied meaning restricted the breadth of applicability of the discipline in clinical practice and research.

In 2017, the American Board of Medical Specialties voted to change the name of the field from *psychosomatic medicine* to *consultation-liaison psychiatry* (14). After this change, the

Academy of Psychosomatic Medicine also transitioned the organization name to the Academy of Consultation Psychiatry (14). *Consultation-liaison* is a more familiar word for most practitioners and psychiatrists. It refers to a subspecialty of psychiatry that functions as an interface between the fields of medicine and psychology; such an interface is essential to understanding and treating psychosomatic conditions even if a definition is not clear.

In the fields of psychology and medicine, the term *psychosomatic disorder* is widely accepted; however, the term does not exist in the Diagnostic and statistical manual of mental disorders, Fourth edition, Text revision (DSM-IV-TR) or the fifth edition (DSM-5) (15, 16). This incompatibility between the DSM and those outside of the DSM makes defining a term that describes psychosomatic conditions very challenging (16). The DSM-IV-TR discusses the somatoform disorders (somatic symptom disorders in DSM-5), which are only psychological in nature but produce medically unexplained symptoms. These disorders include: Somatization disorder, undifferentiated somatoform disorder, conversion disorder, pain disorder, hypochondriasis, body dysmorphic disorder and somatoform disorder NOS.

In primary care, many patients with psychosomatic symptoms may present with legitimate medical conditions. This makes diagnostic clarification difficult and as a result patients with both psychological and medical symptoms get conceptualized very broadly as having a vague array of medically unexplained symptoms accompanied by psychological distress (15). Additionally, almost all illnesses can attribute some function to the role of psychological and/or social factors (17).

Another concern that impacts defining psychosomatic conditions is the literature itself, which often suggests that psychosomatic conditions are linear and one-directional (11). This indicates that a psychological problem is causing medical symptoms, and this view distorts the complexity and holistic nature in which psychosomatic conditions exist.

The confusion regarding defining psychosomatic conditions has led authors to suggest new terminology that takes into account patient acceptability, conceptual clarity, political correctness, etiological neutrality, and compatibility with non-psychiatric professions (15, 16). These terms include functional, subjective health complaints, pseudoneurological disorder, neurologiform, somatic amplification, physiological arousal and reactivity, somatic perception, somatic attention, cognitive elaboration and expression of emotion, and coping with somatic distress.

Psychosomatic conditions will be the primary terminology used for the remainder of this discussion. The term *psychosomatic disorders* does not accurately capture the broad reaching impact of psychosomatic conditions on almost all illnesses and as stated previously, refers to a subspecialty rather than specific category of diagnoses. The term *psychosomatic conditions* appears to be the most representative terminology.

Epidemiology

Describing the epidemiology of psychosomatic conditions is also extremely challenging since most illnesses have psychosomatic influences. However, psychosomatic conditions are often best understood by accepting multiple causal factors that are cognitive-behavioral and bio-psychosocial in nature because the etiology of medically unexplained symptoms is not clear (2). In addition, with the growing incorporation of psychosomatic conditions in health care and research, the cognitive-behavioral and bio-psychosocial dimensions of health may also influence the progression of an illness and can be utilized for possible interventions to optimize patient care (18).

Linear causality does not work while trying to describe the correlation between the mind, body, and environment. Understanding psychosomatic conditions as complex and requiring multiple viewpoints which are "complementary and correlated" is recommended because the connection between the mind, body, and environment cannot be separated (3).

There is no specific etiology that can be attributed to any one psychosomatic condition. Considering that psychosomatic factors can impact almost any illness, utilizing an individualized and integrated approach is often necessary for each patient. Over the past decade, there has been an increasing demand for incorporation of psychosomatic principles and holistic care for pediatric patients due to the evolution of clinical consultation services, an increase in patient acuity, and need for psychosomatic oriented psychiatric care for children onboarding onto inpatient medical services (19).

For many children and adolescents, it is suggested that there is a connection between the development of psychosomatic conditions and stress from social situations and school settings, bullying, family discord, separation from parents, increased number of significant life events and other environmental factors or adverse childhood experiences (7, 20). These concerns increase the incidents of irritable bowel syndrome, headache, hyperventilation syndrome, bronchial asthma, eating disorders, and orthostatic dysregulation. Pre-pubertal children generally have the same prevalence of psychosomatic conditions; however, post-pubertal female children generally have a higher risk of developing psychosomatic conditions than males.

Clinical features

Psychosomatic conditions are common mental health disorders; however, less than half of these patients receive adequate treatment with the average time span between symptom onset and treatment being approximately six years (21). There is an equal prevalence of psychosomatic conditions in pre-pubertal children, however, post-pubertal females had a higher prevalence than males (7). Additionally, a significant majority (75%) of patients who present to primary care with clinically significant symptoms of mental illness often initially report exclusively somatic symptoms. Interestingly, only 10% of these patients denied any relationship to psychological factors suggesting that somatic concerns may be due at least in part to psychological factors. Contrary to popular belief, patients presenting with psychosomatic symptoms present similarly to those with clear psychological symptoms; however, patients with psychosomatic concerns often have a negative attitude toward mental illness and experience an increased sensitivity to bodily sensations (15).

Psychosomatic conditions are rarely diagnosed in children under the age of five years (6). Physical symptoms that cannot be medically explained account for up to 50% of new pediatric outpatient visits (22). Children and adolescents with psychosomatic conditions can present with a very wide range of clinically significant psychological and medical symptoms. This is partly due to the fact that children may find it difficult to verbally express emotional distress, and instead express psychological disturbances with physical symptoms (22). Symptoms of anxiety and depression are very common along with poor insight regarding the connection between psychological and physical symptoms. There is often a strong family component observed in psychosomatic conditions similar to that of eating disorders and diabetes (5).

Some of the most common symptoms among children and adolescents are headache, low energy, sore muscles, loss of appetite, back pain, vague aches and pains, dizziness and fainting, anorexia nervosa, and gastrointestinal symptoms with the most common somatoform disorders (according to DSM-IV-TR criteria) for children and adolescents being pain disorder, conversion disorder, and chronic fatigue disorder, even though it is not in the DSM (5-8). Somatization that causes daily functional impairment or significant distress, characterized in the most recent DSM-5 as Somatic Symptom and Related Disorders, has been reported in up to 13% of children according to previous studies (23).

Symptoms in children can also mimic neurological problems including double vision, poor balance and coordination, paralysis, seizures, and imagined physical deformities (7). Academic problems within school, social withdrawal, anxiety, and behavior problems can also influence psychosomatic conditions (7). Disturbances in daily functioning activities such as dysphagia and breathing abnormalities may also occur (24). Recently, researchers have been shifting the perspective to normalizing somatic experiences and calling them "sensations" instead of "symptoms" grounded from psychological abnormalities (25).

About half of patients experiencing psychosomatic symptoms are also experiencing comorbid illnesses (6). Comorbid psychiatric conditions may present in one third of children with psychosomatic symptoms, with anxiety and depression being the most common culprits in school-aged children (22). In some patients, physical symptoms thought previously to be unexplained by a medical etiology are later found to correlate to pathology of an organ system, which emphasizes a physician's responsibility to keep medical comorbidities on the differential even after diagnosis of a psychosomatic condition (24). Psychosomatic illness is more common in patients from low socio-economic statuses and rural areas; however, prevalence is increasing in urban areas. Common complaints and symptoms include: non-epileptic seizures, fainting, generalized body pain, leg pain, abdominal pain, and tremors with conversion disorder being the most common. Psychosomatic seizures often involve whole body or limb shaking; however, symptoms of typical seizures are not present: frothing from the mouth, tongue biting, and involuntary passage of urine.

Family and socio-culture influences

Factors involving the family are often associated with the development of psychosomatic conditions such as stress as well as family conflict and what is often described as "intolerable predicaments" in which children and adolescents cannot escape. These predicaments often take the form of families creating overwhelming situations that involve parental rejections, anger, hostility, and forced compliance (5, 6). Enmeshed families are the most common family type associated with psychosomatic conditions (17). Parents of patients with psychosomatic conditions are more preoccupied about overall well-being and often possess greater reported symptoms of psychiatric and medical disturbances (24). Psychosomatic conditions are now being viewed as occurring within families such as other illnesses including juvenile diabetes, ulcerative colitis, anorexia nervosa, and bronchial asthma. This does not mean that families are directly causing these illnesses but rather significantly impacting how the patient responds to the illness-- often with somatic symptoms (17). Unfortunately, patients with psychosomatic symptoms rarely seek and often reject psychological treatment (17).

It is popularly understood that stress can cause physical symptoms. However, socio-demographic characteristics can also play a role in eliciting psychosomatic conditions; these include age, sex, marital status, residence, and living conditions (26). For example, Western cultures strongly emphasize muscularity, particularly in men, while many other cultures do not (27).

Considering the complexity of the clinical presentation of psychosomatic conditions and the multiple factors that influence such conditions, conceptualization of these conditions is accomplished best from a holistic perspective. In order to best understand psychosomatic conditions, accepting the complex nature of the condition is necessary as seeking a linear relationship would be to overly simplify the condition (28, 29).

Diagnosis

Diagnosing psychosomatic conditions is more complex than simply identifying unexplained medical symptoms; such complexity is due in part to there being little known about the etiology of unexplained medical symptoms as well as diagnostic criteria often relying on the absence as opposed to presence of symptoms (2). However, with the new guidelines in DSM-5 for somatization symptom and related disorders, the lack of necessity of no known medical etiology for symptoms has made the diagnosis more attainable for psychiatrists (30). Another problem with diagnosing psychosomatic conditions is the tremendous inconsistency between the medical and mental health fields which suggests a need for an accepted, shared, and multi-dimensional conceptual model (1). Considering that most patients with psychosomatic symptoms first present in a medical setting and often do not seek mental health services, the use of pediatric-liaison teams (pediatric and mental health) for accurate and efficient diagnosis is essential (5).

Utilization of a bio-psychosocial model is preferred; in this model, problems are not regarded as physical or psychological but where biological, social, and psychological factors are all considered as contributing factors. For primary care, it is important to understand how psychological factors may trigger and maintain unexplained physical symptoms (5).

For children and adolescents with psychosomatic concerns, evaluation of adverse childhood experiences is necessary. Such experiences include bullying, stress, increased number of significant life events, failure in school, and emotional conflict with parents. These concerns have been found to exacerbate irritable bowel syndrome, headache, hyperventilation, bronchial asthma, eating disorders, and orthostatic dysregulation. Other important factors when diagnosing psychosomatic conditions include feeling powerless, rejected by family, low levels of self-evaluation, distrust, negative life events, psycho-physiological symptoms, mother's health and well-being, and perception of parental love as well as caring (20). More rapid diagnosis and early referral to mental health professionals is needed to avoid unnecessary investigations and delays in diagnosis (6).

This diagnosis should also be acceptable and useful to patients. Patient knowledge about diagnosis has been shown to predict symptomatic remission (21). Parental influences play a huge role in the development and maintenance of somatic symptoms such as familial history of anxiety and depression, parental anxiety during the child's first year of life, and parental somatization (5).

As stated throughout the literature, what was previously known as *psychosomatic medicine* is now known as *consultation-liaison psychiatry*. This supports the idea that the terminology (*consultation-liaison psychiatry*) is more accurate in describing the practice of a specialty as opposed to describing symptoms of disorders. An emphasis on utilizing a holistic approach led to the development of the current DSM-5, which strays away from the diagnosis depending on an absence of a medical cause for somatic symptoms and provides positive diagnostic criteria (31). The DSM-5 thus shifts the focus to the psychological impact somatic symptoms can have rather than a medically or non-medically explained cause (31).

Diagnostics of psychosomatic conditions are still evolving and acceptability of terminology with patients is also important. Terms such as complex somatic symptom disorder more accurately capture what the patient is experiencing. Such a change in terminology could have greater predictive validity, clinical utility, and result in increased treatment efficacy (4, 21).

Diagnosing psychosomatic conditions is also difficult due to the ambiguity of patient presentation. Symptom presentation is often vague and exaggerated with patients often being resistant to psychological intervention; however, psychological factors cannot be overlooked or ignored during any part of treatment. These characteristics are also common to Factitious disorder and are organized around patients trying to meet emotional needs using dysfunctional methods (7, 32). The main difference between Somatoform Disorders and Factitious Disorder is that in the later physical and/or psychological symptoms are intentionally produced.

In psychosomatic conditions there are recurring, multiple, clinically significant physical complaints, symptoms are not produced voluntarily and are usually diagnosed by excluding organic causes for the physical complaints (6). Some clues to diagnose psychosomatic symptoms occur when there is a comorbid illness: no identifiable organic cause, the symptoms and signs do not correlate with damage patterns of known diseases, and the severity, duration and dysfunction of symptoms are disproportionate to the known diseases (6).

DSM-IV-TR somatoform disorders

The DSM-IV-TR provides diagnostic categories for only somatoform disorders. This is problematic because true somatoform disorders are purely psychological in nature while psychosomatic conditions, as stated previously, can impact almost any physical illness. The DSM-IV-TR (33) identifies the following somatoform disorders: Somatization disorder, undifferentiated somatoform disorder, conversion disorder, pain disorder, hypochondriasis, body dysmorphic disorder, and somatoform disorder NOS. However, these labels do not provide nearly enough information to qualitatively understand the patient experiencing psychosomatic symptoms (12).

DSM-5 somatic symptom and related disorders

The DSM-5 changes the terminology from somatoform disorders to *somatic symptom and related disorders* (34). The new classification removes somatization disorder, hypochondriasis, pain disorder, and undifferentiated somatoform disorder. These changes help reduce confusion for physicians while recognizing the complexity of psychosomatic conditions and the interface between mental health as well as medicine. In the DSM-5, there is less emphasis on medically unexplained symptoms and the DSM-5 also defines diagnoses on positive symptoms rather than the absence of symptoms. The potential psychological source of somatic symptoms is less emphasized, and the maladaptive coping mechanism of an individual as a reaction to the somatic symptoms is heavily emphasized (31). The following are the new proposed *somatic symptom and related disorders:*

- Somatic symptom disorder
- Illness anxiety disorder
- Conversion disorder (functional neurological symptom disorder)
- Psychological factors affecting medical condition
- Factitious disorder
- Somatic symptom disorder not elsewhere classified

The DSM 5 work group also noted that somatoform disorders along with psychological conditions affecting medical conditions, and factitious disorders all had in common both physical symptoms and/or concern about medical illness; thus, this led to renaming the category somatic symptom disorder. Due to the mind-body connection found in many psychological and medical conditions and the unreliability of assessing "medically unexplained" symptoms – these symptoms are no longer considered as core features of many of these disorders (34, 35).

Treatment

There is no consensus for treatment; however, it is becoming widely accepted that treatment should be individualized for each patient and that a team approach is often recommended utilizing parents, primary care physicians, pediatricians, psychologists, and psychiatrists (6). Considering that a majority of patients with psychosomatic symptoms first present in a hospital or medical setting, there needs to be an interface within the multidisciplinary team between the mental health and medical fields via co-located work environments or pediatric-liaison teams (36). Shared clinical protocols and a specialty-transcending information system are also necessary for optimal integrated care (36).

Holistic approaches are encouraged in the treatment of psychosomatic conditions; in particular it is important to explore the connections between psychological factors and unexplained medical symptoms (2, 5-8, 10). For children and adolescents, it is important to evaluate self-esteem as health concerns can lead to decreased levels of self-esteem (37). This represents a paradigm shift in the way psychosomatic symptoms are perceived and helps support a holistic and multidimensional view of treatment as opposed to simply responding to reported symptoms.

Treatment should be integrated and focus on the relationship between cognitive, emotional, and behavioral factors. Treatment programs often focus on body relatedness factors such as awareness, acceptance, expression of the self, pain management, and adaptation to impairment.

There needs to be a shift away from negative to more positive factors such as self-regulation, self-care, and integration of mind, body and life context (38).

Cognitive behavioral techniques

Cognitive behavioral interventions and pharmacotherapy are the primary treatment for psychosomatic conditions and are often bio-psychosocial in nature. Techniques suggested are those that involve self-monitoring, diaries, limiting attention given to somatic concerns, relaxation techniques, encouraging routine activities through gradual exposure, and work to help parents understand that their child is not intentionally creating the physical symptoms (2, 5, 6). Acceptance and commitment therapy (ACT) has shown promise in patients with psychosomatic conditions. ACT trains patients to focus on their present bodily sensations to increase mindfulness and develop a new, healthier mind-body relationship (39).

While cognitive behavioral techniques are the preferred interventions for psychosomatic conditions, there are several limitations. For instance, cognitive behavioral therapy often causes patients to challenge their destructive and irrational thoughts; however, the ability to cope with such a challenge may be reduced in psychiatric patients (39). Furthermore, cognitive behavioral therapy does not factor in abnormalities or possess a distinct diagnostic prognosis (39). Accepting multiple causal factors in the development of psychosomatic conditions allows the psychologist and physician the ability to design "hybrid" interventions that meet the complex needs of their patients. Early referral to mental health professionals is required to avoid unnecessary investigations and delays in diagnosis of psychosomatic conditions (2, 6).

Family

Including a strong emphasis on family is critical in the treatment of psychosomatic conditions. Enmeshed families are the most typical of children and adolescents with psychosomatic conditions (17). While working with families, it is recommended that psychosomatic conditions be explained clearly to the parents as many do not accept that psychological factors can cause physical symptoms. Many parents would prefer the diagnosis of an organic illness as it would explain the symptoms more clearly; however, it should be emphasized that the psychosomatic conditions are common, often reversible, and that it does not mean that their child is abnormal (6). In order to facilitate the relationship with the family, the medical team needs to be prepared to discuss with parents that physical disease has been ruled out.

Specific treatment recommendations include a strong emphasis on family treatment utilizing modified techniques to help engage families who are often resistant to treatment. The following are suggested (17):

- Obtain information regarding the family relational system;
- Emphasize positive aspects and resources of the family;
- Do not make early interpretation regarding connection between conflict and illness;
- Understand the illness in its context;
- Build hypothesis through Circular Questioning;

- Few patients are motivated for analytic types of therapy;
- Combine medical and psychological treatment;
- Intervention should be supportive and non-conflict-uncovering;
- Work to develop a long-term, positive, and trusting relationship;
- Utilize a pediatric-liaison model;
- Understand that treatment is often refused in the hospital population.

A professional "assessment" of the following is also recommended and includes the following (7):

- Complete initial workup including physical exam;
- Examine the child without parent;
- Obtain a psychosocial history including information about possible stressors;
- Discuss with family how psychological factors contribute to symptoms;
- Discuss with family the importance of an in-depth psychological evaluation;
- Communication between primary care physician and psychologist is essential;
- Help child learn to interpret bodily sensations;
- Utilization of cognitive behavior therapy, relaxation, and biofeedback techniques;
- Treat any co-occurring diagnoses such as anxiety and depression;
- Consideration of medication management.

Socio-demographics

As mentioned previously, socio-demographic characteristics play a role in eliciting psychosomatic conditions, which suggests that treatment should be grounded in socio-demographic factors (26). Stress does cause psychosomatic symptoms; however, the nature depends on socio-demographics such as age, sex, marital status, residence and economic conditions. Anchoring treatment interventions in socio-demographics allows psychologists and physicians to treat psychosomatic conditions in the context in which they occur.

Conclusion

Psychosomatic conditions are commonly seen in children and adolescents and occur within many illnesses. There remains a sizable amount of confusion regarding the definition, diagnosis, and treatment of psychosomatic conditions with continued research greatly needed in this area. Understanding psychosomatic conditions from a holistic perspective and complex etiology that is grounded in a bio-psychosocial model will aid in early identification, accurate diagnosis, and effective treatment. Pediatric-liaison teams are highly encouraged to help ensure meeting the complex needs of patients with psychosomatic conditions. Cognitive behavioral techniques are the preferred intervention but should also be expanded to include a focus on the relationship between family, socio-cultural factors, and pharmacotherapy.

Acknowledgment

Thank you to Helen D Pratt, PhD, to whom this book is dedicated, for her lifelong commitment to children and adolescents and mentoring of psychologists and physicians. I would also like to thank Donald E Greydanus, MD and Dilip Patel, MD for their ongoing and continued mentorship and support. Thank you also to Natalie K. Anderson, MA, Josephine Parrish, MA and Evan Wouters, MA for their help as research assistants.

References

[1] Löwe B, Mundt C, Herzog W, Brunner R, Backenstrass M, Kronmüller K, et al. Validity of current somatoform disorder diagnoses: Perspectives for classification in DSM-V and ICD-11. Psychopathol 2008;41(1):4-9.

[2] Asper F, Hiller W, Rist F, Bailer J, Witthöft M. Somatic symptom reporting has a dimensional latent structure: Results from taxometric analyses. J Abnorm Psychol 2012; 121(3):725-38.

[3] Onnis L. Psychosomatic medicine: Toward a new epistemology. Fam Syst Med 1993; 11(2):137-48.

[4] Voigt K, Wollburg E, Weinmann N, Herzog A, Meyer B, Langs G, et al. Predictive validity and clinical utility of DSM-5 somatic symptom disorder - Comparison with DSM-IV somatoform disorders and additional criteria for consideration. J Psychosom Res 2012;73(5):345-50.

[5] Garralda ME. Unexplained physical complaints. Child Adolesc Psychiatr Clin Noth Am 2010;19(2):199-209.

[6] Gupta V, Singh A, Upadhyay S, Bhatia B. Clinical profile of somatoform disorders in children. Indian J Pediatr 2011;78(3):283-6.

[7] Oatis MD. Psychosomatic illness in children and adolescents. Child Study Center Letter 2002;6(3):1-4.

[8] Tanaka H, Terashima S, Borres MP, Thulesius O. Psychosomatic problems and countermeasures in Japanese children and adolescents. Biopsychosoc Med 2012;6(1):6.

[9] Herrmann-Lingen C, Melzer J, von Boetticher D. Emotions, bodily changes, and the social environment: How did early psychosomatic medicine consider the social dimension in health and disease? Psychosom Med 2019;81(8):694-703.

[10] Patel KR, Weinrieb RM. Ethical and legal aspects of psychosomatic medicine. J Psychiatry Law 2012;40:63-74.

[11] Stone J, Colyer M, Feltbower S, Carson A, Sharpe M. "Psychosomatic": A systematic review of its meaning in newspaper articles. Psychosomatics 2004;45(4):287-90.

[12] Wise TN. Diagnostic criteria for psychosomatic research are necessary for DSM V. Psychother Psychosom 2009;78(6):330-2.

[13] Gitlin DF, Levenson JL, Lyketsos CG. Psychosomatic medicine: A new psychiatric subspecialty. Acad Psychiatry 2004;28(1):4-11.

[14] Boland RJ, Rundell J, Epstein S, Gitlin D. Consultation-liaison psychiatry vs psychosomatic medicine: What's in a name? Psychosomatics 2018;59(3):207-10.

[15] Kirmayer LJ, Robbins JM, Paris J. Somatoform disorders: Personality and the social matrix of somatic distress. J Abnorm Psychol 1994;103(1):125-36.

[16] Starcevic V. Somatoform disorders and DSM-V: Conceptual and political issues in the debate. Psychosomatics 2006;47(4):277-81.

[17] Wirsching M, Stierlin H. Psychosomatics I. Psychosocial characteristics of psychosomatic patients and their families. Fam Syst Med 1985;(1)4:6-16.

[18] Deter HC, Orth-Gomér K, Wasilewski B, Verissimo R. The European Network on Psychosomatic Medicine (ENPM) - history and future directions. Biopsychosoc Med 2017;11(1):3.

[19] Shaw RJ, Pao M, Holland JE, DeMaso DR. Practice patterns revisited in pediatric psychosomatic medicine. Psychosomatics 2016;57(6):576-85.

[20] Masuda A, Yamanaka T, Hirakawa T, Koga Y, Minomo R, Munemoto T, et al. Intra- and extra-familial adverse childhood experiences and a history of childhood psychosomatic disorders among Japanese university students. Biopsychosoc Med 2007;1:9.
[21] Nagel A, Voigt K, Meyer B, Glaesmer H, Löwe B, Brähler E. Public familiarity with the terms somatoform disorder and functional disorder in Germany: Results from a representative population survey. Prim Care Companion CNS Discord 2012;14(1):e1-5.
[22] Mohapatra S, Deo SJK, Satapathy A, Rath N. Somatoform disorders in children and adolescents. Ger J Psychiatry 2014;17:19-24.
[23] Winarizal AS, Horvath A, Sawyer SM. Measuring functional recovery in somatic symptom and related disorders: a scoping review. Arch Dis Child 2020;105(11):1086-92.
[24] Cottrell DJ. Fifteen-minute consultation: Medically unexplained symptoms. Arch Dis Child Educ Pract Ed 2016;101(3):114-8.
[25] Boerner KE, Green K, Chapman A, Stanford E, Newlove T, Edwards K, et al. Making sense of "somatization": A systematic review of its relationship to pediatric pain. J Pediatr Psychol 2020;45(2):156-69.
[26] Ewhrudjakpor C. Socio-demographics, life event stressors and psychosomatic disorders among public servants in the Niger Delta region of Nigeria. Int J Sociol Anthropol 2009;1(3):55-61.
[27] Kanayama G, Hudson JI, Pope HG. Culture, psychosomatics and substance abuse: the example of body image drugs. Psychother Psychosom 2012;81(2):73-8.
[28] Bergner S. The analytic environment in times of bodily dysfunction: The effect of psychoanalytic psychosomatic theories. Psychoanal Psychol 2009;26(4):362-78.
[29] Boschan PJ. Body, mind and bonds. Am J Psychoanal 2007;67(3):235-48.
[30] Henningsen P. Management of somatic symptom disorder. Dialogues Clin Neurosci 2018;20(1):23-31.
[31] Barsky AJ. Assessing the new DSM-5 diagnosis of somatic symptom disorder. Psychosom Med 2016;78(1):2-4.
[32] Krahn LE, Bostwick JM, Stonnington CM. Looking toward DSM-V: Should factitious disorder become a subtype of somatoform disorder? Psychosomatics 2008;49(4):277-82.
[33] American Psychiatric Association. Diagnostic and statistical manual of mental disorders, Fourth ed, text rev, IV. Washington, DC: American Psychiatric Association, 2000:943.
[34] American Psychiatric Association. Diagnostic and statistical manual of mental disorders, Fifth edition. Washington, DC: American Psychiatric Association, 2013.
[35] American Psychiatric Association. Somatic symptom disorder. American Psychiatric Association, 2013. URL: www.dsm5.org.
[36] Leue C, van Schijndel MA, Keszthelyi D, van Koeveringe G, Ponds RW, Kathol RG, et al. The multidisciplinary arena of psychosomatic medicine – Time for a transitional network approach. Eur J Psychiatry 2020;34(2):63-73.
[37] Hosogi M, Okada A, Fujii C, Noguchi K, Watanabe K. Importance and usefulness of evaluating self-esteem in children. Biopsychosoc Med 2012;6:9.
[38] Kalisvaart H, van Broeckhuysen S, Bühring M, Kool MB, van Dulmen S, Geenen R. Definition and structure of body-relatedness from the perspective of patients with severe somatoform disorder and their therapists. PLoS One 20127(8):e42534.
[39] Sayyar S, Ghanbari MR, Omid A, Eduard Scheidt C, Giveki R, Mohammadian R. Effectiveness of acceptance and commitment therapy on psychosomatic symptoms and mindfulness in patients with psychosomatic disorders. Pract Clin Psychol 2019;7(2):79-86.

Chapter 2

Pediatric sleep disorders

Muhammed Ather, MRCPsych, Nehdia Hashemi, MD, Salma Malik, MD, FAACAP, Finza Latif, MD, FAACAP, Mohammed Al-Breiki, MRCPsych and Ahsan Nazeer*, MD

Sidra Medicine, Doha, Qatar University, Doha, Qatar and Institute of Living/Hartford Healthcare, Hartford, Connecticut, United States of America

Abstract

Patterns of normal sleep are considered, including the circadian cycle, which is considered the body's internal clock, REM, and NREM sleep. Sleep disorders are a prevalent problem in the pediatric population, affecting more than 25-30% of children. Sleep disorders that are discussed include behavioral insomnia, delayed sleep phase disorder (DSPD), disorder of sleep-related rhythmic movement (RMD), nightmares, obstructive sleep apnea (OSA), arousal disorders, sleep disorder secondary to poor sleep hygiene, restless leg syndrome (RLS), and narcolepsy. Clinicians caring for children and adolescents are advised to evaluate the sleep health of their pediatric patients and provide management for sleep problems that may arise.

Introduction

Sleep-related issues are a common source of parental anxiety and concern. It has long been established that adequate sleep is necessary for proper brain and body development. Nonetheless, recent estimates indicate that sleep disorders are a prevalent problem in the pediatric population, affecting more than 25-30% of children (1). Numerous sleep difficulties in childhood can be understood as mild behavioral issues; however, other sleep-related difficulties indicate more severe disorders. Increased understanding of sleep development and disorders is critical for correct diagnosis and successful intervention. Research suggests that sleep problems persist throughout childhood, with up to half of children who experience sleep problems during the first three years also experience them again two to three years later.

* ***Correspondence:*** Email: anazeer@sidra.org.

In: Behavioral Pediatrics II
Editors: Donald E. Greydanus, Dilip R. Patel, Ahsan Nazeer et al.
ISBN: 979-8-88697-019-7

Classification of sleep disorders

In 1979, the "Diagnostic classification of sleep and arousal disorders" tabulated sleep disorders into different groups and served as the foundation for subsequent systems of classification. In 1990, the International Classification of Sleep Disorders (ICSD) was published due to the collaboration of numerous international sleep societies for academic purposes and has since been widely adopted by clinicians. The International classification of sleep disorders (ICSD) was updated and modified slightly in 2005, resulting in version 2 (ICSD-2) and listing 81 major sleep disorders in eight major categories (2). The new ICSD-3 was published in 2014, and the classification scheme was re-evaluated and revised (3).

The third edition of the International Classification of Sleep Disorders (ICSD-3) classified sixty distinct sleep disorders into seven major categories. While the diagnostic guidelines for each condition were updated to be as specific as possible, the fact remains that the current body of research remains unclear about sleep disorders as a whole. The above difficulty is particularly true in clinical practice when a certain level of impairment in functioning is needed to attain therapeutic significance and the best way to measure it.

As a consequence of these limitations, a certain degree of clinical flexibility is needed to diagnose sleep disorders in day-to-day clinical practice. It will be prudent to make a provisional diagnosis while maintaining close monitoring and retesting to clarify the diagnosis further. Like ICSD-2, ICSD-3, with the exception of obstructive sleep apnea (OSA), does not differentiate pediatric conditions from adult diagnoses (4).

In comparison, the DSM-5's new classification classifies sleep-wake disorders into ten broader disorder categories or disorder groups. Common sleep disturbances in children include insomnia, obstructive sleep apnea, parasomnia, narcolepsy, and restless legs syndrome. These disorders impair children's development and functioning in daytime attention, emotion regulation, behavior, and learning. There is mounting evidence that children with medical and psychiatric disabilities, such as attention-deficit/hyperactivity disorder (ADHD), mood disorders, and autism spectrum disorders, are more likely to experience sleep disorders (6). According to current research, 74% to 84% of children and adolescents with psychiatric disabilities suffer from severe sleep problems (7). Other well-known risk factors include asthma, allergic rhinitis, epilepsy, and obesity. Other frequently reported sleep symptoms include bedtime settling issues, restless sleep, shorter sleep, frequent nocturnal awakenings in younger children, and delayed sleep phase syndrome during adolescence.

Patterns of normal sleep

Ongoing research and recent clinical advances have resulted in a greater appreciation for the importance of adequate sleep. We now understand that sleep is a dynamic physiological state involving higher cortical structures and is critical for the overall brain and body development and behavioral and emotional control. Additionally, sleep affects executive functions such as attention, planning, abstract thinking, working memory, and impulse control. As a result, chronically sleep-deprived children are frequently labeled as irritable, aggressive, impulsive, and hyperactive. This may also help to explain why children with a primary sleep disorder are commonly misdiagnosed with ADHD.

The sleep-wake cycle undergoes rapid changes throughout the first year and during infancy. In newborns, sleep cycles are brief and are spread throughout the 24 hours. At three months of age, the circadian rhythm starts to develop, and by implementing consistent feeding and bedtime routines, parents can encourage the development of a sleep pattern that is more rhythmical in nature. Children start taking daytime naps during the early childhood years and can have night awakenings. Whether or not the nighttime disruptions will become troublesome depends on numerous factors. Still, the child's willingness to go back to sleep without assistance is the most critical among those factors. During school years, most children stop taking daytime naps, and the duration of nighttime sleep also decreases steadily through puberty. However, it is essential to note that the above sleep pattern is primarily an academic debate, as in reality, sleep patterns are influenced by cultural norms, parental habits, siblings' practices of sleep, school as well as daycare schedules, and the internal biological plus behavioral rhythms of the children and adolescents (8).

Circadian rhythms

Circadian rhythms involved in the sleep-wake cycle and body temperature regulation are 24-hour repeating physiologic and behavioral cycles regulated by the suprachiasmatic nucleus (SCN), which is located in the anterior hypothalamus (9). The SCN controls the melatonin production via the pineal gland, which starts secreting about two hours before normal sleep time and peaks during the middle of the night. Circadian rhythm and body temperature are also closely related, with deeper sleep occurring around 4 a.m. when the body temperature is lowest and lighter sleep occurring during the late morning hours when the body temperature rises in anticipation of the increased energy demands of impending wakefulness. Any disruptions in these rhythms result in the desynchronization of numerous internal homeostatic cycles, leading to detrimental effects on multiple physiological and behavioral functions.

The circadian cycle, considered the body's internal clock, is one hour longer than a typical 24-hour day and is influenced by light, temperature, noise, bedtime routines, and medications. An ultradian rhythm controls the timing and duration of rapid eye movement (REM) and non-rapid eye movement (NREM) sleep, two distinct types of sleep alternating throughout the sleep period.

REM and NREM sleep

REM sleep is also referred to as active sleep because the active physiological and neurochemical processes and the electroencephalographic patterns are comparable to those of the awake state. It is associated with irregular breathing patterns, decreased muscle tone, increased cerebral blood flow, and increased metabolic rate. While brain activity is at its peak during REM sleep, individuals appear relaxed due to active inhibition of muscle tone via pons signals. As a result, when these inhibitory signals are disrupted, children exhibit abnormal motor activity, a condition known as a REM behavior disorder or parasomnia. The brain increases protein production and stimulates areas of the brain associated with learning during

REM sleep. Infants spend nearly half of their time in REM sleep, which decreases to about 25% during childhood.

Unlike REM sleep, which is characterized by neuronal activation, NREM sleep, or quiet sleep, is characterized by physiological and behavioral inhibition. Breathing and heart rate become rhythmic during this phase, and active inhibition of muscle tone ceases. By six months of age, the differentiation of NREM sleep into four stages is complete, and the stages are identified by sleep spindles, K-complexes, and delta waves.

Common sleep disorders

The following is a brief description of the common sleep disorders encountered in day-to-day clinical practice. Sleep disorders considered now include behavioral insomnia, delayed sleep phase disorder (DSPD), disorder of sleep-related rhythmic movement (RMD), nightmares, obstructive sleep apnea (OSA), arousal disorders, sleep disorder secondary to poor sleep hygiene, restless leg syndrome (RLS), and narcolepsy.

Behavioral insomnia

Nighttime awakening issues are among the most frequently cited reasons for parents to seek help from a health care professional. Bedtime resistance and frequent nighttime awakenings are extremely common in infants, occurring in approximately 20-30% of them (10). Most infants awaken during the night and can self-soothe until they fall back to sleep. The ICSD identifies three subtypes of behavioral insomnia of childhood: sleep-onset association type, limit-setting type, and mixed type. These categories have the common symptoms of difficulty falling asleep on one's own or experiencing repeated night waking.

Negative sleep associations cause insomnia of sleep-onset association type, such as a child's dependence on the parents for rocking, feeding, or having screen time, resulting in delayed sleep onset or repeated night waking. In comparison, insomnia of limit-setting time occurs when children refuse to go to bed or make repetitive demands to postpone bedtime. They may use several tactics, including asking to use the bathroom or "one more story," to defer the bedtime as long as possible. These disorders contrast to the older children's nighttime difficulties, including difficulty going to sleep or repeated waking, which is primarily anxiety-related and are not behavioral.

In order to test children for developmental/behavioral insomnia, it is essential for clinicians to routinely inquire about sleep from parents by asking questions about onset latency, quality and length of sleep, resistance at bedtime, nighttime waking, sleep-related breathing symptoms, and any signs of excessive daytime sleepiness (11). Clinicians can also consider using sleep monitoring questionnaires, including BEARS (bedtime issues, excessive daytime sleepiness, night awakenings, sleep regularity and duration, and snoring). If, after the screening, it is noted that sleep problems need further study, parents should then be encouraged to keep a sleep diary (12). Assessment should also include concerns about the impact of the child's sleep issues on the family to understand the dysfunction that it may be causing in parents' lives. If there is a concern that the child may be struggling with sleep-related breathing disorders, narcolepsy, or periodic limb movement disorder, a referral for polysomnography should be considered.

Behavioral therapies are steadily being accepted as the best first line of defense against behavioral insomnia. These approaches are focused on cognitive-behavioral strategies, including reinforcement. The main goals usually focus on healthy sleeping habits, creating schedules, and incorporating calming skills. Focus is also given to instruct the adults as their responses, in turn, influence the child's behavior; for example, one can encourage them to wait for progressively longer intervals before intervening or allowing the infant to cry for a few nights.

A growing body of research indicates that treatments for childhood insomnia, especially in the first few years of life, are successful (13). One study suggests that behavioral therapies increase children's sleep, attitudes, and maternal well-being (14). Parents are also encouraged to put infants to bed while they are still awake to promote their innate ability to self-soothe. Infants who are rocked or fed until they fall asleep, on the other hand, are more likely to seek parental comfort during nighttime awakenings. Contrary to popular belief, children do not outgrow sleep problems and need parental help and consistency to develop a healthy rhythm.

Delayed sleep phase disorder (DSPD)

Children and adolescents with the delayed sleep-phase disorder have persistent difficulty falling asleep and waking up at socially appropriate times. As a result, they usually display extreme daytime sleepiness. They usually sleep between 1–6 AM (01:00-06:00) and wake in the late morning or early afternoon hours. As a result, they struggle to be on time and are often tardy for morning classes in school. The prevalence of DSPD is estimated to be between 0.2% to 10%. Interestingly, DSPD appears to run in families, pointing to a genetic predisposition (15).

The exact cause of DSPD is unknown, but it possibly develops when the body needs a longer than average time to complete one circadian cycle. Behavioral and psychological influences also influence DSPD. With repeated cycles, the individuals develop a routine in which they function better during the latter part of the day, thus causing further disruptions in circadian cycles (16).

A careful history and a well-kept sleep diary are needed for the diagnosis. Standardized chronotype questionnaires are also effective instruments for determining the associated symptoms, including depression, anxiety, and personality disorders. Treatment is usually with a combination of early morning light therapy and evening melatonin (0.5mg-5mg). Bright light (full spectrum or blue-enriched) is shown to progress circadian patterns; also, melatonin improves sleep and wake-up periods and depression in patients with DSPS. Melatonin can be continued for up to a year; however, up to 90% of people experience relapses after discontinuing melatonin (17-19).

Disorder of sleep-related rhythmic movement (RMD)

This disorder is characterized by repetitive and stereotypical sleep movements involving any body part. Parents may report witnessing questionable behaviors such as head banging and body rocking. RMD is typically a self-limiting, normal physiological phenomenon in a healthy child; however, children with intellectual disabilities and other psychiatric disorders, such as autism and attention deficit hyperactivity disorder, have been observed to present with this disorder as well. These repetitive body movements should always be reported to health care professionals, even more so if they occur during the sleep period. RMD is more likely to persist beyond childhood in these more complex situations and requires specialized treatment; this management may include the use of protective helmets, behavior modification, and medications such as benzodiazepines and atypical antipsychotics. On the other hand, in most cases, reassuring parents and informing them about the benign nature of this physiological variant is sufficient.

Disorder of nightmares

Nighttime fears are most prevalent during the preschool years when children frequently refuse to go to bed. Fears of darkness, being alone, or imaginary creatures in their room are common in this age group's nighttime struggles. Factors contributing to bedtime stalling and disturbed sleep include parental conflict, child anxiety, excessive stimulation during the day, increased emotional arousal, and a desire to spend more time with the parents.

In contrast, nightmares are unpleasant experiences and cause insomnia because of the fear of facing another nightmare after falling asleep. ICSD-3 classifies nightmare disorders as parasomnias that occur during rapid eye movement (REM) sleep and are typically reported by children between the ages of three and six. To make a diagnosis, DSM-5 asks for a frequency criterion to be met: nightmares should occur at least once a week (20). Typically, nightmares occur between the third and fourth hours of the night and cause the child to awaken. Children are distressed and wide awake following the nightmare and typically have vivid memories of the event the following morning, frequently involving loss or abandonment.

While nightmares are a natural occurrence, factors contributing to nightmares and distressing dreams include anxiety, stress, sleep deprivation, posttraumatic stress disorder (PTSD), and medications (e.g., amphetamines). Another cause of REM rebound and nightmares is withdrawal from REM suppressant medications (e.g., clonidine). Numerous other medications can also cause nightmares, including beta-blockers, anti-asthmatics, medications for bronchitis and migraines, and selective serotonin reuptake inhibitors (SSRIs).

A thorough evaluation of the child and the parents are needed as, in most cases, at least one of the parents has a non-restorative sleep issue. It is essential to conduct a thorough sleep history that includes current medication use, sleep hygiene, medications, and recent family traumas, including any ongoing physical or emotional abuse. It is critical to differentiate nightmares from traumatic dreams secondary to traumatic experiences. The subjective quality of nightmares secondary to trauma is different in that after the posttraumatic nightmares' children have more intense symptoms of arousal and feelings of helplessness (21, 22). Polysomnography is usually not needed to diagnose a nightmare disorder; however, it is requested to rule out other sleep disorders, including narcolepsy.

For the nightmares associated with posttraumatic stress disorder (23), prazosin, a centrally-acting antagonist of the alpha 1-adrenergic receptor, is considered the first-line treatment. Non-medication-related treatments are helpful in reducing the repetition of nightmares; these include desensitization and exposure therapy as well as imagery rehearsal therapy (IRT). In IRT, individuals write down their nightmares and then change the ending with a positive twist and desired outcome. In combination with cognitive-behavioral therapy, IRT is also effective in PTSD-induced nightmares (21). Nonpharmacological interventions also need to address maladaptive cognitive schema in older children, including frequent ruminations and catastrophizing about dreams.

Obstructive sleep apnea (OSA)

Obstructive sleep-disordered breathing affects between 3-12% of the children and usually manifests as excessive daytime somnolence. Its prevalence typically peaks during the preschool years. Snoring is found in 3-12% of children and does not necessarily indicate OSA. Affected children display symptoms that suggest OSA but lack associated polysomnographic findings. Compared to occasional snoring that does not have any specific health consequences, children with OSA display behavioral disorders, obesity, hyperactivity, enuresis, and at times cor pulmonale. The American Academy of Pediatrics recommends that all children with habitual snoring be evaluated primarily because of the health-related consequences. Most of these children exhibit only minor symptoms, eventually outgrowing the disease.

OSA is frequently caused by adenotonsillar hypertrophy, neuromuscular dysfunction, or craniofacial anomalies. However, it is essential to note that many children with adenotonsillar hypertrophy never exhibit signs of OSA, which indicates that a combination of adenotonsillar hypertrophy and neuromuscular tone loss may be at the core of OSA. Other risk factors are premature birth, African-American ancestry, and asthma. It is believed that asthma symptoms worsen at night due to circadian changes in lung function. Additionally, young children with asthma have more frequent nocturnal awakenings than non-asthmatic children.

Obesity is increasingly recognized as a risk factor for snoring and sleep apnea in children, contributing to upper airway obstruction during sleep. As childhood obesity rates rise, more attention should be paid to this issue and its mechanisms contributing to sleep problems. OSA causes frequent nighttime awakenings, impairs growth hormone secretion, resulting in growth retardation or failure to thrive syndrome in severe cases.

Children with OSA can present a varied clinical picture. Snoring is the most frequent symptom among children younger than five years of age. At times parents also notice restlessness throughout the night, mouth breathing, apneic episodes, and frequent awakenings. Children older than five years of age usually present with enuresis, inattention during the day, hyperactivity, cognitive difficulties, and inability to succeed in school. In severe cases of OSA, it is not uncommon to see hypertension and pulmonary hypertension. A physical examination of the child suspected of having OSA should focus on craniofacial abnormalities, including midface hypoplasia, micrognathia, septal deviation, nasal polyps, turbinate hypertrophy, and nasal aperture stenosis (24).

Treatment of OSA depends upon the underlying cause. Adenotonsillectomy is usually the treatment of choice; however, continuous positive airway pressure (CPAP) becomes the treatment of choice when it is contraindicated. It is important to note that a six-monthly follow-up is needed to maintain regular face mask adjustments because of the skeletal growth in children. CPAP is an effective treatment; however, about 20% of the children have difficulty tolerating this modality. The underlying cause is chronic tonsillitis or adenoiditis; treatment with antibiotics can be beneficial by reducing post-infectious lymphoid hyperplasia, thus alleviating the obstruction. In children with obesity, weight reduction becomes the primary therapy, and efforts are made to maintain healthy eating habits and exercise.

Maintaining a healthy weight is increasingly becoming one of the mainstays of the treatment, as numerous studies have found that overweight children continue to develop OSA than children with average weight after adenotonsillectomy; this suggests that obesity plays a significant role in the prognosis of the treatment of OSA (25-27).

Arousal disorders (AD)

Arousal disorders include sleep terrors, sleepwalking, sleep talking, and confusional arousal; these are usually considered benign phenomena. In most cases, these disorders do not lead to adverse health outcomes and are mostly a nuisance for the parents and relatives. By definition, these are motor behaviors arising from NREM sleep and are most prevalent between the ages of 3 and 13 years that typically resolve by the age of 10-11 years. Arousals usually occur between the first and second hours of sleep; children simultaneously appear asleep and awake, are sporadic, last between five and fifteen minutes, and typically occur only once a night. During these episodes, the child may exhibit dramatic behavior, be unaware of his or her surroundings, and have a fragmented memory of the events that transpire. These behaviors can be confused with nocturnal epilepsy.

Additionally, the child may experience severe autonomic arousal, manifested by tachypnea, tachycardia, and diaphoresis. Parental attempts to calm and console the child are frequently unsuccessful. Factors that increase the delta sleep augment the probability of AD occurring during the night; these include febrile illness, stress, certain medications, and sleep deprivation (28).

ADs are usually diagnosed by taking a careful history and performing a comprehensive medical, neurological and developmental examination. Parental descriptions and their home recordings on smartphones are usually sufficient to diagnose; in most cases, video-polysomnography (VPSG) is not needed. When evaluating these parasomnias, medical providers must rule out nocturnal frontal lobe seizures (NFLE), nightmares, and PTSD. Careful history-taking to elicit differentiating features is needed. In most cases, ADs start at an early age and usually occur no more than one time per night. The episode is of longer duration. Mostly, they decrease or completely resolve after puberty. In NFLE, the episodes are of a shorter duration, occur between the ages of 10 and 20 years, and often persist into adulthood (29).

Reassuring parents about the benign nature of AD is an essential part of management. Parents are encouraged not to awaken or console their child during the episode, and instead, they should be gently redirected to bed. It is important to maintain regular sleep schedules. Basic protective measures are helpful and provide a sense of safety for the family; these include clearing the clutter in the house, sleeping on the first floor, and installing locks or alarms on the stairs and window (30). Some authors recommend scheduled waking 15-30 minutes before the episode for a few minutes and have noted improvement in the symptoms (31). For severe cases, low-dose clonazepam or imipramine can be recommended.

Sleep disorder secondary to impaired sleep hygiene

The school-age years are characterized by a decline in parental supervision and increased autonomy. Children require at least 10 hours of sleep per night during this phase; however, numerous daily responsibilities may conflict with this requirement, including social, academic, and athletic activities. Electronic communication, which ranges from instant messaging and Internet chat rooms to cyberbullying, competes with sleep and disrupts bedtime routines. Nighttime fears, poor sleep hygiene, parasomnias, and restless leg syndrome are just a few of the prevalent sleep problems in this age group.

Poor sleep hygiene is one of the most common causes of sleep onset problems, affecting approximately 10% of school-aged children. Education of parents about healthy sleeping habits is a critical first step. Sleeping routines assessment and the use of a daily sleep diary aid in the differential diagnosis of sleep-related issues.

Restless leg syndrome (RLS)

Unpleasant sensations typically characterize restless leg syndrome (RLS) in the legs that occur before the sleep onset, an irresistible urge to move the legs, relief after moving, and recurrence of symptoms after the cession of movements. RLS is inherited as autosomal dominant in younger children, and there is typically a positive family history among first-degree relatives. It affects about 2% of children and strongly correlates with ADHD (32). This condition is probably underdiagnosed in children, given that 10% of adults report symptoms beginning before the age of ten years. The diagnosis in children is also challenging primarily because of the inability of the children to describe the typical symptoms; thus, in challenging cases, overnight sleep study and positive family history add to the diagnosis.

The etiology of RLS is not understood well. Low serum ferritin levels are associated with RLS, and those with ferritin levels less than 35g/L may benefit from iron replacement therapy. Some of the current theories guiding its pathophysiology include genetic factors, dopamine dysfunction, shared pathogenesis with ADHD, and indications of chromosome 6p21.1. Numerous medications, including selective serotonin reuptake inhibitors (SSRIs), diphenhydramine, and sleep deprivation, can also cause RLS. Cognitive deficits and ADHD is reported in children with RLS (33). Cardiac complications are common in adults but are not reported in children.

Removing any offending agents is usually the best course at the start of the management. Healthy sleeping habits, avoiding heavy meals at bedtime, and limiting exposure to bright light are also some of the nonpharmacological measures that should be considered. Dopaminergic medication, including carbidopa/levodopa and dopamine agonists (pramipexole, ropinirole), are the preferred choices in adults with RLS; however, no specific approved medications exist for use in children. Sporadic published case reports have shown beneficial effects after using levodopa, ropinirole, pramipexole, and pergolide in youth and adolescents (34, 35).

Narcolepsy

Narcolepsy is a chronic neurodegenerative condition that manifests as excessive daytime sleepiness accompanied by cataplexy, hypnagogic hallucinations, and sleep paralysis. The onset of symptoms is around 16 years of age, and children usually present with poor academic performance, social difficulties, parent-child conflicts, depression, and hopelessness. Genetic factors are significant, and between 8% and 10% of affected individuals report having a first-degree relative with a similar disorder. Because of the comorbidity with psychiatric symptoms, there is a serious risk of misdiagnosis, and in one recent study, almost 60% of the participants received an alternate diagnosis before the diagnosis of narcolepsy (36). To improve on the diagnosis, it is recommended to use validated measures, including Epworth Sleepiness Scale-child and adolescent version (EPP-CHAD), to identify sleepiness (37).

Narcolepsy is associated with hypocretin ligand deficiency in the brain and cerebrospinal fluid, as well as a specific human leukocyte antigen (HLA-DQB1*0602). The differential diagnosis includes chronic sleep deprivation, Kleine-Levin syndrome, and psychiatric disorders such as depression and attention-deficit/hyperactivity disorder. The diagnosis is aided by polysomnography and multiple sleep latency testing.

The treatment of narcolepsy should be tailored individually by both pharmacological and nonpharmacological interventions. Medications are usually used to treat excessive daytime sleepiness. Sodium oxybate, methylphenidate, and dextroamphetamine are wake-promoting agents approved by the FDA for use in children seven years and older. SSRI, selective norepinephrine reuptake inhibitor (SNRI), and atomoxetine are the most frequently prescribed agents for cataplexy. Among the SNRIs, venlafaxine is usually the one that is most favored. Educating parents and teachers about this disorder helps reduce stigma and dispels the myth that the child is rebellious, slothful, or bored. Nonpharmacological strategies are also helpful; these include yoga, mindfulness, support groups, small meals that are low in carbohydrates, and temperature regulation (preference for cold temperatures) in the environment (38).

Conclusion

Children's sleep disturbances are common during childhood and are a significant cause of parental concern. They are, however, sometimes misdiagnosed. Due to the high incidence of behavioral comorbidities in children with sleep disorders, most children with sleep disorders receive an initial evaluation in a mental health clinic. Essential tools for timely diagnosis and delivering adequate care to children with sleep disorders include suspicion, a multidisciplinary clinical plan that considers developmental factors, and coordination with a pediatric sleep specialist.

References

[1] Owens J. Classification and epidemiology of childhood sleep disorders. Prim Care 2008; 35(3):533-46.

[2] American Academy of Sleep Medicine: International Classification of Sleep Disorders: Diagnostic and Coding Manual, 2nd edition. Westchester: American Academy of Sleep Medicine, 2005.

[3] American Academy of Sleep Medicine. International classification of sleep disorders. 3rd edition. Darien, IL: American Academy of Sleep Medicine, 2014.

[4] Sateia MJ. International classification of sleep disorders, Third Edition. Chest 2014; 146(5):1387–94.

[5] Gregory AM, Sadeh A. Sleep, emotional and behavioral difficulties in children and adolescents. Sleep Med Rev 2012;16(2):129-36.

[6] Gau SSF, Kessler RC, Tseng W-L, Wu Y-Y, Chiu Y-N, Yeh C-B, et al. Association between sleep problems and symptoms of attention-deficit/hyperactivity disorder in young adults. Sleep 2007;30(2):195–201.

[7] Cortesi F, Giannotti F, Ivanenko A, Johnson K. Sleep in children with autistic spectrum disorder. Sleep Med 2010;11(7):659–64.

[8] Galland BC, Taylor BJ, Elder DE, Herbison P. Normal sleep patterns in infants and children: A systematic review of observational studies. Sleep Med Rev 2012;16(3):213–22.

[9] Golombek DA, Rosenstein RE. Physiology of circadian entrainment. Physiol Rev 2010; 90(3):1063–102.

[10] Vriend J, Corkum P. Clinical management of behavioral insomnia of childhood. Psychol Res Behav Manag 2011;4:69-79.

[11] Fallone G, Owens JA, Deane J. Sleepiness in children and adolescents: clinical implications. Sleep Med Rev 2002;6(4):287–306.

[12] Moore M, Meltzer LJ, Mindell JA. Bedtime problems and night wakings in children. Sleep Med Clin 2007;2(3):377–85.

[13] Mindell JA, Kuhn B, Lewin DS, Meltzer LJ, Sadeh A. Behavioral treatment of bedtime problems and night wakings in infants and young children. Sleep 2006;29(10):1263–76.

[14] Mindell JA, Telofski LS, Wiegand B, Kurtz ES. A nightly bedtime routine: impact on sleep in young children and maternal mood. Sleep 2009;32(5):599–606.

[15] Archer S.N., Carpen JD, Gibson M, Lim GH, Johnston JD, Skene DJ, et al. Polymorphism in the PER3 promoter associates with diurnal preference and delayed sleep phase disorder. Sleep 2010;33(5):695–701.

[16] Crowley SJ, Carskadon MA. Modifications to weekend recovery sleep delay circadian phase in older adolescents. Chronobiol Int 2010;27(7):1469-92.

[17] Paul MA, Gray GW, Lieberman HR, Love RJ, Miller JC, Trouborst M, et al. Phase advance with separate and combined melatonin and light treatment. Psychopharmacology (Berl) 2011;214(2):515-23.

[18] Crowley SJ, Acebo C, Fallone G, Carskadon MA. Estimating dim light melatonin onset (DLMO) phase in adolescents using summer or school-year sleep/wake schedules. Sleep 2006;29(12):1632–41.

[19] Rahman SA, Kayumov L, Shapiro CM. Antidepressant action of melatonin in the treatment of delayed sleep phase syndrome. Sleep Med 2010;11(2):131–6.

[20] American Psychiatric Association, Diagnostic and statistical manual of mental disorders, DSM-5, fifth edition. Arlington, VA: American Psychiatric Association, 2013.

[21] Gieselmann A, Ait Aoudia M, Carr M, Germain A, Gorzka R, Holzinger B, Aetiology and treatment of nightmare disorder: State of the art and future perspectives. J Sleep Res 2019;28(4):e12820.

[22] Germain A, Nielsen TA. Sleep pathophysiology in posttraumatic stress disorder and idiopathic nightmare sufferers. Biol Psychiatry 2003;54(10):1092-8.

[23] Aurora RN, Zak RS, Maganti RK, Auerbach SH, Casey KR, Chowdhuri S, et al. Best practice guide for the treatment of REM sleep behavior disorder (RBD). J Clin Sleep Med 2010;06(01):85–95.

[24] Chan J, Edman JC, Koltai PJ. Obstructive sleep apnea in children. Am Fam Physician 2004;69(5):1147-54.

[25] Mitchell RB, Kelly J. Outcome of adenotonsillectomy for obstructive sleep apnea in obese and normal-weight children. Otolaryngol Head Neck Surg 2007;137(1):43-8.

[26] O'Brien LM, Sitha S, Baur LA, Waters KA. Obesity increases the risk for persisting obstructive sleep apnea after treatment in children. Int J Pediatr Otorhinolaryngol 2006; 70(9):1555-60.

[27] Marcus CL, Moore RH, Rosen CL, Giordani B, Garetz SL, Taylor HG, et al. A randomized trial of adenotonsillectomy for childhood sleep apnea. N Engl J Med 2013; 368(25):2366–76.

[28] Moore M, Allison D, Rosen CL. A review of pediatric nonrespiratory sleep disorders. Chest 2006;130(4):1252–62.

[29] Tinuper P, Provini F, Bisulli F, Vignatelli L, Plazzi G, Vetrugno R, et al. Movement disorders in sleep: Guidelines for differentiating epileptic from non-epileptic motor phenomena arising from sleep. Sleep Med Rev 2007;11(4):255–67.

[30] Kotagal S. Parasomnias in childhood. Sleep Med Rev 2009;13(2):157–68.

[31] Lask B. Sleep disorders. "Working treatment" best for night terrors. BMJ 1993; 306(6890):1477.

[32] Picchietti D, Allen RP, Walters AS, Davidson JE, Myers A, Ferini-Strambi L. Restless legs syndrome: Prevalence and impact in children and adolescents The Peds REST Study. Pediatrics 2007;120(2):253–66.

[33] Pearson VE, Allen RP, Dean T, Gamaldo CE, Lesage SR, Earley CJ. Cognitive deficits associated with restless legs syndrome (RLS). Sleep Med 2006;7(1):25–30.

[34] Walters AS, Mandelbaum DE, Lewin DS, Kugler S, England SJ, Miller M. Dopaminergic therapy in children with restless legs/periodic limb movements in sleep and ADHD. Dopaminergic Therapy Study Group. Pediatr Neurol 2000;22(3):182-6.

[35] Konofal E, Arnulf I, Lecendreux M, Mouren M-C. Ropinirole in a child with attention-deficit hyperactivity disorder and restless legs syndrome. Pediatr Neurol 2005;32(5):350–1.

[36] Ohayon M, Thorpy M, Black J, Williams MJ, Pasta DJ, Hyman D, et al. Misdiagnoses and comorbidities among participants in the Nexus Narcolepsy Registry. Neurology 2019;92(15 Suppl):P3.6-037.

[37] Johns, M. The assessment of sleepiness in children and adolescents. Sleep Biol Rhythm 2015;13 (Suppl 1):97.

[38] Morse AM. Narcolepsy in children and adults: a guide to improved recognition, diagnosis and management. Med Sci 2019;7(12):106.

Chapter 3

Tic disorders in children and adolescents: Principles of psychopharmacologic management

Donald E. Greydanus*, MD, DrHC(Athens)

Department of Pediatric and Adolescent Medicine, Western Michigan University Homer Stryker MD School of Medicine, Kalamazoo, Michigan, United States of America

Abstract

Tics are one of the most common neuropsychiatric disturbances in children and adolescents. This chapter reviews tic disorder definition, epidemiology, differential diagnosis, and co-morbidity. The major emphasis is on current principles of psychopharmacologic management of tic disorders in children and adolescents. Chronic motor tic disorder and Tourette's syndrome typically require the use of psychopharmacologic agents that traditionally have included haloperidol, pimozide, and clonidine. Risperidone and aripiprazole are now preferred by many to haloperidol. A variety of other medications have been used to ameliorate tics, but with less anecdotal and research support. The safe and effective treatment of Tourette's disorder, and other tic disorders, is based on a logical hierarchy of interventions, from cognitive and behavioral therapies to pharmacologic agents. Thus, it is important for clinicians caring for pediatric patients to have knowledge of the various medications used to ameliorate tics.

Introduction

Because tics are one of the most common neuropsychiatric disturbances in children and adolescents, it is important for clinicians dealing with the pediatric population to understand basic concepts of tics disorders and underlying treatment concepts (1-6). One theory regarding etiology of tics involves central nervous system (CNS) circuitry dysfunction linking various CNS areas, such as the frontal lobe, thalamus, striatum, and globus pallidus. The possibility of dopaminergic abnormality is also supported by finding of a therapeutic response to neuroleptics. The negative reinforcement model proposes that tics are associated with relief in

---

* *Correspondence:* Professor Donald E Greydanus, MD, Pediatric and Adolescent Medicine, Western Michigan University Homer Stryker MD School of Medicine, 1000 Oakland Drive, Kalamazoo, MI 49008-1284, United States. Email: Donald.Greydanus@med.wmich.edu.

In: Behavioral Pediatrics II
Editors: Donald E. Greydanus, Dilip R. Patel, Ahsan Nazeer et al.
ISBN: 979-8-88697-019-7

urges that continues the tic behavior; thus, if the annoying premonitory urges are taken away, tics are negatively reinforced (7, 8).

Research data also suggest that there is an increase in the number of dopamine receptors and elevated levels of dopamine transporters. There is also a proposed prefrontal-dopaminergic abnormality. The safe and effective treatment of Tourette's disorder, and other tic disorders, is based on a logical hierarchy of interventions, from cognitive and behavioral therapies to pharmacologic agents. The major emphasis in this review is on current principles of psychopharmacologic management of tic disorders in children and adolescents.

A more recent and controversial theory looks at the potential role of Group A beta-hemolytic streptococcal infection leading to conditions called PANDAS (pediatric autoimmune neuropsychiatric disorders associated with streptococcal infections) (9,10). The place of PANDAS in the taxonomic order of tics or obsessive-compulsive disorders continued to be debated as it suggests that potential treatment for these conditions may involve antibiotics or immune-specific drugs. Revised acronyms have been suggested for PANDAS in the 21st century, including CANS (childhood acute neuropsychiatric syndrome and PANS (11-13).

Clarifying such a set of conditions is important to provide the correct treatment and avoid excessive, unnecessary treatments with potential adverse effects. The role of cefdinir has been identified as being beneficial in those with recent onset of pediatric neuropsychiatric disorders that includes obsessive-compulsive disorder and/or tics (14). One therapeutic proposal is to look at the role of tonsillectomy in those with PANDAS/CANS/PANS who do not improve with antibiotics (15).

Definitions

Tic or habit spasms are movements that are sudden, brief, highly stereotyped, involuntary, and purposeless. Tics are usually listed as motor tics, vocal tics, and, a rare third type, sensory tics. Uncomfortable premonitory sensations or urges are sensory phenomena (premonitory urge to tic) and have been measured with a nine-item self-report scale (PUTS: Premonitory Urge to Tic Scale) that noted correlation with intelligence (IQ) and severity of tics; they do not correlate with use of medication nor severity of comorbid conditions such as OCD or ADHD (16). Difficulties in understanding tic disorders include problems in reliable tic rating by patients as well as observers (17).

Classification of tic disorders is often divided into transient tic disorder, chronic motor/vocal tic disorder and Tourette's syndrome. Psychogenic tics are uncommon, present in adulthood, and usually occur without accompanying motor tics (18, 19). Views of tics have changed and continued to evolve over time. For example, some experts recommend that the terms psychogenic and habit cough not be used and recommend the terms somatic cough syndrome (for psychogenic cough) and tic cough (for habit cough) (20).

Tic disorders were first included in the American Psychiatric Association's Diagnostic and statistical manual of mental disorders (DSM) schemata in the 1980 DSM-III. The 1994 DSM-IV modifications to tic disorders involved changing the age of onset from under 21 years of age to under 18 years of age and impairment criteria were added as well as required for the diagnosis of tic disorder. The 2000 DSM-IV-TR changes involved removal of the impairment criteria because of concern about those with essential features of Tourette's disorder (i.e., chronic motor and vocal tics) who did not experience impairment.

In the DSM-IV-TR, tic disorders involved transient tic disorder, chronic tic disorder, Tourette syndrome, and tic disorder (NOS: not-otherwise specified) (see Table 1) (6). Transient tic disorder consisted of multiple motor and/or phonic tics with a duration of at least four weeks, but less than 12 months. Chronic tic disorder involved either single or multiple motor or phonic tics but not both, which were present for less than a year. The diagnosis of Tourette's syndrome involved having both motor and phonic tics being present for over a year; it is seen in 3-8 per 1,000 children. Tic disorder NOS was seen in those with tics but not meeting specific criteria of any specific tic disorder.

In the 2013 DSM-5, tics are identified as motor movements or vocalizations that are sudden, rapid, recurrent, and non-rhythmic---this definition is consistent for all tic disorders; tics can be simple or complex (21, 22). The word stereotyped was deleted from the tic definition to help distinguish between stereotypies (common in autism spectrum disorder) and tic disorders. Stereotypies and stereotypic movement disorder are commonly misdiagnosed as tics or Tourette syndrome. Stereotypies are repetitive or ritualistic movement, posture, or utterance; they can be simple movements (i.e., body rocking) or complex (i.e., marching in place, crossing/uncrossing of legs, or self-caressing).

Table 1. DSM-IV-TR diagnostic criteria for tic disorders (6)

Transient tic disorder: A. Single or multiple motor and/or vocal tics. B. Tics lasting for at least 4 weeks but for no longer than 12 consecutive months. C. Age of onset before 18 years. D. Tics are not the result of substances such as stimulants or illnesses such as Huntington's disease or post-viral encephalitis E. Criteria for Tourette's syndrome have never been met.
Chronic motor or vocal tic disorder: A. Single or multiple motor or vocal tics, but not both, have been present at some time during the illness. B. Duration of tics longer than a year without any period longer than 3 months free of tics. C. Age of onset before 18 years. D. Tics are not the result of substances such as stimulants or illnesses such as Huntington's disease or post-viral encephalitis. E. Criteria for Tourette's syndrome have never been met.
Tourette's disorder: A. Multiple motor tics and one or more vocal tics. B. Duration of tics longer than a year without any period longer than 3 months free of tics. C. Age of onset before 18 years. D. Tics are not the result of substances such as stimulants or illnesses such as Huntington's disease or post-viral encephalitis.
Tic disorder not otherwise specified: Presentations that do not meet criteria to be classified as Tourette's syndrome, transient tic disorder or chronic motor or vocal tic disorder. Examples include tics lasting less than 4 weeks, or with age of onset above 18 years or cases with only one motor and one vocal tic.

See the Text for 2013 DSM-5 changes (21).

In the DSM-5 changes in Tic Disorders include differentiation of chronic motor or vocal tic disorder in which a specifier is added to differentiate between vocal and motor tics that are chronic. This analysis was made because increased rates of comorbid diagnoses are present with vocal tics relative to motor tics. Stimulant use as a cause of tic disorder was removed in the DSM-5 because there is no evidence that use of stimulants is etiologic in the development of tics.

In the DSM-5 taxonomic system, Tourette's and tic disorders are placed in a motor disorder listing in the neurodevelopmental disorder category. Tic disorders are identified in this listing in order of severity: Other specified tic disorder (specify reason; 307.20), unspecified tic disorder (307.20), provisional tic disorder (307.21), persistent (chronic) motor or vocal tic disorder (specify motor or vocal; 307.22), and Tourette's disorder (307.23).

This new category of other specified and unspecified tic disorder (307.20) was added for tic disorders that can result in significant impairment to a person yet do not meet the full criteria for other tic disorders. These new groups account for tics triggered by illicit drug use, tics with onset in adulthood and tics triggered by other medical conditions. In unspecified tic disorder, the clinician chooses not to or cannot identify the trigger for the tics.

Epidemiology

Transient tic disorder is noted in 4-20% of children, including young adolescents (23). There is a 2-3:1 male to female ratio and a positive family history for tics is often present. Voluntary suppression of these tics may occur for minutes to hours, and stress may worsen these tics. There may be eye blinking, shoulder shrugging, facial grimacing and others. Vocal tics are not present and multiple motor tics may occur in uncommon situations. The tics usually disappear spontaneously, often within weeks of their onset.

Chronic motor tic disorder (chronic tic disorder) is noted in 1-2% of the general population and may be related to Tourette's syndrome; a positive family history is often found and the etiology is related to central nervous system dopamine metabolism dysfunction. Tourette syndrome is named after French neurologist Georges Albert Gilles de la Tourette (1857-1904) after an 1885 paper that described this condition; his famous teacher, Jean-Martin Charcot (1825-1893; father of modern clinical neurology) suggested that his student receive the honor of calling this condition the Tourette syndrome (24,25).

Gilles de la Tourette's syndrome (Tourette's syndrome) is noted in 5 per 10,000 and is ten times more common in children versus adults (1). There is a 3-4:1 male to female ratio and its onset is usually between 2 and 15 years of age; the average age of onset is seven years and, by definition, the end age of onset is age 21 years. There is often a positive family history for tic disorder, Tourette's syndrome, and/or chronic tic disorder. Tourette's syndrome typically improves in adulthood after starting in childhood (26).

Differential diagnosis/comorbidity

Table 2 provides a differential diagnosis of involuntary muscle movements. One must also consider obsessive-compulsive (spectrum) disorders and various genetic syndromes such as Huntington's disorder. Tics are not the result of stimulants or illnesses, such as post-viral encephalitis. The diagnosis is made in the patient with classic features, as noted in Table 1 and as modified by DSM-5 (21).

Tic disorders can be comorbid with a variety of conditions including Sydenham's chorea, ADHD, autism spectrum disorder, affective disorders, executive function disorders, impulse control disorders, rage attacks, sleep disorders and even psychosis (27-29). Different subtypes can be seen including persons with tic disorder, ADHD, and OCD. Research has noted an increased risk for tic disorders in children with epilepsy (30).

These co-morbid conditions may be even more influential on the person's quality of life than even the tics themselves (31). However, the combination of tics with obsessive-compulsive disorder ("Tic-related obsessive-compulsive disorder") does not mean that the tics nor the OCD are worse in this co-morbid state (32, 33). Tic severity may worsen when found with ADHD, oppositional defiant disorder and rage attacks (29). Quality of life in adults with tic disorders is particularly influenced by the presence or absence of depression and/or anxiety (34).

A wide variety of tics are noted in Tourette's syndrome (see Table 3) (1). Motor tics usually start before vocal tics and a single tic is the presenting symptom in 50%; multiple tics are also seen in 50% of patients (35, 36). The presenting tic is the eye tic in 37%, the head tic in 16%, and a vocal tic in 18% (1, 2). Eye tics can consist of eye rolling, blinking, and eye widening (37). Coprolalia is the presenting feature in 0.1%, though one-third of patients with Tourette's syndrome eventually develop this classic swearing feature. A sensory tic is noted in 3% in which an unpleasant sensation develops about a joint or muscle group that is relieved with a tic. Voluntary suppression of tics is characteristic for a brief period of time; however, a feeling of unpleasantness develops, leading to the tic.

Table 2. Involuntary muscle movements*

1. Athetosis
Slow, sinuous, writhing, involuntary movement that most frequently involves distal extremities; frequently increased by voluntary movements.
2. Ballismus
Wild, flinging, coarse, irregular, involuntary movements beginning in proximal limb muscles.
3. Chorea
Rapid, irregular, non-repetitive, sudden movement that may involve any muscle or muscle group; these movements generally interfere with voluntary movements.
4. Dystonia
Slow, twisting, involuntary movements associated with changes in muscle tone; movements generally involve trunk and proximal extremity muscles.
5. Myoclonus
Involuntary rapid, shock-like muscular contractions that are generally non-repetitive; can be increased by voluntary actions.
6. Spasm
Slow and prolonged involuntary contraction of a muscle or group of muscles.
7. Tic
Involuntary, repetitive movement of related groups of muscles; movements do not interfere with voluntary muscle movements.
8. Tremor
Involuntary movement that may be a slow or rapid vibration of the involved body part; tremors may get worse with movement (intentional tremor) or may occur only at rest.

*Used with permission from S Kuperman. Tic disorders in children and adolescents. In: Greydanus DE, Wolraich ML, eds. Behavioral pediatrics. New York: Springer, 1992:452.

Table 3. Tics noted in Tourette's syndrome

Simple or complex tics involving
Head
Neck
Trunk
Extremities (upper or lower)
Motor Tics
Eye blinking
Lip smacking
Shoulder shrugging
Head Tossing
Grimacing
Others
Simple Vocal Tics
Coughing
Grunting
Shouting
Crying
Barking
Throat clearing
Sniffing
Complex Vocal Tics
Echolalia (repeating words)
Palilalia (repeating the last sound)
Coprolalia (swearing)

Table 4. Conditions associated with Tourette's syndrome

Condition	Frequency (estimated %)
Attention-deficit/hyperactivity disorder	50-60
Obsessive-compulsive disorder	25-50
Other anxiety disorders	30-40
Mood disorders	30-40
Learning disorders (± ADHD)	20-30
Disruptive behavior disorders	Common, but more related to ADHD
Explosive anger ("rage"), including Intermittent explosive disorder	Common, related to ADHD & mood disorders
Substance use disorders	Unknown, but increases with age
Pervasive developmental disorders	Unknown, but likely low

Table 4 lists conditions associated with Tourette's Syndrome (10, 11). For example, attention-deficit/hyperactivity disorder is noted in 30% to 50% of children and adolescents with Tourette's syndrome (TS); obsessive-compulsive disorder is found in 30% to 60% (23, 29, 38). TS is usually seen as an autosomal recessive disorder and brain GABA dysfunction has been noted (26).

Genetic studies are occurring to explore the complexities of a phenotypic structure with potentially shared etiologic features that results in as many as 60% of persons with Gilles de la Tourette's syndrome having symptoms of obsessive-compulsive disorder, ADHD, and autism spectrum disorder (39). There appears to be more than one TS phenotype (40). The complexities of Tourette's syndrome is that it likely has some rare mutations and as yet unknown epigenetic and environmental influences (41, 42). Epigenetic mechanisms of tic disorders are under current research that include the importance of DNA methylation (43).

Patient education about Tourette syndrome can be obtained at the web site of the Tourette Syndrome Association from the United States at http://www.tsa-usa.org. Patients may become confused with various medical terminology. For example, in the International Cclassification of headache disorders 3 beta (ICHD-3 beta), "Tics' refers to trigeminal neuralgia in contrast to "TACs" which refers to SUNCT and SUNA that are primary headache disorders that include trigeminal autonomic cephalalgias (44).

Psychopharmacology of tic disorders

Tic disorders often require a wide range of treatment from education of the patient to intensive behavioral therapy as well as actual use of psychotropic medications (1-4, 45-47). Treatment of tics does not change the natural history of the person's disorder. Severity of tics tends to improve in adulthood (though severe tics may continue in 10-20% of adults) and tics do not need to be treated unless quality of life is considerably worsened (48). It may be more important to treat co-morbid conditions (i.e., OCD, ADHD, others) than the tics themselves. The focus of treatment revolves around the person with a tic disorder having a good quality of life (29).

Transient tic disorder often disappears spontaneously within one year, often within several weeks. In general, pharmacotherapy for tic disorders is reserved for tics that are functionally disabling. Thus, specific medical management is often not necessary, unless tic progression develops in unusual situations. Chronic motor tic disorder and Tourette's syndrome typically require the use of psychopharmacologic agents (see Table 5) that traditionally have included haloperidol, pimozide, and clonidine (1, 2, 45-50). Risperidone and aripiprazole are now preferred by many to haloperidol. A variety of other medications have been used to ameliorate tics, but with less anecdotal and research support (1, 48-54). Changes are occurring as noted later in this section.

A variety of behavioral therapies are available as well and these are viewed positively by many parents and patients (41, 54, 55). Such therapy should be "Comprehensive behavioral intervention for tic disorders" (CBIT) that includes habit reversal training (HRT); this can be done for mild to moderate tic disorders and can be applied via telemedicine technology (55). There should be no punishment for children having tics. When considering either behavioral or pharmacological treatment for tic disorders, it should be recognized that there is natural variability and waxing and waning of tics, a large placebo response to treatment, and influences of co-existing psychopathology on the outcome. Tics can be worsened with stress, fatigue and anxiety; thus, actions that improve anxiety and/or increase concentration on specific tasks can be beneficial including relaxation, exercise, music activity, others (56, 57).

Therapeutic compliance by persons with tic disorders can be limited by adverse effects of various anti-tic medications and this may be improved over time with research utilizing effective animal models of tic disorders (58). The best overall approach for tic disorders is often a combination of behavioral therapy with judicial application of state-of-the art psychopharmacology in an individualized manner (59, 60). Treatment of co-morbid conditions is important as noted, for example, by research that suggests cognitive function in persons with

TS is influenced by the presence of ADHD and the combination of TS with ADHD can strongly influence the presence of acquiring a disruptive disorder (61).

Table 5. Medications used in persons with Tourette's syndrome and comorbid disorders, and ages at which use may be appropriate

Class	Agent (A-C) ‡	Doses*	Ages**
Antipsychotics			
First-generation			
Phenothiazines	Fluphenazine (B)	1.5-10 mg/d	≥ 18
Butyrophenones	Haloperidol (A)	1-4 mg/d	≥ 18; ≥ 3†
Other	Pimozide (A)	0.05-0.2 mg/kg/d	≥ 12
Second-generation	Risperidone (A)	0.25-2 mg, 1-2x/d	≥ 18
	Ziprasidone (B)	5-40 mg/d	≥ 18
	Olanzapine (C)	2.5-12.5 mg/d	≥ 18
	Quetiapine (C)	25-150 mg/d	≥ 18
Partial DA agonist	Aripiprazole (C)	10-20 mg/d	≥ 18
Alpha-agonists	Clonidine (B)	0.05-0.3 mg/d	≥ 12
	Guanfacine (B)	0.5-1 mg, 3x/d	≥ 12
Anticonvulsants	Topiramate	50-200 mg/d	≥ 2
	Levetiracetam	1-2 g/d	≥ 16
Antidepressants			
SSRIs (for OCD)	Fluoxetine (A)	10-60 mg/d	≥ 7
	Sertraline (A)	50-250 mg/d	≥ 6
	Fluvoxamine (A)	50-350 mg/d	≥ 6
	Paroxetine (B)	10-60 mg/d	≥ 18
	Citalopram (B)	20-60 mg/d	N/A
	Escitalopram (B)	10-20 mg/d	N/A
Other (for ADHD)	Atomoxetine	0.5-1.2 mg/kg/d	≥ 6
DA receptor agonists	Pergolide (B)	0.1-0.4 mg/d	≥ 18
Muscle relaxants	Baclofen (C)	5-20 mg, 3x/d	≥ 12
Miscellaneous	Nicotine patch (C)	7-21 mg/d	≥ 18
	Mecamylamine (C)	2.5-7.5 mg/d	≥ 18
	Tetrabenazine (C)	12.5-25 mg, 1-3x/d	≥ 18

Psychostimulants: See Chapter 1 for details.

‡ = Empirical support categories

* Dosing is clinically-based, unless stated otherwise.

** Ages (years) are for FDA-approved indications; use for other indications and/or at other ages is based on clinical judgment.

† For "severe behavioral problems."

DA = Dopamine

Category A denotes good supportive evidence for efficacy and safety (based on ≥ 2 randomized, placebo-controlled studies); Category B denotes fair supportive evidence (based on a minimum of one placebo-controlled study); and Category C represents minimal supportive evidence, based on less rigorous sources (such as open-label studies, case reports, others).

Alpha agonists

These medications (36, 49, 62-65) are suggested as the first-line agents when pharmacotherapy is needed to treat the tics of Tourette's syndrome. This group of medications helps to reduce adrenergic outflow from the central nervous system CNS; how this lowers tic activity is uncertain. There are no known specific contraindications to their use. Data has suggested that alpha-2 adrenergic agonists have minimal effect in persons with tic disorders and no comorbid ADHD (66).

Clonidine is a presynaptic, central-acting alpha-2 adrenergic agonist that is used to improve tic symptoms. Its daily dose range is 0.05 to 0.3 mg/day; depending on its use, clonidine is provided 2 to 4 times a day or only at bedtime. Common side effects include dry mouth, drowsiness, dizziness, constipation, and sedation. Children may experience orthostatic hypotension, but it is uncommon. Children may be more susceptible to the rebound hypertension associated with the abrupt discontinuation of the alpha agonist. Gradual build-up and withdrawal when using clonidine are recommended; rapid withdrawal may lead to rebound hypertension. Sedation is a major limiting factor in using this medication.

When prescribing clonidine, take some baseline data (blood pressure, pulse, blood sugar, electrocardiogram); follow this data on a regular basis, including a repeat electrocardiogram every six months. A few cardiac-related deaths have been reported in children and adolescents taking both methylphenidate and clonidine simultaneously.

Guanfacine is an alpha2A adrenergic agonist related to clonidine, and is also used to reduce tic frequency. Its daily dosage range is 0.5 mg to 1 mg, three times a day. Guanfacine use may result in less blood pressure problems and sedation than seen with clonidine. Adverse reactions are similar to clonidine, but there may be more agitation and headaches, so patients should be monitored closely. Long-acting guanfacine is being used for treatment of persons with ADHD and tic disorders.

Antipsychotics

If tics are severe or bothersome to the patient, and they have not responded to the alpha agonists or behavioral interventions, a trial of an antipsychotic is warranted (47, 65, 66). Even with aggressive treatment, complete tic suppression may not be possible, thus reduction in tic frequency may be the management goal along with education about the tic disorder itself.

Two common medications which have traditionally been used for tic suppression are haloperidol and pimozide (47); however, risperidone and aripiprazole are now more commonly prescribed in place of haloperidol than in the past (67-69). Tiapride is a selective blocker of D2 and D3 dopamine receptors and has studies noting its beneficial effect in those with tic disorders (70).

Also, quetiapine has been studied for use in persons with tic disorders (71). Also being evaluated are newer antipsychotic medications such as paliperidone and sertindole. No matter which agent is chosen, a general rule in using these agents in children and adolescents is to start with a low dose and titrate slowly upwards to seek the best balance between tic amelioration and minimization of adverse effects.

Approximately one fourth of patients placed on haloperidol experience a 70% reduction in tics at a dose that avoids major side effects; 50% note a reduction in tics only at a dose that leads to major side effects, and 25% do not respond to haloperidol. Pimozide can lead to a 70-80% reduction in tics, often without development of serious side effects. Risperidone has been used to suppress tics at an oral dose that ranges from 0.25 mg a day to 2 mg twice a day.

It is unclear exactly how the antipsychotics work in reducing the tics of Tourette's syndrome and other tic disorders. However, it is presumed that a major part of the mechanism involves dopamine blockade of post-synaptic receptors somewhere in the cortico-striato-thalamic-cortical circuitry.

For haloperidol, one should start with 0.25 mg each day, and increase to 2 mg, two times per day orally, as tolerated. Although higher doses may be used (e.g., 5 mg twice daily), tics generally respond to doses lower than those used to treat psychosis. Dosing for risperidone is similar to that of haloperidol. For pimozide, starting with 1 mg daily and increasing up to 4 mg two times per day is one approach. A safer strategy may be to dose by weight, 0.05-0.2 mg/kg/d, with dosing not to exceed 10 mg daily. Haloperidol and fluphenazine are contraindicated in patients with blood dyscrasias, hepatic disease, subcortical brain damage, and mental obtundation.

The antipsychotics haloperidol, pimozide, and risperidone are the most effective at treating the tics of Tourette's syndrome. They are also the most likely to cause extrapyramidal symptoms (EPS) and neuroleptic malignant syndrome (NMS). Pimozide can also prolong the QTc interval. The atypical antipsychotics (AAs) risperidone, quetiapine, and olanzapine (in increasing order) tend to cause weight gain, and all of the AAs can elevate blood glucose to varying degrees. With the exception of quetiapine and aripiprazole, the newer antipsychotics used in Tourette's syndrome can elevate serum prolactin. In a recent study in England, aripiprazole was the most positively viewed medication as seen by young people with TS and their parents (53).

Pimozide should not be used in tic disorders other than Tourette's syndrome. Concurrent use with stimulant medications is discouraged if there is suspicion that the stimulant, and not Tourette's, is the cause of the tics. Pimozide should not be used with any other medications that may combine to prolong the QTc interval, including the psychotropics thioridazine, chlorpromazine, nefazodone, fluvoxamine, fluoxetine, sertraline, ziprasidone, and citalopram.

The patient's height, weight, and BMI (body mass index) should be measured before starting antipsychotic medications and at each subsequent visit. Blood pressure and pulse should be checked at baseline, and then at least every three months. Fasting glucose and lipids should be measured before starting treatment, after three months, and then every six months thereafter. A baseline examination for extrapyramidal signs should be recorded, and re-checked during dosage escalations, and then once every three months. The use of the pimozide or ziprasidone requires baseline and follow-up ECGs, particularly during dosage titrations. Prolactin should be checked at any point if menstrual or sexual dysfunction develop.

Dopamine receptor agonists

The use of these medications to treat Tourette's syndrome seems counterintuitive, given that the effective antipsychotic agents are dopamine antagonists. These medications, at low doses, do seem to reduce the frequency of tic activity. The hypothesized mechanism of action involves agonism at pre-synaptic dopamine receptors.

Pergolide is used cautiously, starting at 0.1 mg daily, with a gradual increase to a maximum of 0.4 mg daily. The most common side effects with pergolide refer to the nervous system. Other frequently experienced side effects include gastrointestinal upset, dry mouth, anemia, weight changes, dyspnea, cough, sweating, diplopia, and urinary frequency. Pergolide should not be used in patients who are hypersensitive to this drug or other ergot derivatives.

As the use of this medication in Tourette's is experimental, extreme caution should be taken when used in children and adolescents. Pergolide may cause somnolence and the possibility of falling asleep during activities of daily living; therefore, patients should be cautioned about certain activities (e.g., bike riding, skateboarding, roller skating) until there is reasonable certainty that the medication does not affect them adversely. Caution should be used when patients are taking other central nervous system (CNS) depressants in combination with pergolide.

No specific laboratory tests are necessary for the management of patients on pergolide. Periodic routine evaluation of all patients should be carried out at appropriate times. Blood pressure and pulse should be checked at home and during clinical visits.

Baclofen

Baclofen may also be helpful, and may involve inhibition via gamma-aminobutyric acid (GABA) of which baclofen is an analogue. Baclofen is started at 5 mg, three times daily, with increases every five days, as needed, to a maximum of 20 mg, three times daily (lower than the 80 mg/d maximum in adults).

Baclofen produces a transient somnolence in over half of the patients who take it. Other common side effects include dizziness, weakness, fatigue, confusion, headache, nausea, and urinary frequency. In a few patients receiving baclofen, laboratory testing has disclosed increased SGOT, alkaline phosphatase, and blood sugar. There is no specific contraindication to the use of baclofen. The clinical approach to use of baclofen- and the associated cautions- are similar to those of pergolide. For patients on baclofen, periodic laboratory testing for serum glutamic oxaloacetic transaminase (SGOT), alkaline phosphatase, and blood sugar should be ordered.

Stimulants

Stimulants (36, 38, 63) increase availability of dopamine and norepinephrine at post-synaptic neurons, likely via reuptake blockade, or increased release, at pre-synaptic neurons. As noted, ADHD is found in 50% or more of patients with Tourette's syndrome. Children and adolescents with both ADHD and Tourette's may be given both stimulant medications (if effective) and anti-tic medications (such as pimozide, haloperidol or other neurleptic as noted above) if tics develop.

Research does not suggest that stimulant medications cause Tourette's; however, these medications should be used in a "start low and go slow" manner. If the tics are worsened by the stimulant drugs, other anti-ADHD medications may be tried that do not typically worsen tics; these include alpha2 agonists (such as clonidine or guanfacine) or atomoxetine, a selective norepinephrine reuptake inhibitor. In those with ADHD and Tic disorders, an alpha-2 adrenergic agonist can be the first choice of medication; some experts recommend sustained release psychostimulants as the second choice and then, atomoxetine as the third-line (64).

Antidepressants

These medications exert their effects by increasing catecholamine availability via reuptake inhibition, pre-synaptic antagonism, post-synaptic antagonism, or a combination of mechanisms. The most commonly used antidepressants in patients with Tourette's syndrome are the selective serotonin reuptake inhibitors, or SSRIs.

The SSRIs have been used to improve various co-morbidities of Tourette's syndrome, such as phobias, obsessive-compulsive disorder, and generalized anxiety disorder (see Table 4). Anxiety may worsen tics and thus, anxiety reduction may lead to tic reduction as well. All antidepressants with serotonergic activity (except mirtazapine and venlafaxine) are contraindicated for use with pimozide, the combination of which can greatly prolong the QTc interval.

Table 5 lists the SSRIs that have been used to improve the symptoms of obsessive-compulsive disorder associated with Tourette's syndrome. Of the listed agents, citalopram and escitalopram are less likely to lead to behavioral activation and agitation; thus, their use is preferred by some experts. No matter which antidepressant is used for obsessive-compulsive disorder, there is a tendency for successful treatment to require high doses, sometimes above the range recommended for the treatment of depression. Close monitoring is necessary to prevent or minimize medication side effects. No routine laboratory tests are required for any of the SSRIs.

Anticonvulsants

Hypothesized mechanisms of action include neuronal membrane stabilization, the inhibition of excitatory amino acids (e.g., glutamate and aspartate), and the increase of GABA, a known inhibitory neurotransmitter. There is little data to guide dosing of the anticonvulsants topiramate and levetiracetam to treat Tourette's syndrome. However, topiramate has been used at oral doses ranging from 50-200 mg once per day and levetiracetam has been used at 1000-2000 mg once per day (72, 73). Some studies note that levetiracetam is not efficacious for persons with tic disorder and other research notes that sodium valproate has not been shown to be efficacious for persons with tic disorders (74). Carbamazepine has also been used but with limited research support. Clinicians should also keep in mind research showing that anticonvulsant medications can also induce tic disorders in some persons (75).

Topiramate can produce sedation, fatigue, cognitive slowing, behavioral changes, word finding difficulty, precipitation of glaucoma, anemia, dehydration, and renal stones. Levetiracetam's most common side effects include weakness, headache, dizziness, and somnolence. There are no specific contraindications to the use of topiramate or levetiracetam. The use of topiramate and levetiracetam is strictly clinical, so the previous caution of "start low and go slow" applies to these agents as well. This is especially relevant in the presence of renal impairment. Patients on topiramate should have a periodic complete blood count (CBC), blood urea nitrogen (BUN) and creatinine. The medication infrequently causes increases of liver function tests. No routine laboratory tests are recommended for patients on levetiracetam.

Other management options

A variety of other pharmacologic agents are under study for management of tic disorders (73). Nicotine receptor agonism (via a nicotine patch) and antagonism (with mecamylamine) have shown limited success in reducing the symptoms of Tourette's syndrome. Nicotine patches are available without prescription in the United States. They come in dosages of 7, 14, and 21 mg/patch (76). The lowest effective dose should be used.

The use of the nicotine patch is guided by clinical response and tolerance. It should be applied in the morning and taken off in the late afternoon or early evening. Acute adverse effects from nicotine are increases in pulse, blood pressure, psychomotor activity, headache, and nausea. The concern for longer-term use is addiction to the nicotine.

Mecamylamine

Mecamylamine is a secondary aliphatic amine that is started at 2.5 mg daily, with a maximum of 2.5 mg, 3 times daily. The time between dosage increases should probably be longer than the 2 days recommended for adults. Mecamylamine may cause constipation (and occasionally ileus), orthostatic hypotension, seizures, abnormal movements, urinary retention, blurred vision, weakness, fatigue, and sedation. Both nicotine and mecamylamine are contraindicated in patients with hypertension.

For patients on the nicotine patch or mecamylamine, blood pressure and pulse should be checked routinely at home and during clinical visits. Mecamylamine should also not be used if the patient has renal insufficiency, glaucoma, or is taking antibiotics. Mecamylamine absorption improves when taken with food, and sedation can be better tolerated if it is given later in the day.

Tetrabenazine

Some experts prefer using tetrabenazine to classic neuroleptic medications and it is used in Canada, New Zealand, and some countries in Europe (55). Known since the 1950s this medication is not sold in the United States, but can be purchased legally from Canada (with a valid prescription), as the Food and Drug Administration has classified tetrabenazine as an orphan drug, with fast-track status. It is approved by the US FDA for management of chorea found in persons with Huntington's disease.

Tetrabenazine has two main mechanisms of action; one is depletion of catecholamines from presynaptic neurons, the other is postsynaptic dopamine antagonism. Tetrabenazine is absorbed unevenly after oral dosing. It should therefore be taken 2-3 times daily for greatest effect. Tetrabenazine is started with one-half of a 25 mg tablet daily, and titrated by 12.5 mg weekly; maximum dosage in children would likely not exceed 75 mg daily.

Tetrabenazine may cause drowsiness, nervousness, anxiety, restlessness, insomnia, parkinsonism, akathisia, and depression. Tetrabenazine may cause a recurrence or exacerbation of depression in patients with a prior or current episode, respectively, of depression. Tetrabenazine-induced oculogyric crisis has been reported (77). Patients treated with tetrabenazine should be screened at each visit for symptoms of depression.

Miscellaneous

The evidence of cannabinoids (i.e., tetrahydrocannabinol) for tic disorders remains limited at this time (78). Also under study is the use of histamine H3R antagonist for Tourette syndrome based on theorized dysfunction of the brain's histaminergic modulatory system (79).

Other medication under study for treatment of tic disorders include steroid 5alpha-reductase, lithium, norepinephrine, naloxone, buspirone, metoclopramide, phytostigmine, and spiradoline mesylate. As with all such chemicals, strict adherence to potential adverse effects should occur both known to the clinician and also phenominologically experienced by the patient.

Botulinum toxin has been used successfully in treating motor and vocal tics with response within 5-6 days lasting for about three months. The most common side effect is hypophonia. Streptococcal infection in a person with Tourette's syndrome may be seen with various cytokine and immunological abnormalities and in theory may improve with immunomodulator treatment (80). The literature has reported Gilles de la Tourette syndrome induced by Mycoplasma pneumoniae that was effectively managed with use of macrolide antibiotics (81).

Deep brain stimulation

In addition to electroconvulsive therapy (ECT), surgery has also been utilized in severe situations and includes deep brain stimulation (23, 41). Repetitive transcranial magnetic stimulation (rTMS) applied to the supplementary motor area in persons with Tourette syndrome that involves tics and obsessive-compulsive comorbidity have shown safe improvement in tic severity (82, 83). Ancient humans attempted trephination in the Stone Age and modern humans utilize deep brain stimulation on areas dealing with emotional circuitry that is under study to improve severe, refractory tic disorders by stimulation to motor and limbic pathways (i.e., globus pallidus internus, thalamic nuclei, and nucleus accumbens) (84, 85). Clinicians seeking the use of such therapy for persons under age 18 years of age should seek consultation with local ethics committee(s) (86).

Conclusion

Transient tic disorder can be seen in as many as 20% of children while chronic tic disorder can occur in 1-2%; Gilles de la Tourette's syndrome (Tourette's syndrome) is noted in 5 per 10,000 and is ten times more common in children versus adults (23, 60). DSM-5 2013 changes in tic disorders are reviewed (21). The basis for a Tourette syndrome spectrum is emerging that is involves both concepts of neurology and psychiatry (87-89).

The effect of co-morbid conditions on tic disorders continues to be analyzed especially with respect to ADHD as well as ODC (89-91) and affects the quality of life in these persons (92). Co-morbid conditions may be seen before the clinical appearance of the tic disorder (28, 93). The frequency and severity of tics tend to abate with ageing into adulthood in up to 85% of persons with tic disorders though this can be reversed in those with severe childhood tics and limited fine motor control (94).

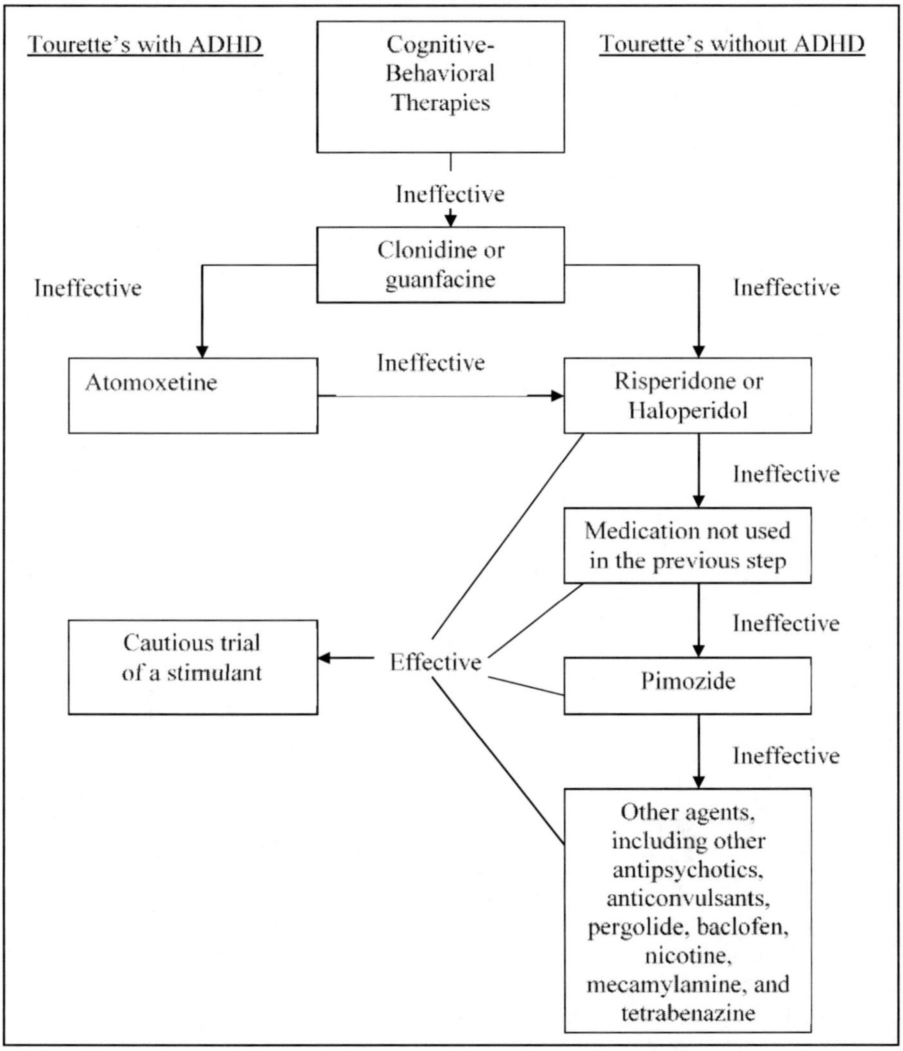

Figure 1. Treatment algorithm for Tourette's syndrome, with/without ADHD.

Education and support of the pediatric person with a tic disorder and the family are important parts of the management program (95). The safe and effective treatment of Tourette's disorder, and other tic disorders, is based on a logical and personalized hierarchy of interventions, from cognitive and behavioral therapies to pharmacologic agents that focus on comorbid conditions as well as the tics (23, 56, 60, 96-101). Some persons with tics may not need to be treated. Behavior therapy can also consider that life events can have considerable impact on person with tic disorders as for example the presence of friends, anxiety, depression, aggression, impact of vocal versus motor tics and other complexities of living (102, 103).

Management of persons with tic disorders does vary from clinician to clinician and from country to country (104, 105). Figure 1 illustrates one example of a treatment algorithm (106); other approaches may be found in the medical literature (55, 73, 90, 98, 108). The potential use of tetrahydrocannabinol (THC) remains under research (107). Management of persons with tic disorders and multiple comorbid conditions (i.e., triad of tics, ADHD, OCD) can be challenging (109-115). Deep brain stimulation is used for refractory and severe (malignant) TS (55, 110-118). Research continues in the 21st century on etiologic factors in tic disorders and it is important that all persons with tic disorders have access to primary care and specialty services to help them deal with the effects of this neurological condition (119-124).

Acknowledgments

This chapter is modified and updated with permission from: Greydanus DE, Calles JLJr, Patel DR, eds. Pediatric and adolescent pharmacology. Cambridge: Cambridge Univ Press, 2008:223-40.

References

[1] Greydanus DE, Tullio J. Tourette's disorder in children and adolescents. Transl Pediatr 2020;9 (Suppl 1):S94-S103.

[2] Jones KS, Saylam E, Ramphul K. Tourette syndrome and other tic disorders. In: StatPearls. Treasure Island, FL: StatPearls Publishing, 2021 Jan–.

[3] Ueda K, Black KJ. A comprehensive review of tic disorders in children. J Clin Med 2021;10(11):2479.

[4] Kuperman S. Tic disorders in the adolescent. Adolesc Med 2002;13:537-51.

[5] Black KJ, Kim S, Yang NY, Greene DJ. Course of tic disorders over the lifespan. Curr Dev Disord Rep 2021;8(2):121-32.

[6] American Psychiatric Association. Diagnostic and statistical manual of mental disorders, 4th ed, text rev. Washington, DC: APA, 2000.

[7] Capriotti MR, Brandt BC, Turkel JE, Lee HJ, Woods DW. Negative reinforcement and premonitory urges in youth with Tourette syndrome: an experimental evaluation. Behav Modif 2014;38(2):276-96.

[8] Brandt VC, Beck C, Sajin V, Baaske MK, Bumer T, Beste C, et al. Temporal relationship between premonitory urges and tics in Gilles de la Tourette syndrome. Cortex 2016;77:24-37.

[9] Swedo SE, Leonard HL, Garvey M, Mittleman B, Allen AJ, Perlmutter S, et al. Pediatric autoimmune neuropsychiatric disorders associated with streptococcal infections: clinical description of the first 50 cases. Am J Psychiatry 1998;155:264-71.

[10] Swedo SE. Pediatric autoimmune neuropsychiatric disorders: associated with streptococcal infections (PANDAS). Mol Psychiatry 2002;7:S24-5.

[11] Singer HS, Gilbert DL, Wolf DS, Mink JW, Kurlan R. Moving from PANDAS to CANS. J Pediatr 2011;160(5):725-31.

[12] Swedo SE, Leckman JF, Rose NR. From research subgroup to clinical syndrome: modifying the PANDAS criteria to PANS (pediatric acute- onset neuropsychiatric syndrome). Pediatr Therapeut 2012;2:113. doi: 10.4172/2161-0665.1000113.

[13] Dop D, Marcu IR, Padureanu R, Niculescu CE, Padureanu V. Pediatric autoimmune neuropsychiatric disorders associated with streptococcal infections. Exp Ther Med 2021;21(1):94.

[14] Murphy TK, Parker-Athill EC, Lewin AB, Storch EA, Mutch PJ. Cefdinir for recent-onset pediatric neuropsychiatric disorders: A pilot randomized trial. J Child Adolesc Psychopharmacol 2015; 25(1):57-64.
[15] Demesh D, Virbalas JM, Bent JP. The role of tonsillectomy in the treatment of pediatric autoimmune neuropsychiatric disorders associated with streptococcal infections (PANDAS). JAMA Otolaryngol Head Neck Surg 2015;141(3):272-5.
[16] Reese HE, Scahill L, Peterson Al, Crowe K, Woods DW, Piacentini J, et al. The premonitory urge to tic: measurement, characteristics, and correlates in older adolescents and adults. Behav Ther 2014;45(2):177-86.
[17] Müller-Vahl KR, Riemannn L, Bokemeyer S. Tourette patients' misbelief of a tic rebound is due to overall difficulties in reliable tic rating. J Psychosom Res 2014;76(6):472-6.
[18] Janik P, Milanowski L, Szejko N. Psychogenic tics: clinical characteristics and prevalence. Psychiatr Pol 2014;48(4):835-45.
[19] Karakaya I, Sismanlar SG. Tic disorders in the differential diagnosis of chronic cough in children in relation to four cases. Turk Pediatri Ars 2015;5 0(3):176-9.
[20] Vertigan AE, Murad MH, Pringsheim T, Feinstein A, Chang AB, Newcomb PA, et al. Somatic cough syndrome (previously referred to as psychogenic cough) and tic cough (previously referred to as habit cough) in adults and children: CHEST guidelines and expert panel report. Chest 2015;148(1):24-31.
[21] American Psychiatric Association. Diagnostic and statistical manual of mental disorders, 5th edition (DSM-5). Arlington, VA: Amercan Psychiatric Association, 2013.
[22] Eapen V, Crncec R. DSM 5 and child psychiatric disorders: what is new? What has changed? Asian J Psychiatr 2014;11:114-8.
[23] Greydanus DE. Tic disorders. In: Greydanus DE, Patel DR, Pratt HD, Calles Jr JL, Nazeer A, Merrick J, eds. Behavioral pediatrics, 4th edition, New York: Nova Biomedical Science, 2015:341-52.
[24] Gilles de la Tourette G. Etude sur une affection nerveuse caracterisee par de l'incoordination motrice accompagnee d'echolalie et de coprolalie. Arch Neurol 1885;9:158-200. [French]
[25] Trivet HA, Chien HF, Munhoz RP, Barbosa ER. Charcot's contribution to the study of Tourette syndrome. Arq Neuropsiquiatr 2008;66:918-21.
[26] Hallett M. Tourette syndrome: Update. Brain Dev 2015;37(7):651-5.
[27] Punukollu M, Mushet N, Linney M, Hennessy C, Morton M. Neuropsychiatric manifestations of Sydenham's chorea: a systematic review. Dev Med Child Neurol 2016;58(1):16-28.
[28] Mol Debes NM. Co-morbid disorders in Tourette syndrome. Behav Neurol 2013;27(1):7-14.
[29] Lorentzos MS, Heyman I, Baig BJ, Coughtrey AE, McWilliams A, Dossetor DR, et al. Psychiatric comorbidity is common in dystonia and other movement disorders. Arch Dis Child 2021;106(1):62-67.
[30] Weng WC, Huang HL, Wong LC, Jong YJ, Yin YJ, Chen HA, et al. Increased risks of tic disorders in children with epilepsy: a nation-wide population-based case-control study in Taiwan. Res Dev Disabil 2016;51-52:173-80.
[31] Eapen V, Snedden C, Crncec R, Pick A, Sachdev P. Tourette syndrome, co-morbidities and quality of life. Aust NZ J Psychiatry 2016;50(1):82-93.
[32] Conelea CA, Walther MR, Freeman JB, Garcia AM, Sapyta J, Khanna et al. Tic-related obsessive-compulsive disorder (OCD): phenomenology and treatment outcome in the Pediatric OCD Treatment Study II. J Am Acad Child Adolesc Psychiatry 2014;53(12):1308-16.
[33] Lewin AB, Chang S, McCracken J, McQueen M, Piacentini J. Comparison of clinical features among youth with tic disorders, obsessive-compulsive disorder (OCD), and both conditions. Psychiatry Res 2010;178(2):317-22.
[34] Evans J, Seri S, Cavanna AE. The effects of Gilles de la Tourette syndrome and other chronic tic disorders on the quality of life across the lifespan: a systematic review. Eur Child Adolesc Psychiatry 2016 Feb 15.
[35] Jankovic J. Tourette's syndrome. N Engl J Med 2001;345:1184-92.
[36] Leckman JF. Tourette's syndrome. Lancet 2002;360:1577-86.
[37] Bisker ER, McClelland CM, Brown LW, Liu GT. The long-term outcomes of ocular tics in a pediatric neuro-ophthalmology practice. J AAPOS 2014;18(1) :31-5.

[38] Greydanus DE, Pratt HD, Patel DR: Attention deficit hyperactivity disorder across the lifespan. Disease a Month 2007;53(2):65-102.

[39] Huisman-van Dijk HM, Schoot RV, Rijkeboer MM, Mathews CA, Cath DC. The relationship between tics, OC, ADHD and autism symptoms: A cross-disorder symptom analysis in Gilles de la Tourette syndroms patients and family-members. Psychiatry Res 2016;237:138-46.

[40] Cavanna AE, Termine C. Tourette syndrome. Adv Exp Med Biol 2012:724:375-83.

[41] Serajee FJ, Mahbubul Hug AH. Adances in Tourette's syndrome: diagnoses and treatment. Pediatr Clin North Am 2015;62(3):687-701.

[42] El Malhany N, Gulisano M, Rizzo R, Curatolo P. Tourette syndrome and comorbid ADHD: causes and consequences. Eur J Pediatr 2015;174(3):279-88.

[43] Zilhao NR, Padmanabhuni SS, Pagliaroli L, Barta C, BIOS Consortium, Smith DJ et al. Epigenome-wide association study of tic disorders. Twin Res Hum Genet 2015;18(6):699-709.

[44] VanderPluym J, Richer L. Tic versus TAC: differentiating the neuralgias (trigeminal neuralgia) from the cephalalgias (SUNCT and SUNA). Curr Pain Headache Rep 2015;19(2):473. doi: 10.1007/s11916-014-0473-9.

[45] Besag FM, Vasey MJ, Lao KS, Chowdhury U, Stern JS. Pharmacological treatment for Tourette syndrome in children and adults: What is the quality of the evidence? A systematic review. J Psychopharmacol 2021; 35(9):1037-1061.

[46] Tourette Syndrome Study Group. Treatment of ADHD children with tics: A randomized controlled trial. Neurology 2002;58:527-36.

[47] Sallee FR, Nesbitt L, Jackson C, Sine L, Sethuraman, G. Relative efficacy of haloperidol and pimozide in children and adolescents with Tourette's disorder. Am J Psychiatry 1997;154:1057-62.

[48] Leivonen S, Sourander A, Voutilainen A, Leppämäki S. Tourette's syndrome—diverse group of patients, individual need for treatment. Duodecim 2015;131(11):1058-64. [Finnish].

[49] Cohen DJ, Young JG, Nathanson JA, Shaywitz BA. Clonidine in Tourette's syndrome. Lancet 1979;2:551-3.

[50] Gilbert D. Treatment of children and adolescents with tics and Tourette syndrome. J Child Neurol 2006;21:690-700.

[51] Wehr AM, Namerow LB. Citalopram for OCD and Tourette's syndrome. J Am Acad Child Adolesc Psychiatry 2001;40:740-1.

[52] Gaffney GR, Perry PJ, Lund BC, Bever-Stiller KA, Arndt S, Kuperman S. Risperidone versus clonidine in the treatment of children and adolescents with Tourette's syndrome. J Am Acad Child Adolesc Psychiatry 2002;41:330-6.

[53] Cuenca J, Glazebrook C, Kendall T, Hedderly T, Heyman I, Jackson G et al. Perceptions of treatment for tics among young people with Tourette syndrome and their parents: a mixed methods study. BMC Psychiatry 2015;15:46. doi: 10.1186/s12888-015-0430-0.

[54] Bennett SM, Keller AE, Walkup JT. The future of tic disorder treatment. Ann NY Acad Sci 2013;1304:32-9. doi: 10.1111/nyas.12296.

[55] Gunduz A, Okun MS. A review and update on Tourette syndrome: Where is the field headed? Curr Neurol Neurosci Rep 2016;16(4):37. doi: 10.1007/s11910-016-0633-x.

[56] Cohen SC, Leckman JF, Bloch MH. Clinical assessment of Tourette syndrome and tic disorders. Neurosci Biobehav Rev 2013;37(6):997-007.

[57] Bodeck S, Lappe C, Evers S. Tic-reducing effects of music in patients with Tourette's syndrome: self-reported and objective analysis. J Neurol Sci 2015;352(1-2):41-7.

[58] Godar SC, Mosher LJ, Di Giovanni G, Bortolato M. Animal models of tic disorders : a translational perspective. J Neurosci Methods 2014; 238:54-60.

[59] Fourneret P, Desombre H, Broussolle E. From tic disorders to Tourette syndrome: current data, comorbidities, and therapeutic approach in children. Arch Pediatr 2014;21(60 :646-51. [French]

[60] Chadehumbe MA, Greydanus DE, Feucht C. Psychopharmacology of tic disorders in children and adolescents. Pediatr Clin North Am 2011; 58(1):259-72.

[61] Martino D, Madhusudan N, Zis P, Cavanna AE. An introduction to the clinical phenomenology of Tourette syndrome. Int Rev Neurobiol 2013;112:1-33.

[62] Yasaei R, Saadabadi A. Clonidine. 2021 Aug 6. In: StatPearls. Treasure Island, FL: StatPearls Publishing, 2021 Jan–.

[63] Zinner SH, Coffey BJ: Developmental and behavioral disorders grown up: Tourette's disorder. J Dev Behav Pediatr 2009;30:560-73.

[64] Rizzo R, Gulisano M. Clinical pharmacology of comorbid attention deficit hyperactivity disorder in Tourette syndrome. Int Rev Neurobiol 2013;112:415-44.

[65] Tamara P. Tourette syndrome and other tic disorders of childhood. Handb Clin Neurol 2013;112:853-6.

[66] Weisman H, Qureshi IA, Leckman JF, Scahill L, Bloch MH. Systematic review: pharmacological treatment of tic disorders—efficacy of antipsychotic and alpha-2 adrenergic agonist agents. Neurosci Biobehav Rev 2013;37(6):1162-71.

[67] Cothros N, Medina A, Pringsheim T. Current pharmacotherapy for tic disorders. Expert Opin Pharmacother 2020;21(5):567-580.

[68] Yang CS, Huang H, Zhang LL, Zhu DR, Guo Q. Aripiprazole for the treatment of tic disorders in children: a systematic review and meta-analysis. BMC Psychiatry 2015;15:179. doi: 10. 1186/s12888-015-0504-z.

[69] Zheng W, Li XB, Xiang YQ, Zhong BL, Chiu HF, Ungvari GS, et al. Aripiprazole for Tourette's syndrome: A systematic review and meta-analysis. Hum Psychopharmacol 2016;31(1):11-8.

[70] Roessner V, Schoenefeld K, Buse J, Bender S, Ehrlich S, Münchau A. Pharmacological treatment of tic disorders and Tourette syndrome. Neuropharmacology 2013;68(143-9.

[71] Lan CC, Liu CC, Chen YS. Quetiapine and clozapine combination treatment for tourette's syndrome in an adolescent boy: Potential role of dopamine supersensitivity in loss of treatment response. J Child Adolesc Pschopharmacol 2015;25(2):188-90.

[72] Kruer MC. Pediatric movement disorders. Pediatr Rev 2015;36(3):104- 15.

[73] Yang CS, Zhang LL, Zeng LN, Huang L, Liu YT. Topiramate for Tourette's syndrome in children: A meta-analysis. Pediatr Neurol 2013;49(5):344-50.

[74] Yang CS, Zhang LL, Lin YZ, Guo Q. Sodium valproate for the treatment of Tourette's syndrome in children: A systematic review and meta-analysis. Psychiatry Res 2015;226(2-3):411-7.

[75] Peters J, Vijiaratnam N, Angus-Leppan H. Tics induced by antiepileptic drugs: A pragmatic review. J Neurol 2021;268(1):321-336.

[76] Greydanus DE, Patel DR: The adolescent and substance abuse: Current concepts. Disease-a-Month 2005;51(7):387-432.

[77] Janik P, Figura M. Tetrabenazine-induced oculogyric crisis- a rare complication in the treatment of Gilles de la Tourette syndrome. Neuropsychiatr Dis Treat 2016;12:497-9.

[78] Whiting PF, Wolff RF, Deshpande S, Di Nisio M, Duffy S, Hernandez AC, et al. Cannabinoids for medical use: A systematic review and meta-analysis. JAMA 2015;313(24):2456-73.

[79] Rapanelli M, Pittenger C. Histamine and histamine receptors in Tourette syndrome and other neuropsychiatric conditions. Neuropharmacology 2015 Aug 14. pii: S0028-3908(15)30065-4.

[80] Li E, Ruan Y, Chen Q, Cui X, Lv L, Zheng P et al. Streptococcal infection and immune response in children with Tourette's syndrome. Childs Nerv Syst 2015;31(7):1157-63.

[81] Schuhfried G, Schuhfried G, Stanek G. Gilles de la Tourette syndrome caused by Mycoplasma pneumoniae successfully treated with macrolides. Klin Padiatr 2014;226(5):295-6.

[82] Bloch Y, Arad S, Levkovitz Y. Deep TMS add-on treatment for intractable Tourette syndrome: A feasibility study. World J Biol Psychiatry 2016;17(7):557-61.

[83] Fu M, Wei H, Meng X, Chen H, Shang B, Chen F, et al. Effects of low- frequency repetitive transcranial magnetic stimulation of the bilateral parietal cortex in patients with Tourette syndrome. Front Neurol 2021; 12:602830.

[84] Cleary DR, Ozpinar A, Rasian AM, Ko AL. Deep brain stimulation for psychiatric disorders; where are we now? Neurosurg Focus 2015;38(6):E2. doi: 10.3171/2015.3FOCUS1546.

[85] Israelashvili M, Loewenstern Y, Bar-Gad I. Abnormal neuronal activity in Tourette syndrome and its modulation using deep brain stimulation. J Neurophysiol 2015;114(1):6-20.

[86] Schrock LE, Mink JW, Woods DW, Porta M, Servello D, Visser- Vandewalle V, et al. Tourette syndrome deep brain stimulation: A review and updated. Mov Disord 2015;30(4):448-71.

[87] Lebowitz ER, Motlagh MG, Katsovich L, King RA, Lombroso PJ, Grantz H et al. Tourette syndrome in youth with and without obsessive compulsive disorder and attention deficit hyperactivity disorder. Eur Child Adolesc Psychiatry 2012;21(8):451-7.
[88] Eddy CM, Cavanna AE, Guilsano M, Cali P, Robertson MM, Rizzo R. The effects of comorbid obsessive-compulsie disorder and attention-deficit hyperactivity disorder on quality of life in Tourette syndrome. J Neuropsychiatry Clin Neurosci 2012;24(4):458-62.
[89] Cavanna AE, Rickards H. The psychopathological spectrum of Gilles de la Tourette syndrome. Neurosci Biobehav Rev 2013;37(6):1008-15.
[90] Grant JE, Fineberg N, van Ameringen M, Cath D, Visser H, Carmi L, et al. New treatment models for compulsive disorders. Eur Neuropsychopharmacol 2016;26(5):877-84. pii: S0924-977X(15)00358-2.
[91] Rizzo R, Gulisano M, Pellico A, Cali PV, Curatolo P. Tourette syndrome and comorbid conditions: A spectrum of different severities and complexities. J Child Neurol 2014;29(10):1383-9.
[92] Eddy CM, Rizzo R, Gulisano M, Agodi A, Barchitta M, Cali P, et al. Quality of life in young people with Tourette syndrome: A controlled study. J Neurol 2011;258(2):291-301.
[93] Oluwabusi OO, Parke S, Ambrosini PJ. Tourette syndrome associated with attention deficit hyperactivity disorder: the impact of tics and psychopharmacological treatment. World J Clin Psychiatry 2016;5(1):128-35.
[94] Hassan N, Cavanna AE. The prognosis of Tourette's syndrome: implications for clinical practice. Funct Neurol 2012;27(1):23-7.
[95] Kurlan RM. Treatment of Tourette syndrome. Neurotherapeutics 2014;11(1):161-5.
[96] Greydanus DE, Pratt HD. Attention-deficit/hyperactivity disorder in children and adolescents: Interventions for a complex costly clinical conundrum. Pediatr Clin North Am 2003;50:1049-92.
[97] Shaw ZA, Coffey BJ. Tics and Tourette syndrome. Psychiatr Clin North Am 2014;37(3):269-86.
[98] Murphy TK, Lewin AB, Storch EA, Stock S, American Academy of Child and Adolescent Psychiatry (AACAP), Committee on Quality Issues (CQI). Practice parameter for the assessment and treatment of children and adolescents with tic disorders. J Am Acad Child Adolesc Psychiatry 2013;52(12):1341-59.
[99] Rizzo R, Gulisano M, Cali PV, Curatolo P. Tourette syndrome and comorbid ADHD: current pharmacological treatment options. Eur J Paediatr Neurol 2013;17(5):431-8.
[100] Tagwerker Gloor F, Walitza S. Tic disorders and Tourette syndrome: current concepts of etiology and treatment in children and adolescents. Neuropediatrics 2016;47(2):84-96.
[101] Pringsheim T, Steeves T. Pharmacological treatment for attention deficit hyperactivity disorder (ADHD) in children with comorbid tic disorders. Cochrane Database Syst Rev 2011;4:CD007990.
[102] Cavanna AE, Luoni C, Selvini C, Biangiardo R, Eddy CM, Silvestri PR, et al. Disease-specific quality of life in young patients with Tourette syndrome. Pediatric Neurol 2013;48(2):111-4.
[103] Steinberg T, Shmuel-Baruch S, Horesh N, Apter A. Life events and Tourette syndrome. Compr Psychiatry 2013;54(5):467-73.
[104] Rickards H, Cavanna AE, Worrall R. Treatment practices in Tourette syndrome: the European perspective. Eur J Paediatr Neurol 2012;16(4):361-4.
[105] Bachmann CJ, Roessner V, Glaesk0e G, Hoffmann F. Trends in psychopharmacologic treatment of tic disorders in children and adolescents in Germany. Eur Child Adolesc Psychiatry 2015;24(2):199-207.
[106] Greydanus DE, Calles JR JL, Patel DR. Pediatric and adolescent psychopharmacology. Cambridge: Cambridge Univ Press, 2008:223-40.
[107] Shprecher DR, Kious BM, Himle MH. Advances in mechanistic understanding and treatment approaches to Tourette syndrome. Discov Med 2015;20(111):295-301.
[108] Huss M, Chen W, Ludolph AG. Guanfacine extended release: a new pharmacologic treatment option in Europe. Clin Drug Investig 2016;36(1):1-25.
[109] Rice T, Coffey B. Pharmacotherapeutic challenges in treatment of a child with "the triad" of obsessive compulsive disorder, attention-deficit/hyperactivity disorder and Tourette's disorder. J Child Adolesc Psychopharmacol 2015;25(2):176-9.
[110] Yang C, Hao Z, Zhu C, Guo Q, Mu D, Zhang L. Interventions for tic disorders: An overview of systematic reviews and meta analyses. Neurosci Biobehav Rev 2016;63:239-55.

[111] Macerollo A, Martino D. What is new in tics, dystonia and chorea? Clin Med (Lond) 2016;16(4):383-9.
[112] Hauseux PA, Cyprien F, Cif L, Gonzalez V, Boulenger JP, Coubes P, et al. Long-term follow-up of pallidal deep brain stimulation in teenagers with refractory Tourette syndrome and comorbid psychiatric disorders: about three cases. Eur J Paediatr Neurol 2017;21(1):214-7.
[113] Ganos C. Tic and Tourette's: update on pathophysiology and tic control. Curr Opin Neurol 2016;29(4):513-8.
[114] Robinson S, Hedderly T. Novel psychological formulation and treatment of "tic attacks" in Tourette syndrome. Front Pediatr 2016;4:46. doi: 10.3389/fped.2016.00046.
[115] Whittington C, Pennant M, Kendall T, Glazebrook C, Trayner P, Groom M, et al. Practitioner review: treatments for Tourette syndrome in children and young people-a systematic review. J Child Psychol Psychiatry 2016;57(9):988-1004.
[116] Godeiro C, França C, Carra RB, Saba F, Saba R, Maia D, et al. Use of non-invasive stimulation in movement disorders: A critical review. Arq Neuropsiquiatr 2021;79(7):630-46.
[117] Rothenberger A, Heinrich H. Electrophysiology echoes brain dynamics in children and adolescents with Tourette syndrome: A developmental perspective. Front Neurol 2021;12:587097.
[118] Bruce AB, Yuan W, Gilbert DL, Horn PS, Jackson HS, Huddleston DA, et al. Altered frontal-mediated inhibition and white matter connectivity in pediatric chronic tic disorders. Exp Brain Res 2021;239(3):955-65.
[119] Bhikram T, Elmaghraby R, Abi-Jaoude E, Sandor P. An international survey of health care services available to patients with Tourette syndrome. Front Psychiatry 2021;12:621874.
[120] Andrén P, de la Cruz LF, Isomura K, Lenhard F, Hall CL, Davies EB, et al. Efficacy and cost-effectiveness of therapist-guided internet-delivered behaviour therapy for children and adolescents with Tourette syndrome: study protocol for a single-blind randomised controlled trial. Trials. 2021; 22(1):669. doi: 10.1186/s13063-021-05592-z.
[121] Li F, Cui Y, Li Y, Guo L, Ke X, Liu J, et al. Prevalence of mental disorders in school children and adolescents in China: diagnostic data from detailed clinical assessments of 17,524 individuals. J Child Psychol Psychiatry 2022; 63(1):34-46.
[122] Vermilion J, Augustine EF, Adams HR, Vierhile A, Collins AT, McDermott MP, et al. Risk behaviors in youth with and without Tourette syndrome. Pediatr Neurol 2022;126:20-5.
[123] Xin X, Feng Y, Zang Y, Lou Y, Yao K, Gao X. Multivariate classification of brain blood-oxygen signal complexity for the diagnosis of children with Tourette syndrome. Mol Neurobiol 2022 Jan 3. doi: 10.1007/s12035-021- 02707-0.
[124] Edelsohn GA, Abright AR. Editorial: Safer use of antipsychotics in youth (SUAY): Should treatment be guided by symptoms? J Am Acad Child Adolesc Psychiatry 2022;61(1):34-6.

Chapter 4

Enuresis: Current concepts and conundrums

Donald E. Greydanus*, MD, DrHC(Athens) and Mahesh Shrestha, MD

Department of Pediatric and Adolescent Medicine, Western Michigan University
Homer Stryker MD School of Medicine, Kalamazoo, Michigan, United States of America

Abstract

Incontinence disorders are an important group of problems clinicians manage in children and adolescents. This chapter reviews the physiology of micturition, the epidemiology of enuresis, general clinical approach to enuresis, laboratory evaluation, and general principles of management.

Introduction

Enuresis which is defined as intermittent urinary incontinence is a common problem in children affecting about 15% of children who are five years and older (1-3). Various behavioral problems may be seen in children with urinary incontinence that can include low self-esteem, inability to socilalize with peers, fear of doing nightovers and others (4). Many parents who have not experienced nocturnal enuresis themselves may find fault in their children and develop frustation as well as anger towards these children. It is therefore imortant for clinicians to understand the pathophysiology and overall management of pediatric enuresis (5, 6).

Physiology of micturition

Normal function of the lower urinary tract relies on the complex coordination of a number of inhibitory and stimulatory inputs (1, 2). These inputs, both automatic and volitional in nature, originate in the central nervous system and travel over nerves of the peripheral nervous system

---

* **Correspondence:** Professor Donald E Greydanus MD, DrHC(Athens), Department of Pediatric and Adolescent Medicine, Western Michigan University Homer Stryker MD School of Medicine, 1000 Oakland Drive, Oakland Drive Campus, Kalamazoo, MI 49008, United States. Email: donald.greydanus@med.wmich.edu.

In: Behavioral Pediatrics II
Editors: Donald E. Greydanus, Dilip R. Patel, Ahsan Nazeer et al.
ISBN: 979-8-88697-019-7

to specific end organs. Continence relies heavily on the integrity of the autonomic nervous system. Intentional bladder emptying requires that input from the cortex be transmitted to somatic peripheral nerves and be integrated with appropriate changes in the basal state of the autonomic nervous system. While a number of supraspinal inputs and local reflex mechanisms contribute to the fine tuning and full conscious control of micturition, a more simplified approach may facilitate the present discussion.

Urine storage

As the bladder fills and stretches, a mechanism to prevent urination must be in place. Afferent impulses travel through the pelvic nerves to the spinal column and result in a synapse with efferent neurons in two places: 1) With alpha motor neurons (at the same level) in the anterior horn of the spinal gray matter, sending excitatory impulses via the pudendal nerve to the striated muscle of the external urethral sphincter (contraction of the urethral sphincter); 2) After ascending briefly near the site of entry into the spinal column with cell bodies of the lumbar intermediolateral cell column (site of sympathetic outflow), sending impulses via the hypogastric nerve to inhibit detrusor (bladder) contraction and facilitate contraction of the smooth muscle of the internal urethral sphincter.

Bladder sensation

While afferent fibers that run through the pelvic nerve are part of the involuntary reflex described above, the message regarding bladder distention is also carried up through the spinal cord to the cortex where the sensation of bladder fullness is realized.

Voiding mechanism

Afferent fibers carry the message of bladder distention not only to the cortex, but also to the pontine micturition center in the brainstem. Synapses here give rise to interneurons that 1) stimulate contraction of the detrusor muscle and 2) inhibit firing of neurons that facilitate urethral sphincter contraction. Bladder emptying then follows. This reflex, however, is governed by input from the cortex, hypothalamus, and other supraspinal structures. Thus, voluntary control requires the integrity of structures above the level of the brainstem.

Normal development

Bladder control is a developmental, as well as a social milestone that in the Western world, parents and society expect the child to achieve by 5 years of age age (1-3). There is a chronologic progression of bladder control that matures with the individual's age. Voiding in fetuses and infants is an automatic process triggered by bladder distention to functional capacity. Voluntary control is clearly not present in infancy and urination occurs frequently in the newborn. Frequency diminishes during the first 12-24 months of life and awareness of the sensation of bladder fullness develops. Willful retention normally develops and appears to be practiced before voluntary voiding is mastered. Day time bladder control is obtained earlier than night time bladder control. The term enuresis is used in reference to the involuntary voiding by a child who has reached an age in which bladder control is expected.

It is now clear that the traditional concept that voiding in the fetus and in the infant is simply a sacral, automatic response to bladder distention is an oversimplification. Intrauterine voiding is more frequent when the fetus is awake, as demonstrated by ultrasound and can be triggered by other stimuli such as vibration or auditory stimulation indicating the participation of higher neurologic centers in the process even at these early states of development. In newborns, during sleep, the bladder is quiescent and there is no detrusor activity. When the bladder is distended, there is electroencephalographic evidence of cortical arousal. Such evidence along with animal studies indicate a complex fetal and postnatal development of bladder functions simultaneously at different levels.

After the normal diuresis observed in the first day, the number of voiding decreases to a few times a day in the first week of life only to increase up to around one per hour by the first month of life; then it decreases to 10 to 15 times a day by six months. By 2 to 3 years, the frequency of voiding is 8 to 10 times a day and by 12 years of age, the frequency is similar to that of an adult. The bladder capacity can be estimated by several formulas including the frequently used Hjalmas' formula: bladder capacity in ml = 60 + (age in years X 30) (1, 2). The evaluation of the bladder capacity by non-invasive methods, such as ultrasonography, has practical implications for the treatment of enuresis, as noted later.

Definitions

The American Psychiatry Association's Diagnostic and Statistical Manual for Mental Disorders, 5th edition, Text Revision (DSM-5) defines enuresis as repeated intentional or involuntary voiding of urine into bed or clothes, with a frequency of at least twice a week for not less than three consecutive months or associated with significant social or academic impairment; the child should be five years of age or older (or of equivalent developmental level); also, the voiding behavior is not due to underlying medical conditions or physiologic effect of any substance (7, 8). The impact on the person's quality of life may be considerable (4, 9). The International Children's Continence Society terminology related to enuresis is listed in Table 1.

Table 1. International children's continence society terminology

Enuresis	Intermittent incontinence of urine while sleeping
Enuresis, monosymptomatic	Enuresis without any (other) lower urinary tract symptoms
Enuresis, non-monosymptomatic	Enuresis with (other) lower urinary tract symptoms
Enuresis, primary	Enuresis in a child who has previously been dry for less than 6 months
Enuresis, secondary	Enuresis in a child who has previously been dry for at least 6 months

Based on Neveus T, von Gontard A, Hoebeke P, et al. The standardization of terminology of lower urinary tract function in children and adolescents: Report from the Standardization Committee of the International Children's Continence Society. J Urology 2006;176:314-324.

The majority of nocturnal enuresis are *primary monosymptomatic nocturnal enuresis* (PMNE) without any lower urinary tract symptoms and without a history of bladder dysfunction. Another important terminology is *secondary enuresis* who develop enuresis after a dry period of at least six months. It is important to understand these different definitions as management and success rates varies among them (10).

Epidemiology

Research continues to explore the epidemiology of urinary incontinence in the pediatric population (11). By 2 1/2 years of age 90% of the girls and 80% of the boys know the need to micturate (1, 2). Certainly by three years of age, boys and girls, with help and understanding, are able to be dry during the day. By 3-5 years of age 75% of the children will obtain night time bladder control. By five years of age between 15 to 20% of children will continue to have nocturnal enuresis. The number decreases to around 7% by 10 years of age.

Approximately 3%-4% have enuresis by 12 years of age. The incidence of nocturnal enuresis continues to decline so that by 15 years of age and older still, about 1% of individuals will continue to have nocturnal enuresis. Sixty percent of the cases have been present from early childhood without interruption. Approximately 40% are "secondary," developing 3-6 months after the appearance of continence. Ninety percent of the cases of enuresis present only at night (nocturnal enuresis). Diurnal enuresis occurs more commonly in females while nocturnal enuresis is noted more commonly in males. The genetic basis for nocturnal enuresis continues to be identified in 21st century research (12).

Clinical features

Parents generally bring the child for evaluation because of bed wetting (9). Bed wetting may or may not be associated with day time incontinence or other behavioral symptoms.

History

The history should include specific questions regarding the frequency and severity of the enuresis. The parents may be able to answer the clinician's questions for the shy or embarrassed younger child. They will also be able to tell you if the child has ever been continent, thereby differentiating between primary and secondary enuresis. Questions that help differentiate between isolated nocturnal enuresis and incontinence in children are listed in Table 2. A medical history may reveal drug-induced enuresis such as seen with methylphenidate, clomazine, aripiprazole and others in unusual cirumstances (13-15).

Table 2. Questions that help differentiate between isolated nocturnal enuresis and incontinence

1)	The severity of the daytime voiding is evaluated by the size of the wet spot in the clothing.
2)	Is the length of time between voiding greater than or less than 30 minutes?
3)	Is the frequency of voiding more than 8 times during the day time?
4)	Is the frequency of voiding during the day less than three times?
5)	Is the child unable to hold back urine?
6)	Does the child squat down or squeeze to hold back urine?
7)	Does the child strain when voiding?
8)	Does the child have an interrupted, staccato or weak stream? Keeps on dribbling?
9)	Has periods when urinating is painful?
10)	Once had blood in the urine?
11)	Once had a urinary tract infection?
12)	Gets out of bed at night to drink regularly?
13)	Has a day without defecation? Does the child soil the underwear with feces?
14)	Only a wet spot in bed (not a soaking wet bed)?
15)	Has he/she been wetting the bed since infancy?
16)	Has he/she been dry for at least 6 months in a row?
17)	When were other children in the family older than 6 years dry?
18)	When were the parents dry?
19)	What has been done to stop the bed wetting?
20)	How wet is he/she at night?
21)	How many times does he/she wet at night?
22)	Is the child easy to rouse at night?
23)	How is the child doing in school?
24)	Are there problems at school or at home?
25)	Is the child also wet during the day?
26)	If the child is wet during the day time: since when has he/she been wet during the day?
27)	How does the wetting during the day relate to interrupting play? Laughing, giggling?
28)	How wet is he/she during the day?

Physical examination

A complete physical examination should be done with particular emphasis on the genitourinary exam (external genitalia, palpation of bladder, odor of urine), neurologic examination (sensory and motor function of the lower extremities, reflexes, anal wink, fundoscopic eye exam for increased intracranial pressure), and musculoskeletal examination (spinal abnormalities such as tufts of hair, hemangiomas, masses, scoliosis, and lower extremity abnormalities [clubfoot, tone or gait abnormalities]) (1-3, 10). The abdominal examination includes evaluation of the flanks for enlarged kidneys, enlarged bladder or masses, and severe constipation, the gluteal areas and back looking for asymmetry or midline defects.

Diagnosis

Diagnosis of enuresis is primarily based on a detailed history and physical examination (1, 2, 16-21). Laboratory studies are indicated based on findings of the history and physical examination to exclude any underlying organic causes for enuresis.

Urinalysis and urine cultures are necessary; infection must be considered and ruled out. Other studies including renal and bladder ultrasonography or VCUG (voiding cystourethrogram) are to be requested only when clearly indicated (21). Imaging studies are seldom indicated for monosymptomatic nocturnal enuresis, but may be valuable in patients with significant dysfunctional voiding or associated with neurologic abnormalities. Usually the nocturnal enuresis resolves itself once the day time voiding problem has been successfully treated.

Most children with monosymptomatic enuresis do not require image studies and cystometrographic studies are of no additional value in the evaluation and management of these patients. Cystomethographic evaluation as well as imaging studies are reserved for patients that have symptomatic enuresis, recurrent UTI or evidence of neurological compromise (1-3). Patients with Hinman syndrome or those with suspected motor neuron abnormalities should undergo thorough neurologic evaluation. It is often recommended that patients with the Hinman syndrome (non-neurogenic neurogenic bladder) also undergo a psychiatric evaluation (22).

Also, those with enuresis may have comorbid conditions such as obesity, constipation and sleep disorders such as obstructive sleep apnea (23-27). Each co-morbidity needs to be managed with its specific issues and management, for example, of sleep apnea obstuction does not correct the co-morbid primary nocturnal enuresis (28). The presence of nocturnal enuresis in female children may indicate pelvic floor disorders and urinary tract symptomatology later in their lives as adult women (29). Various psychiatric co-morbidities can be seen as well (30, 31).

Treatment

Standards of management have been developed by various groups including the International Children's Continence Society (ICCS), European Society for Paediatric Urology (ESPU), the European Association of Urology (EAU), and the National Institute for Health and Care Excellence (NICE) (32, 33). In evaluating the enuretic child, the physician must know how to answer two crucial questions: When to treat, and how to treat? Nocturnal enuresis (enuresis nocturna) in children has traditionally motivated very little interest in terms of research, evaluation, and treatment.

This attitude is based on the observation that treatment is not always curative and most children with nocturnal enuresis will, with time, outgrow their condition. However, it had become increasingly evident that children with enuresis suffer from lack of self-esteem and embarrassment, potentially leading to stress and depression. It has been demonstrated that when the enuresis is successfully treated, the self-esteem of the child is normalized. Failure of treatment is associated with increasing stress and anger. Low self-esteem is a risk for psychiatric disorders and problems with social adjustment. Treatment needs to be instituted early, when the child expresses the desire to be dry at night.

Treatment of nocturnal enuresis

Though the timing for initiation of active treatment is variable, most physicians and families are comfortable starting treatment when the child is around five years of age. However, the most important consideration is the time when the child is ready to receive treatment. In the

United States there are several well accepted treatments for monosymptomatic nocturnal enuresis (1-3). These include:

- Lifestyle changes and motivation therapy
- Enuresis alarm
- Pharmacological treatment

Lifestyle changes and motivation therapy

It is important to obtain the cooperation of the patient and the family for the treatment of enuresis to be successful. The family and child need to be educated at the appropriate level of communication and the use of visual aids about the causes of enuresis, how the different methods of treatment work, and the side effects of medications. The goals of the treatment need to be clearly established. The contributing effects of modern technology for comunication as well as entertainment before bedtime must be explained to the patient and family (34).

Parents should be educated that enuresis is a common issue that usually resolves as children get older. It is important to understand that nocturnal enuresis does not happen at a conscious level and thus, children are not at fault. Criticism and punishment for wet nights should be avoided (35). It is important to encourage the child to keep a chart of dry and wet nights. Parents need to support and praise the achievement and efforts of the child. Children should void regularly during the day and before going to bed. Fluid intake should be limited before going to bed to about 200 ml or roughly 20-30% of total daily fluid intake after 5 pm. Parents should discourage pullups and diapers unless the children are staying away from home.

Motivation therapy is helpful for children aged 5-7 years who do not wet every night and those who accept some responsibility for treatment (1-3). These children should be rewarded for any success by giving awards; this can include a sticker for every dry night and a book for 7 consecutive dry nights. Initial rewards should be given for some agreed–upon behaviour such as going to toilet before bed rather than having a dry night and increased slowly. Complete success is achieved once the child has 14 consecutive dry nights. Relapse is more than 2 wet nights in 2 weeks. Lifestyle changes and motivation therapy should be tried for 3-6 months before additions interventions occur. Psychological and behavioral interventions can reduce parental punishment of children with enuresis (35).

Enuresis alarm and other non-pharamacological management

Most pharmacologic treatment of enuresis is combined with one of several behavior modification programs in order to improve bladder capacity and sphincter control (9, 36-38). Enuresis alarms are first line management for long term therapy with minimal side effects (39-41). It is helpful for motivated children and parents with children who have frequent bed wetting. A number of operant conditioning devices are available, such as the Enurotone. The Bell-Pad conditioning devise is based on the principle that urine will complete an electric circuit that triggers an alarm. The patient learns to awaken to the sensations of bladder fullness and micturition and rises to complete voiding on a voluntary basis.

The newer models of these systems are safe and relatively inexpensive. The use of the conditioning device is associated with a change in the awakening response by EEG, as well as a significant increase in the nocturnal bladder capacity in those patients that become dry. The success rate of this treatment is over 70%, and is clearly related to the patient's age, with better results obtained in children 7 years and older. It is necessary to continue treatment until the child is dry for one month and s/he is able to tolerate normal fluid intake. Relapses are less frequent with this method of treatment. In case of a relapse, treatment with the alarm may be restarted. The exact benefit of the alarm system for management of enuresis remains under research (40).

It is important that the child (and not parents) should turn off the alarm himself/herself, get up and void in toilet, change underwear if needed, reset the alarm and sleep. Initially if child does not wake up, parents could wake the patient but should not turn off the alarm by themselves. If there is some improvement by 2-3 weeks, treatment should be continued for 3-4 months till child achieves 14 consecutive dry nights. If no improvement by 2-3 weeks, oral desmopression could be added or alarm should be discontinued till the child gets mature (1-3).

Bladder retention exercises have been employed with occasional success. The patient is instructed to try to hold his or her urine for increasingly longer periods of time after experiencing the urge to micturate. Some individuals respond to a timed voiding program in which they learn to void "by the clock" every two hours rather than waiting for a sensation of fullness which may come too late. Fluid restriction in the evening and rousing the patient to void when the last family member goes to bed may be helpful. However, these adjunctive measures alone are generally futile in themselves.

Current thinking often concludes that counseling, per se, will not ameliorate enuresis, but is helpful in improving secondary emotional distress. Hypnosis, dietary manipulations, allergy therapies and other treatments have been suggested, but controlled studies are needed to confirm the effectiveness of these concepts as potential management tools. Reassurance that enuresis does not adversely affect sexual function is an important component of counseling for enuretic teenagers. If the child snores and has enlarged adenoids, adenoidectomy may correct the enuresis.

Pharmacologic treatment

Desmopressin (DDAVP) is a derivative of AVP. It is frequently used for the treatment of monosymptomatic nocturnal enuresis (17, 42-53). The rational for the use of this medication is the observation that in some patients with nocturnal enuresis, the nocturnal levels of AVP are low, the osmotic pressure is low, and the urine volume is large in relation to the nocturnal bladder capacity resulting in bladder overflow and enuresis.

Desmopression is is best suited for children whose parents need rapid improvement of enuresis or those who need short–term improvement but replases are common. Desmopression works best in children with normal functional bladder capacity and nocturnal polyuria (>130% night time urine production than expected bladder capacity for age). The dosage guideline is summarized in Table 3. Current recommendation is to start oral desmopressin tablet with initial dose of 0.2 mg and increase to 0.4 mg in 2 weeks if needed (54). The therapeutic response usually occurs during the first 48 hours.

One has to be careful and clearly advise the parents and the patient about the importance of limiting the fluid intake during the evening (<240 ml). Symptomatic hyponatremia, including seizures has been reported in patients on DDAVP that do not limit fluid intake; this was more common in intranasal route and thus was discontinued.

If there is improved response within 2 weeks, the treatment is continued for 3 months until the patient remains dry at night; then, the dose is gradually decreased by decreasing to half the dose in 2 weeks and stopped. If used daily, desmopression should be withheld 1 week every 3 months to determine if treatment needs to be continued.The therapeutic response is greater than 70% and the relapse rate as high as 40%. The medication may be restarted in cases of relapse.

Table 3. Drugs used in neurogenic bladder dysfunction

Bladder Dysfunction	**Drug**	**Mechanism**	**Dosage**	**Comments**
Impaired Urine Storage				
Decreased Bladder Capacity	Proprantheline	Anticholinergic	2-3 mg/kg/day divided every 4-6 hrs & at bedtime	Administer 30 minutes before meals & at bedtime
	Flavoxate	Direct smooth muscle relaxation	6-12 yrs: 100-200mg at bedtime >12 yrs: 100-200mg 3-4 times daily	Administer 1 hour before or 2 hours after a meal
	Oxybutynin	Anticholinergic	Immediate release: 1-5 yrs: 0.2 mg/kg/dose 2-3 times daily >5 yrs: 5mg twice daily; maximum 15mg/day Extended release: ≥6 yrs: 5mg daily; increase in 5mg increments to maximum of 20mg daily	Administer on an empty stomach for immediate release formulation
	Tolterodine	Anticholinergic	Immediate release: ≥5 yrs: 1mg twice daily Extended release: ≥5 yrs: 2mg once daily	May require lower doses if patient concurrently taking CYP 450 3A4 inhibitors
	Hyoscyamine	Anticholinergic	Drops <2 yrs: 2.3kg: 3 drops every 4h as needed (max. 18 drops) 3.4kg: 4 drops every 4h as needed (max. 24 drops) 5kg: 5 drops every 4h as needed (max. 30 drops) 7kg: 6 drops every 4h as needed (max. 36 drops) 10kg: 8 drops every 4h as needed (max. 48 drops) 15kg: 11 drops every 4h as needed (max. 66 drops) 2-12 yrs: 0.25-1ml every 4h as needed (max. 6ml/day) >12 yrs: 1-2ml every 4h as needed (max. 12ml/day)	Oral drop concentration: 0.125 mg/ml Elixir concentration: 0.125mg/5ml Administer before meals

Table 3. (Continued)

Bladder Dysfunction	**Drug**	**Mechanism**	**Dosage**	**Comments**
Impaired Urine Storage				
			Elixir: 2-12yrs: 10kg: 1.25ml every 4h as needed (max. 30ml/day) 20kg: 2.5ml every 4h as needed (max. 30ml/day) 40kg: 3.75ml every 4h as needed (max. 30ml/day) 50kg: 5ml every 4h as needed (max. 30ml/day) >12 yrs: 5-10ml every 4h as needed (max. 60ml/day) Oral/Sublingual: 2-12 yrs: 0.0625-0.125mg every 4h as needed (max. 0.75mg/day) >12 yrs: 0.125-0.25mg every 4 hours as needed (max. 1.5mg/day) Extended release: ≥12 yrs: 0.375-0.75mg every 12h (max. 1.5mg/day)	
	Desmopressin	Enhanced water reabsorption in the kidneys	Oral: ≥6 yrs: 0.2mg at bedtime; maximum 0.6mg daily	Restrict fluid intake 1 hour prior to dose until the following morning or for at least 8 hours after administration Intranasal no longer indicated for primary nocturnal enuresis due to multiple reports of hyponatremia -related seizures
Decreased Outflow Resistance	Imipramine	Anticholinergic & Sympathomimetic	4-12 yrs: 10-25mg at bedtime; maximum 2.5 mg/kg/day or 50mg/day (the lesser of the two) >12 yrs: 10-25mg at bedtime; maximum 75mg/day	Administer 1 hour prior to bedtime May increase by 25mg increments each week Overdose can be fatal
Impaired Bladder Emptying				
Increased Bladder Capacity	Bethanechol	Cholinergic	0.3-0.6 mg/kg/day divided in 3-4 doses	Administer 1 hour before or 2 hours after meals
Increased Outflow Resistance	Phenoxybenzamine	Alpha-adrenergic antagonist	0.6-1.5 mg/kg/day	
	Doxazosin	Alpha$_1$-adrenergic antagonist	Immediate release: ≥3 years & adolescents: 0.5mg at bedtime; maximum 2mg/day	Dose may be titrated to effect

For monosymptomatic patients with nocturnal enuresis that have failed to respond to maximal doses of desmopressin, the addition of a long-acting anticholinergic medication results in improvement in the risk of bed wetting by 66% compared with controls (43). Patients with nocturnal enuresis associated with low bladder capacity (as assessed by ultrasound) respond better to treatment with a combination of desmopressin and a long-acting anticholinergic medication than with desmopressin alone. Patients with normal bladder capacity, as assessed by ultrasound, who are treated with desmopressin alone have a positive response to this treatment; also, those children with a large bladder capacity benefit from treatment with desmopressin, and utilization of a double voiding technique and scheduled voiding.

Tricyclic antidepressants

Tricyclic antidepressants (TCAs), particularly imipramine pamoate, are classic medications in the treatment of children with enuresis (44). The dosage of imipramine is summarized in table 3. The clinical effects may be seen within 1-2 weeks of therapy initiation. When the patient responds and remains dry for 2 weeks or more, the medication is given every other day, and then decreased or discontinued. The response rate is between 43-80%. The drug has anticholinergic effects that have been associated with urinary retention, delayed micturation, and dilatation of the urinary tract. The use of TCAs has been associated with arousal changes in the EEG. The medication has also been implicated in an increase in the secretion of anti-diuretic hormone (ADH).

The use of DDAVP and imipramine as a combination medication for treatment of enuresis should be avoided. Other side effects with TCAs include severe cardiac arrhythmias with accidental overdose or suicide attempts (55). It is critical to keep this in mind if there are small children in the home who may ingest the medication. Granulocytopenia and bone marrow suppression have also been described.

Given the risk profile of the medication and other suitable alternative options, tricyclic antidepressants are now considered third line agents in the treatment of nocturnal enuresis. If they are prescribed, the medication needs to be prescribed in small quantities and a responsible adult needs to give the medication to the patient due to the severity of complications with overdose (including cardiac arrhythmias). It should not be used in the child or adolescent who is at risk for suicide.

Anticholinergics

Some of the children who have nocturnal enuresis may also have daytime voiding syndrome (DVS) (1-3). These symptoms include urinary frequency, urgency, urge incontinence, and urine withholding. Many of these children have developed poor toilet habits, resulting in abnormal patterns of defecation, including severe encopresis. Many of these children also have recurrent urinary tract infections as well as daytime and nighttime bladder control problems. Important issues in management include addressing the psychological factors involved in these situations as well as developing a program of bladder-bowel retraining and treatment of urinary tract infections.

Children with nocturnal enuresis and daytime voiding symptoms without urinary tract infections are otherwise asymptomatic. The treatment should be directed, initially, to the daytime enuresis with a program that involves timed voiding every 2 hours and anticholinergic medications such as oxybutynin; this may be given as a single nighttime dose or as frequently as twice or three times daily for daytime enuresis associated with an unstable bladder. Children should be alerted to the common side effects of anti-cholinergic medications, including sedation, constipation, dry mouth, flushing, and others. It is important to avoid over-heating on hot days.

While oxybutynin is the only oral anticholinergic approved by the Food and Drug Administration (FDA) for use in children, tolterodine has been used to treat enuresis including nonneurogenic daytime urinary incontinence and for enuresis when oxybutynin has failed (56-58). Side effects include blurred vision, constipation, abdominal pain, and others. See Table 3 for details regarding dosing.

Newer anticholinergics such as darifenacin and solifenacin are thought to have greater bladder specificity (M3 receptor) and would therefore have less risk for anticholinergic side effects (59-61). Several small studies have evaluated solifenacin (1.25-10 mg daily) in children with neurogenic and nonneurogenic detrusor overactivity (59, 60). These open-label studies demonstrated overall good efficacy and tolerability with solifenacin despite prior intolerance or lack of efficacy with tolterodine/oxybutynin.

A recent agent to be introduced and in a class by itself is mirabegron which was approved in the United States in 2012 for overactive bladder in adults (62-65). It has a unique mechanism of action by stimulating the beta-3 adrenergic receptor in the bladder resulting in relaxation of the detrusor muscle. While not yet evaluated in pediatric patients, it may offer a tolerability advantage due to its lack of anticholinergic properties.

Refractory nocturnal enuresis and referral

Some children may be refractory to treatment with alarms and even medications such as desmopressin and lead to multi-modal management (66). It is important for a clinician to find the causes and do referral if needed. Constipation is a frequent cause of treatment failure so a bowel regimen should be started if the history or medical examination is indicative of retained stools. Referral to urology should occur for children and adolescents who have clinical or radiographic findings of renal/urologic abnormailties; these include daytime incontinence, urgency, weak stream, proteinuria, increased or decreased frequency, and polydipsia.

Careful evaluation of urodynamics of enuresis should occur in refractory situations (67). Children with secondary enuresis should be particularly evaluated for major life stressors that include birth of a sibling, death or divorce of parents and recent migration; referral to a behavioral specialist may be needed. Referral to a pediatric neurosurgeon should be done in cases of occult spinal dysraphism. Children should be evaluated for snoring, enlarged adenoids and tonsils or sleep disorders; referral to a sleep specialist may be needed.

Conclusion

Enuresis is a common conundrum seen in pediatric practice but also seen in adult practice as well (1-3, 68-73). Although most children tend to have decreasing frequency of nocturnal episodes of bed wetting as they get older and have an excellent prognosis, some need active management because of the impact of enuresis on their academic and social functioning as well as their overall quality of life (74). The diagnosis of enuresis is primarily based on clinical evaluation and behavioral management is effective in many children (69, 70, 75-77). The field of urotherapy has been developed to provide non-pharmacologic management for various lower urinary tract disorders including nocturnal enuresis, datytime urinary incontinuence, functional constipation and others (78).

Some children who do not respond adequately to behavioral management will benefit from the addition of pharmacotherapy (1-3, 39, 79-81). Desmopressin, oxybutynin and imipramine are the most widely used drugs (39, 81-84). A variety of antimuscarinic drugs have been developed to deal with the overactive bladder in adults; these include oxybutynin, tolterodine, solifenacin, darifenacin, propiverine, fesoterodine, trospium, and imidafenacin (85). Some have been applied to pediatrics as noted in the text and research continues to evaluate their overall use in children and adolescents (86). The role of telemedicine for follow-up of patients with enuresis continues to be explored (87). The research into various areas of pediatric urology in the 21st century remains exciting and includes investigations for new technologies (i.e., electrical nerve stimulation, altering sleep architecture, bladder-bowel training, others) in the management of enuresis and related conditons (88-98).

Acknowledgment

This chapter is modified and updated with permission from Greydanus DE, Torres AD, O'Donnel DM, Feinberg AN. Enuresis: Current concepts. Indian J Pediatr 1999;66:425-38.

References

[1] Greydanus DE, Torres AD, Wan JH. Genitourinary and renal disorders. In: Greydanus DE, Patel DR, Pratt HD, eds. Essential adolescent medicine. New York: McGraw-Hill Medical, 2006:329-59.
[2] Greydanus DE, Feinberg AN, Patel DR, Homnick DN, eds. The pediatric diagnostic examination. New York: McGraw-Hill Medical, 2008:616, 663,684.
[3] Greydanus DE, Calles Jr JL, Patel DR. Pediatric and adolescent psychopharmacology: A practical manual for pediatricians. Cambridge: Cambridge University Press, 2008.
[4] Hamed SA, Fawzy M, Hamed EA. Behavioral problems in children with primary monosymptomatic nocturnal enuresis. Compr Psychiatry 2021;104:152208. doi: 10.1016/j.comppsych.2020.152208.
[5] Gomez Rincon M, Leslie SW, Lotfollahzadeh S. Nocturnal enuresis. In: StatPearls. Treasure Island, FL: StatPearls Publishing, 2021.
[6] Wilson M, Gupta V. Enuresis. 2021 Feb 6. In: StatPearls [Internet]. Treasure Island, FL: StatPearls Publishing, 2021.
[7] American Psychiatric Association. Diagnostic and statistical manual of mental disorders, 5th ed (DSM-5). Arlington, VA, American Psychiatric Association, 2013:355-7.

[8] Nevéus T, von Gontard A, Hoebeke P, Hjälmås K, Bauer S, Bower W, et al. The standardization of terminology of lower urinary tract function in children and adolescents: Report from the Standardisation Committee of the International Children's Continence Society. J Urol 2006;176(1):314-24.
[9] Kilicoglu AG, Mutlu C, Bahali MK, Adaleti H, Gunes H, Metin Duman H, et al. Impact of enuresis nocturna on health-related quality of life in children and their mothers. J Pediatr Urol 2014;10(6):1261-6.
[10] Bayne AP, Skoog SJ. Nocturnal enuresis: an approach to assessment and treatment. Pediatr Rev 2014;35(8):327-34.
[11] Shrestha N, Sahukhala S, K C D, Sandalcidi D, Adhikari SP. Prevalence of urinary incontinence in school going children: A cross-sectional Study. J Nepal Health Res Counc 2021;18(4):676-80.
[12] Jørgensen CS, Horsdal HT, Rajagopal VM, Grove J, Als TD, Kamperis K, et al. Identification of genetic loci associated with nocturnal enuresis: a genome-wide association study. Lancet Child Adolesc Health 2021;5(3):201-9.
[13] Uzun N, Akinci MA, Karatoprak S. Methylphenidate-induced enuresis: 3 case reports. Clin Neuropharmacol 2021;44(1):37-8.
[14] Naguy A. A comment on clozapine-induced enuresis: An underrecognized and undertreated problem. Prim Care Companion CNS Disord 2021; 23(1):20lr02678.
[15] Özdemir YE, Tanir Y. Low-dose aripiprazole-induced nocturnal enuresis in a 9-year-old boy: A case report and the possible underlying mechanism. Clin Neuropharmacol 2021 Mar 13. doi: 10.1097/WNF.0000000000000450.
[16] Goessaert AS, Everaert K, Hoebeke P, Kapila A, Walle JV. Nocturnal enuresis and nocturia, differences and similarities-lessons to learn? Acta Clin Belg 2014 Nov 6:2295333714Y0000000055.
[17] Roth EB, Austin PF. Evaluation and treatment of nonmonosymptomatic enuresis. Pediatr Rev 2014;35(10):430-6.
[18] Feldman AS, Bauer SB: Diagnosis and management of dysfunctional voiding. Curr Opin ediatr 2006;18:139-47.
[19] Ghoniem GM and Sakr MA: Bladder dysfunciton syndromes. State Art Rev Adolesc Med 1996;7(1):35-46.
[20] Vande Walle J, Rittig S, Bauer S, Eggert P, Marschall-Kehrel D, Tekgul S; American Academy of Pediatrics; European Society for Paediatric Urology; European Society for Paediatric Nephrology; International Children's Continence Society. Practical consensus guidelines for the management of enuresis. Eur J Pediatr 2012;171(6):971-83.
[21] Naseri M. Lower urinary tract urological abnormalities and urodynamic findings of physiologic urinary incontinence versus non-mono symptomatic nocturnal enuresis in children. Nephrourol Mon 2014;6(2):e15360. doi:10.5812/numonthly.15360.
[22] Mannemuddhu SS, Bayne CE, Tufan Pekkucuksen N, Shoemaker LR. Attention to detail: not simple bed wetting-Hinman-Allen syndrome. J Nephrol 2021;34(1):247-50.
[23] Karaci M. Obesity contributes to lower urinary system voiding dysfunction in childhood. Ir J Med Sci 2021 Jan 12. doi: 10.1007/s11845-020-02461-7.
[24] Wright AJ. Nocturnal enuresis: a comorbid condition. J Pediatr (Rio J) 2020;96(3):276-8.
[25] Hsiao YC, Wang JH, Chang CL, Hsieh CJ, Chen MC. Association between constipation and childhood nocturnal enuresis in Taiwan: a population-based matched case-control study. BMC Pediatr 2020;20(1):35. doi: 10.1186/s12887-020-1939-z.
[26] Pedersen MJ, Rittig S, Jennum PJ, Kamperis K. The role of sleep in the pathophysiology of nocturnal enuresis. Sleep Med Rev 2020;49:101228. doi: 10.1016/j.smrv.2019.101228.
[27] Shafiek H, Evangelisti M, Abd-Elwahab NH, Barreto M, Villa MP, Mahmoud MI. Obstructive sleep apnea in school-aged children presented with nocturnal enuresis. Lung 2020;198(1):187-94.
[28] Davaro F, Kaba A, Osei H, Joshi P, Hamilton Z, Phillips T. Treatment of obstructive sleep apnea does not treat primary nocturnal enuresis. J Pediatr Urol 2021;17(2):182-2.
[29] Othman JA, Åkervall S, Molin M, Gyhagen M. Childhood nocturnal enuresis-a marker for pelvic floor disorders and urinary tract symptoms in women? Int Urogynecol J 2021;32(2):359-65.
[30] Gizli Çoban Ö, Önder A, Sürer Adanır A. Psychiatric comorbidities of children with elimination disorders. Arch Pediatr 2021;28(1):59-63.

[31] Mohammadi MR, Hojjat SK, Ahmadi N, Alavi SS, Hooshyari Z, Khaleghi A, et al. Prevalence of elimination disorders and comorbid psychiatric disorders in Iranian children and adolescents. J Pediatr Rehabil Med 2021;14(1):19-29.

[32] Bogaert G, Stein R, Undre S, Nijman RJM, Quadackers J, 't Hoen L, et al. Practical recommendations of the EAU-ESPU guidelines committee for monosymptomatic enuresis-Bedwetting. Neurourol Urodyn 2020;39(2):489-97.

[33] Nevéus T, Fonseca E, Franco I, Kawauchi A, Kovacevic L, Nieuwhof-Leppink A, et al. Management and treatment of nocturnal enuresis-an updated standardization document from the International Children's Continence Society. J Pediatr Urol 2020;16(1):10-9.

[34] Sürmeli Döven S. The effect of using entertainment and communication devices before sleep on nocturnal enuresis. Pediatr Int 2020;62(4):492-5.

[35] Sá CA, Martins de Souza SA, Villela MCBVA, Souza VM, de Souza MHF, de Figueiredo AA, et al. Psychological intervention with parents improves treatment results and reduces punishment in children with enuresis: A randomized clinical trial. J Urol 2021;205(2):570-6.

[36] Caldwell PH, Nankivell G, Sureshkumar P. Simple behavioural interventions for nocturnal enuresis in children. Cochrane Database Syst Rev 2013;7:CD003637.

[37] Fazeli MS, Lin Y, Nikoo N, Jaggumantri S, Collet JP, Afshar K. Biofeedback for nonneuropathic daytime voiding disorders in children: a systematic review and meta-analysis of randomized controlled trials. J Urol 2015;193(1):274-80.

[38] Ebiloglu T, Ergin G, Irkilata HC, Kibar Y. The biofeedback treatment for non-monosymptomatic enuresis nocturna. Neurourol Urodyn 2016;35(1):58-61.

[39] Sundaram V. Urologic conditions in infants and children: Toilet training and nocturnal enuresis. FP Essent 2020;488:21-4.

[40] Caldwell PH, Codarini M, Stewart F, Hahn D, Sureshkumar P. Alarm interventions for nocturnal enuresis in children. Cochrane Database Syst Rev 2020;5:CD002911.

[41] Baird D, Atchison R. Effectiveness of alarm therapy in the treatment of nocturnal enuresis in children. Am Fam Physician 2021 Jan 1;103(1):Online.

[42] Van Herzeele C, De Bruyne P, Evans J, Eggert P, Lottmann H, Norgaard JP, Vande Walle J. Safety profile of desmopressin tablet for enuresis in a prospective study. Adv Ther 2014;31(12):1306-16.

[43] Austin PF, Ferguson G, Yan Y, Campigotto MJ, Royer ME, Coplen DE. Combination therapy with desmopressin and an anticholinergic medication for nonresponders to desmopressin for monosymptomatic nocturnal enuresis: A randomized, double-blind, placebo-controlled trial. Pediatrics 2008;122(5):1027-32.

[44] Glazener CM, Evans JH, Petro RE: Tricyclic and related drugs for nocturnal enuresis in children. Cochrane Database Sys Rev 2003;3: CD002117.

[45] Lane W, Robson M: Current management of nocturnal enuresis. Curr Opin Urol 2008;18:425-30.

[46] Caldwell PH, Deshpande AV, Von Gontard A. Management of nocturnal enuresis. BMJ 2013;347:f6259. doi: 10.1136/bmj.f6259.

[47] Deshpande A, Caldwell P. Medical management of nocturnal enuresis. Pediatr Drugs 2012;14(2):71-7.

[48] Reiner WG. Pharmacotherapy in the management of voiding and storage disorders, including enuresis and encopresis. J Am Acad Child Adolesc Psychiatr 2008;47(5):491-8.

[49] Glazener CM, Evans JH. Desmopressin for nocturnal enuresis in children. Cochrane Database Sys Rev 2002;3:CD002112.

[50] Gasthuys E, Dossche L, Michelet R, Nørgaard JP, Devreese M, Croubels S, et al. Pediatric pharmacology of desmopressin in children with enuresis: A comprehensive review. Paediatr Drugs 2020;22(4):369-83.

[51] Dossche L, Michelet R, De Bruyne P, Van Herzeele C, Gasthuys E, Rittig S, et al. Desmopressin oral lyophilisate in young children: new insights in pharmacokinetics and pharmacodynamics. Arch Dis Child 2020; 106(6):597-602. doi: 10.1136/archdischild-2019-318225.

[52] McCarty TS, Shah AD. Desmopressin. In: StatPearls. Treasure Island, FL: StatPearls Publishing, 2021.

[53] Kasamo S, Matsumoto S, Kawasaki Y, Inoue H, Tasaki Y. Changes in prescribing trends and initial pharmacotherapy of children with nocturnal enuresis in Japan: a large-scale medical claims database analysis. World J Urol 2021 Mar 22. doi: 10.1007/s00345-021-03664-y.

[54] National Clinical Guideline Centre (UK). Nocturnal enuresis: The management of bedwetting in children and young people. London: Royal College of Physicians, 2010.
[55] Khalid MM, Waseem M. Tricyclic Antidepressant Toxicity. In: StatPearls. Treasure Island, FL: StatPearls Publishing, 2021.
[56] Deshpande AV, Caldwell PH, Sureshkukmar P. Drugs for nocturnal enuresis in children (other than desmopressin and tricyclics). Cochrane Database Syst Rev 2012;12:CD002238.
[57] Humphreys MR, Reinberg YE: Contemporary and emerging drug treatments for urinary incontinence in children. Paedatr Drugs 2005;7:151-62.
[58] Nijman R, Borgstein N, Ellsworth P, Siggaard C. Long-term tolerability of tolertodine extended release in children 5-11 years of age: Results from a 12-month, open-label study. Eur Urology 2007;52:1511-7.
[59] Hoebeke P, DePooter J, Caesteckeer K, Raes A, Dehoorne J, VanLaecke E, et al. Solifenacin for therapy resistant overactive bladder. J Urology 2009;182:2040-4.
[60] Nadeau G, Schroder A, Moore K, Genois L, Lamontagne P, Hamel M, et al. Long-term use of solifenacin in pediatric patients with overactive bladder: extension of a prospective open-label study. Can Urol Assoc J 2014;8:118-23.
[61] Samir M, Mahmoud MA, Elawady H. Can the combined treatment of solifenacin and imipramine has a role in desmopressin refractory monosymptomatic nocturnal enuresis? A prospective double-blind randomized placebo-controlled study. Urologia 2021;88(4):369-73.
[62] Soebadi MA, Hakim L, Van der Aa F, De Ridder D. Real-Life data on mirabegron in neurogenic bladder dysfunction. Urol Int 2019;103(2):195-201.
[63] Gratzke C, van Maanen R, Chapple C, Abrams P, Herschorn S, Robinson D, et al. Long-term safety and efficacy of mirabegron and solifenacin in combination compared with monotherapy in patients with overactive bladder: A randomised, multicentre Phase 3 Study (SYNERGY II). Eur Urol 2018;74(4):501-9.
[64] Wada N, Watanabe M, Banjo H, Tsuchida M, Hori J, Tamaki G, et al. Long-term persistence with mirabegron in a real-world clinical setting. Int J Urol 2018;25(5):501-6.
[65] Ness TJ, McNaught J, Clodfelder-Miller B, Su X. Medications used to treat bladder disorders may alter effects of neuromodulation. Neurourol Urodyn 2020;39(5):1313-20.
[66] Meyer SIR, Jørgensen CS, Kamperis K, Andersen RF, Pedersen MJ, Faerch M, et al. Efficacy and safety of multimodal treatment in nocturnal enuresis: A retrospective cohort study. J Pediatr Urol 2021;17(4):447.e1-7.
[67] Jia ZM, Wen JG, Zhu W, Zhang RL, Wang Y, Zhang CY, et al. [Evaluation of refractory monosymptomatic nocturnal enuresis with ambulatory urodynamics monitoring and conventional urodynamics]. Zhonghua Yi Xue Za Zhi 2021;101(2):142-6. [Chinese]
[68] DiBianco JM, Morley C, Al-Omar O. Nocturnal enuresis: A topic review and institution experience. Avicenna J Med 2014;4(4):77-86.
[69] Ferrara P, Franceschini G, Bianchi Di Castelbianco F, Bombace R, Villani A, et al. Epidemiology of enuresis: a large number of children at risk of low regard. Ital J Pediatr 2020;46(1):128. doi: 10.1186/s13052-020-00896-3.
[70] Katz EG, MacLachlan LS. Nocturnal enuresis in the adult. Curr Urol Rep 2020;21(8):31. doi: 10.1007/s11934-020-00983-2.
[71] Song QX, Wang L, Cheng X, Hao Y, Liu Z, Abrams P. The clinical features and predictive factors of nocturnal enuresis in adult men. BJU Int 2020;126(4):472-80.
[72] Ural ÜM, Gücük S, Ekici A, Topçuoğlu A. Urinary incontinence in female university students. Int Urogynecol J 2021;32(2):367-73.
[73] Hu HJ, Zhang ZW, Liang Y, Luo YY, Dou QF, Song CP, et al. Prevalence, risk factors, and psychological effects of primary nocturnal enuresis in Chinese young adults. Int Neurourol J 2021;25(1):84-92.
[74] Rangel RA, Seabra CR, Ferrarez CEPF, Soares JL, Choi M, Cotta RG, et al. Quality of life in enuretic children. Int Braz J Urol 2021;47(3):535-41.
[75] Hamed SA, Fawzy M, Hamed EA. Behavioral problems in children with primary monosymptomatic nocturnal enuresis. Compr Psychiatry 2021;104:152208.

[76] Radhakrishnan Pillai R, Sara B. Conquering bedwetting: Non pharmacologic methods for managing nocturnal enuresis. Creat Nurs 2020;26(1):23-7.
[77] Hussain Shah SS, Aalia B, Raza A, Najeeb S, Rehman AU. An outcome of conservative management of primary nocturnal enuresis in children. J Ayub Med Coll Abbottabad 2021;33(1):71-4.
[78] Nieuwhof-Leppink AJ, Hussong J, Chase J, Larsson J, Renson C, Hoebeke P, et al. Definitions, indications and practice of urotherapy in children and adolescents: - A standardization document of the International Children's Continence Society (ICCS). J Pediatr Urol 2020; S1477-5131(20)30630-6.
[79] Kiddoo D. Nocturnal enuresis: non-pharmacologic treatments. BMJ Clin Evid 2015;2015:0305.
[80] Ma Y, Shen Y, Liu X. Self-concept in children with primary nocturnal enuresis and related influencing factors. Iran J Public Health 2020; 49(4):805-7.
[81] Sundaram V. Urologic conditions in infants and children: Toilet training and nocturnal enuresis. FP Essent 2020;488:21-4.
[82] Önol FF, Guzel R, Tahra A, Kaya C, Boylu U. Comparison of long-term efficacy of desmopressin lyophilsate and enuretic alarm for monosymptomatic enuresis and assessment of predictive factors for success: a randomized prospective trial. J Urol 2015;193(2):655-61.
[83] Prince E, Heys M. Nocturnal enuresis: An update on management. Drug Ther Bull 2020;58(2):25-9.
[84] Liu J, Ni J, Miao Q, Wang C, Lin F, Cao Q, et al. Exploration of the optimal desmopressin treatment in children with monosymptomatic nocturnal enuresis: Evidence from a Chinese cohort. Front Pediatr 2021;8:626083.
[85] Yamada S, Ito Y, Nishijima S, Kadekawa K, Sugaya K. Basic and clinical aspects of antimuscarinic agents used to treat overactive bladder. Pharmacol Ther 2018;189:130-48.
[86] Ghanavati PM, Khazaeli D, Amjadzadeh M. A comparison of the efficacy and tolerability of treating primary nocturnal enuresis with Solifenacin Plus Desmopressin, Tolterodine Plus Desmopressin, and Desmopressin alone: A randomized controlled clinical trial. Int Braz J Urol 2021;47(1):73-81.
[87] Smith E, Cline J, Patel A, Zamilpa I, Canon S. Telemedicine versus traditional for follow-up evaluation of enuresis. Telemed J E Health 2021;27(2):213-7.
[88] Monaghan TF, Delanghe JR, Agudelo CW, Alwis US, Pauwaert K, Weiss JP, et al. Toward a dry tomorrow: Novel technologies in the treatment of nocturnal enuresis. J Pediatr Urol 2020;16(5):733-4.
[89] Souza TMP, de Lima GS, Pasqualini LB, Melleiro V, Glina FPA, Serra MJR, et al.. Electrical nerve stimulation therapy in refractory primary monosymtomatic enuresis: A systematic review. J Pediatr Urol 2021;17(3):295-301.
[90] Matsumoto T. Suvorexant improves intractable nocturnal enuresis by altering sleep architecture. BMJ Case Rep 2021;14(3):e239621. doi: 10.1136/bcr-2020-239621.
[91] Ghijselings L, Renson C, Van de Walle J, Everaert K, Spinoit AF. Clinical efficacy of transcutaneous tibial nerve stimulation (TTNS) versus sham therapy (part I) and TTNS versus percutaneous tibial nerve stimulation (PTNS) (part II) on the short term in children with the idiopathic overactive bladder syndrome: protocol for part I of the twofold double-blinded randomized controlled TaPaS trial. Trials 2021;22(1):247. doi: 10.1186/s13063-021-05117-8.
[92] de Abreu GE, de Souza LA, Fonseca MLVD, Barbosa TBC, de Mello ERD, Nunes ANB, et al. Parasacral transcutaneous electrical nerve stimulation for the treatment of children and adolescents with bladder and bowel dysfunction: A randomized clinical trial. J Urol 2021;205(6):1785-91.
[93] Petros PE, Garcia-Fernandez A. Cure of enuresis/bowel dysfunction in children may provide insights for adult dysfunctions. Tech Coloproctol. 2021;25(3):351-3.
[94] Hussong J, Mattheus H, Wachs S, Equit M, von Gontard A. Evaluation of a bladder and bowel training program for therapy-resistant children with incontinence. J Pediatr Urol 2021 Feb 2:S1477-5131(21)00073-5.
[95] Canning DA. Pediatric urology. J Urol 2021;205(1):292-4.
[96] Sivakumar CT, Rajan M, Pasupathy U, Chidambaram S, Baskar N. Effect of sleep habits on academic performance in schoolchildren age 6 to 12 years: a cross-sectional observation study. J Clin Sleep Med 2022; 18(1):145-9.
[97] Kapoor P, Chowdhry A, Sengar P, Mehta A. Development, testing, and feasibility of a customized mobile application for obstructive sleep apnea (OSA) risk assessment: A hospital-based pilot study. J Oral Biol Craniofac Res 2022;12(1):109-15.

[98] Che YH, Xu ZR, Ni LL, Dong XX, Yang ZZ, Yang ZB. Isolation and identification of the components in Cybister chinensis Motschulsky against inflammation and their mechanisms of action based on network pharmacology and molecular docking. J Ethnopharmacol 2022;285:114851.

Chapter 5

Encopresis

Jocelyn DeLeon, MD, Mahesh Shrestha, MD, Zainab Mahmood, MD and Dilip R. Patel*, MD, MPH, MBA

Department of Pediatric and Adolescent Medicine, Western Michigan University Homer Stryker MD School of Medicine, Kalamazoo, Michigan, United States of America

Abstract

Functional fecal incontinence or encopresis is a condition commonly seen in children, and as such, pediatricians and health care providers who care for children should be familiar with this diagnosis. Encopresis refers to the passage or leakage of feces in inappropriate settings. There is a high prevalence of associated behavioral symptoms in children who have encopresis. Treatment involves patient and family education, behavioral strategies for stool regulation, disimpaction of stool in children who have constipation, and long-term maintenance of regular bowel habits. This discussion reviews the definition, epidemiology, clinical presentation, and treatment of children who have encopresis.

Introduction

There is a wide range of practices and attitudes towards child rearing and bowel training across cultures, but the majority of children cross-culturally are successfully toilet trained by 3 to 4 years of age (1-3). A study of different cultures reported that bowel training in most cultures was primarily the role of mothers; this study looked at a primitive Kenyan community, an Indian farming community, a Japanese rural community, and a United States urban community (1-3). Most children in this study achieved bowel control at about the same age regardless of rearing method, suggesting a significant role of maturational factors (1-8).

* ***Correspondence:*** Dilip R Patel, MD, MPH, MBA, Department of Pediatric and Adolescent Medicine, Western Michigan University School of Medicine, 1000, Oakland Drive, Kalamazoo MI, United States. Email: Dilip.patel@med.wmich.edu.

In: Behavioral Pediatrics II
Editors: Donald E. Greydanus, Dilip R. Patel, Ahsan Nazeer et al.
ISBN: 979-8-88697-019-7

Definition

Encopresis is defined as repeated voluntary and involuntary passage of feces in inappropriate places by a child, who is chronologically at least four years old (or of equivalent mental age or developmental level); at least one such event must occur every month over a period of 3 months (9-13). Functional fecal incontinence is classified as retentive, if it is associated with functional constipation (i.e., a history of retentive posturing, history of hard, painful stools, presence of large fecal mass in rectum or history of passing large diameter stool) and non-retentive, if not associated with functional constipation (9-10).

Pathophysiology

Functional constipation can result from either intentional or unintentional withholding of stool (6, 9, 10). Withholding of stool leads to retention of stool in the rectum. The water is further absorbed and the stool becomes firm and hard; also, this stool is difficult and painful to pass, further leading to withholding by the child. As the rectum continues to accommodate increasing amounts of stool mass, the rectal walls are stretched, and the urge or the sensation to defecate is diminished or lost, further leading to retention. When the mass is large enough, the anal sphincter loses competency, leading to leakage of unformed or watery stool around the impacted mass. The leakage is involuntary and cannot be controlled by the child, leading to fecal soiling.

Epidemiology

Encopresis is 3 to 6 times more common in boys than in girls; the prevalence at age four years is estimated to be between 2-8% in boys and between 1-3% in girls (3, 11, 14). The prevalence from preschool years through early adolescence is reported to be 2-4% in boys and 1-2% in girls (2, 4, 5). It is most prevalent between the ages of 3 and 7 years, with time from symptoms onset to diagnosis being between 1 to 5 years. There is no significant correlation between encopresis and socio-economic factors, family dynamics, or a child's relation within a family. Particular interest is given to studying the association between attention-deficit/ hyperactivity disorder (ADHD) and encopresis, as both have an impact on psychosocial functioning (14, 15). One study found that children with ADHD were more likely to have encopresis than children without ADHD (14). Children with ADHD are significantly more likely to have constipation and fecal incontinence. Medical therapy for ADHD does not impact visit rates for defecation disorders. About 80-90% of functional fecal incontinence is retentive in nature and thus is associated with constipation (5, 6, 8,-10).

Clinical presentation

Problems with defecation, however common, can be distressing for a child and the parents. This distress and embarrassment from fecal soiling may deter the child from bringing to attention these occurrences to parents. Some parents may think soiling in underwear as diarrhea. Parents may also find it difficult to seek external guidance from anyone, including the physician, and may feel guilty for failing to adequately toilet train their child. Unfortunately, without proper guidance and attention, the problem may continue to worsen, leading to tension within the family. The child may refuse to go to school and may be teased by other children, resulting in isolation and adjustment problems for the child. The child may also be at an increased risk for punishment and physical abuse by parents who may assume their child is defiant. They may not fully understand that these occurrences of fecal soiling are not the child's fault. In a significant number of cases, the time from symptom onset to diagnosis can take up to 5 years.

Infants and pre-school children may present with a history of gradually worsening constipation and withholding maneuvers. An infant may extend the body and contract the anal and gluteal muscles. A toddler may stand on his or her toes, hold their legs stiff, cross them, or rock back and forth. A school-aged child may present after having had the problem for some years. The child may have fecal incontinence more than once daily or intermittently with periods of no stools or soiling. Such periods will generally follow passage of a large bowel movement. The child may deny foul odor and may hide the soiled clothes. Children may also present with intermittent acute as well as moderate to severe abdominal pain or chronic non-specific abdominal pain preceding the passage of a large bowel movement. Some children may present with non-specific symptoms of headaches and not feeling well. There is associated enuresis in 20-30% of children with encopresis, and in approximately 10% of girls, there is associated urinary tract infection (7, 16-18).

Diagnosis

Ninety percent of encopresis is functional, meaning without an anatomical or physiological defect or illness (4-9). About 5-10 percent of children have an underlying organic cause that may be neurologic, anatomic, metabolic, or iatrogenic (2, 3, 8). Several specific areas of history and physical examination may yield findings that would guide appropriate course of evaluation, including imaging studies or laboratory tests (1-8, 16-18). The history should specifically include information on the usual pattern of bowel habits, and description of the stool---its character, odor, consistency, and amount. Additional questions should ascertain a triggering event, associated symptoms, and medical history of known gastrointestinal disorder or surgical procedure in the past. Passage of recurrent, small pellet like stool suggests incomplete evacuation, whereas intermittent massive stools are suggestive of functional fecal retention. A thorough dietary history should also be obtained.

The general examination should include the growth and developmental parameters, height as well as weight progression, and signs of malnutrition. Many children with encopresis present with palpable stool mass due to constipation. Severe abdominal distension may raise concern for organic disease. Anterior displacement of anus is suggestive of anorectal anomaly. Soiled underwear could be a sign of overflow incontinence due to large stool burden and constipation. Anal fissures could be also due to constipation. Hard stool felt during digital exam is more indicative of large stool burden with constipation; whereas increased tone with soft stool suggests anorectal dysfunction including Hirschsprung disease (named after the first Danish professor of pediatrics, Harald Hirschsprung, 1830-1916). Explosive stool coming out after digital exam could also suggest Hirschsprung disease. The presence of tuft of hair or sacral dimple could be due to spina bifida occulta that could lead to incontinence due to neurologic dysfunction. Absent anal wink elicited points to neurologic impairment.

A urinalysis and plain film of the abdomen are useful initial studies though they are not routinely indicated. Urinalysis and urine culture are more appropriate if the child also has enuresis. Plain abdominal radiograph could be helpful to document large stool burden in an uncooperative child for exam or in children who did not have large stool mass on exam. Barium studies of the bowel, anorectal manometry, endoscopy, and biopsy may be indicated in some children to exclude organic causes of fecal incontinence. Laboratory tests are usually not indicated; however, in selected cases tests for celiac disease, blood lead level, thyroid function tests, calcium, or electrolytes could help to distinguish organic causes of constipation.

The prevalence of other behavioral disorders is higher in children who have encopresis. The most common co-morbid behavioral disorders seen in children with encopresis are oppositional defiant disorder, attention-deficit/hyperactivity disorder, separation anxiety disorder, and depression (3, 5, 11, 14, 15). A high association between encopresis and sexual abuse has been reported. Encopresis has been reported in between 20% and 30% of children who have learning disability; the more severe the disability, the higher the prevalence (3, 5, 11, 14, 15). As such, further work-up should include a holistic approach, ensuring this child is properly cared for from a psychosocial aspect as well.

It is important to consider in practice that initial presentation of encopresis could be at a visit primarily for behavioral concerns. Primary care physicians should routinely inquire about urinary and bowel habits at such visits. The child's age at time of onset of encopretic symptoms may be difficult to ascertain, as initially the child may not tell parents. Later, the parents may be reluctant to seek medical advice. The family may be experiencing significant stress, and it is essential to assess parental emotions, family functioning, and how parents are dealing with the child.

Pharmacologic treatment

Successful treatment of fecal encopresis requires a team approach—family members, health care providers, and the patient. They work as a team for better treatment outcomes. Before instituting the treatment regimen for encopresis, any specific organic obstructive or non-obstructive etiology for chronic constipation should be ruled. General measures should be implemented to achieve stool regulation. These include adequate fluid intake, appropriate modification of the diet, including high fiber intake and behavioral measures. Education of the family is the essential first step in the overall management of the encopresis. It is essential to clarify to the family that fecal incontinence is caused by rectal impaction and is beyond the child's control. Parents need to understand that there is no quick solution to this condition. Parents should be reassured that recovery is possible with adequate, often protracted treatment. Pharmacotherapy is a primary and integral component of overall management approach for children with encopresis (5, 6, 16-24).

Disimpaction

The next step in children who have encopresis with constipation is to achieve complete evacuation of the bowels. The physician should explain that constipation often leads to a vicious cycle that results in stool withholding, fecal retention, and eventually fecal incontinence. Polyethylene glycol-based solutions have become the mainstay of therapy. Other options such as osmotic or stimulant laxatives are available. Disimpaction of the fecal mass can be achieved by several methods and may take from 2 to 5 days. Initially polyethylene glycol (PEG) given orally should be tried (Table 1). If oral PEG fails to achieve disimpaction, rectal enemas containing phosphates such as sodium hydrogen phosphate and sodium monohydrogen phosphate are administered.

In some cases, a child may have to be hospitalized to achieve complete disimpaction. In most children, 1 -2 enemas should achieve this state. Excessive use of hypertonic phosphate enema may cause hypernatremia, hypokalemia, hypovolemia, and dehydration. Soap water enemas should be avoided as they may result in perforation and necrosis of the bowel. Tap water enemas should be avoided; they may cause water intoxication, hyponatremia, and seizures. If oral PEG and rectal phosphate enemas fail to achieve disimpaction and bowel evacuation, other methods are considered preferably in consultation with a pediatric gastroenterologist.

Table 1. Commonly used oral and rectal laxative drugs for disimpaction

Laxative	Dosage	Comments
Rectal Administration		
Mineral oil	2–11 y: 30–60 mL once per day >11 y: 60–150 mL once per day	
Sodium phosphate enema	1–18 y: 2.5 mL/kg, maximum 133 mL/dose	Usual 1-2 per day for 1-2 days May result in metabolic abnormalities
Bisacodyl suppository	2–10 y: 5 mg once per day >10 y: 5–10 mg once per day	May be used up to 4 days
Glycerin suppository	Infant: 1 gm Children: 2gm	Safe for use in infants
Milk-of-molasses	10 ml/kg up to 240 mls per dose	1:1 concentration
Oral/Nasogastric Administration		
Mineral oil	1-18 y/o: 1–3 mL/kg/d, once or divided, maximum 90 mL/d	Do not use in infants <12 mos Can mix with chocolate milk or ice cream to improve taste
Polyethylene glycol 3350	Fecal disimpaction: 1–1.5 g/kg/d (up to 6 consecutive days)	Lack of taste
Bisacodyl	3–10 y: 5 mg/d >10 y: 5–10 mg/d	
Senna	2–6 y: 2.5–5 mg once or twice per day 6–12 y: 7.5–10 mg/d >12 y: 15–20 mg/d	Give at bedtime for once daily administration
Milk of magnesium	2–5 y: 0.4–1.2 g/d, once or divided 6–11 y: 1.2–2.4 g/d, once or divided 12–18 y: 2.4–4.8 g/d, once or divided	

Maintenance

Once disimpaction and complete evacuation is achieved, the next step in the treatment is to prevent reaccumulation of the stool. This is achieved by regular use of stool softeners and laxatives (Table 2). The most widely used and recommended laxatives are PEG and lactulose. The goal of this phase is to allow sufficient time for the colon to return to normal caliber and tone; this may take up to 6 months or longer. In addition to the use of laxatives, dietary fiber should be appropriately increased. One can also use fiber supplements containing cellulose, psyllium, or polycarbophil. Use of laxatives and stool softeners may have to be continued for months in order to maintain regular bowel movements and prevent reaccumulation of stools. The child should be followed regularly in the office. Relapses may occur and evacuation may be needed with use of enemas. Lactulose and glycerin suppositories may be used. PEG 3350 in infants at doses of 0.8 g/kg/day, is well tolerated, effective and safe in the management of constipation in infants younger than 18 months of age (5, 20, 21).

Table 2. Stool softeners and laxatives for maintenance therapy

Laxative	Dosage	Comments
Lactulose	> 6 mos: 1-3 ml/kg/day in divided doses	
Sorbitol (70% solution)	1-3 ml/kg/day in divided doses	Limited data available. May be mixed with prune, pear or apple juices
Mineral oil	> 1 yr: 1-3 ml/kg/day in 1-2 divided doses	Avoid use in infants due to risk of aspiration Do not give with docusate
Magnesium hydroxide (milk of magnesia)	2–5 y: 0.4–1.2 g/d 6–11 y: 1.2–2.4 g/d 12–18 y: 2.4–4.8 g/d	Administer in 1-2 divided doses Increased risk of electrolyte abnormalities in infants & renal dysfunction
Polyethylene glycol 3350	0.2–0.8 g/kg/d	Mix with water or juice Well tolerated
Docusate sodium	6 mo-2 yrs: 12.5 mg 3x a day 3-12 yrs 50-360 mg/day in divided doses 13-21 yrs: up to 500 mg/day	Can cause rash, bitter taste and throat irritation Do not give with mineral oil

A child undergoing treatment should be weaned from the laxative regimen gradually at the same time. He or she should be encouraged to sit on the toilet after breakfast or the evening meal to take advantage of the gastrocolic reflex. The goal is to create a positive experience with the child, without a struggle, coercing, or forcing in order to help develop a habit.

Behavioral treatment

A number of behavioral techniques have shown to be effective in the management of encopresis and associated behavioral symptoms (1-18, 23-31). Most patients referred for behavioral or biofeedback therapies have failed to obtain bowel control from primary treatment interventions (e.g., laxatives, suppositories, enemas, education, dietary changes, or toilet training). Prerequisites for treating children with behavioral interventions or biofeedback for fecal incontinence include intact sphincter function, ability to follow instructions, presence of discriminate rectal sensations, and parental motivation to engage in toilet training. Both behavioral and biofeedback interventions are most effective when used as adjuncts to the medical treatment. Children with a history of treatment failures may require psychological interventions to address specific fears and toilet phobias.

Clinicians rely heavily on parental data collection to measure treatment outcomes in a child's control of feces, bowel habits, and fecal staining. Parents are asked to complete survey instruments, participate in face-to-face or telephone interviews, and maintain behavioral charts or diaries; these involve recording data on the presence/absence and intensity of pain at elimination, food intake, and number of laxatives or enemas required to prevent or eliminate constipation.

Behavioral treatment of fecal incontinence requires the clinician to maintain a good working relationship with parents and their children to access information and enlist cooperation for treatment interventions as well as data collection. The most effective behavioral approaches combine education, toilet training, incentive programs, and positive reinforcement using reward/response system. These techniques are time intensive for parents but are inexpensive and do not rely on technology.

Enhanced toilet training

Enhanced toilet training (ETT) is a behavioral management program that involves behavioral modification techniques, education, and training about appropriate defecation dynamics; these include breathing technique, abdominal muscle training and relaxation. This treatment may also contain a contingency-based reward program, such as a star chart. In a randomized trial of 87 children 6–15 years of age, one study demonstrated that ETT significantly benefited more children than biofeedback (30). In addition, ETT required fewer laxatives and fewer treatment sessions at a lower cost (30). Incentive programs are designed according to the developmental stage and motivational level of a child. The goal is to reward the child for spontaneous trips to the toilet and for having clean pants. Children are shown how to appropriately strain to defecate using a structured procedure.

Toilet time should be structured. Fifteen to thirty minutes after a meal, the child is required to sit on the toilet for a 12-minute session. During the first four minutes, the child is encouraged to practice tensing and relaxing his or her sphincter. This procedure is designed to help the child localize control of as well as fatigue the sphincter and to mechanically stimulate the rectum. The second four minutes is designed to desensitize the child to toilet sitting. Parents are taught how to engage their child in fun activities (those that motivate the child – being read to or playing games). The last four minutes are spent encouraging the child to strain and attempt to have a bowel movement.

A reward/response cost system is integral component of ETT. Parents provide rewards for their child when he or she engages in specific activities that lead to appropriate control of feces (i.e., clean pants, defecating in the toilet, drinking water, asking to go to the toilet, etc). Parents make the child wash or assist in washing his or her soiled underpants and to clean his or her own soiled body.

Biofeedback

The purpose of biofeedback therapy is to restore a normal pattern of defecation using visual and verbal feedback techniques. It is another method to aid in training a child to void appropriately. This form of therapy consists of using a probe with a balloon on the end. It is inserted into a child's anus (manometric procedure) and is designed to create, maintain, and measure the amount of pressure a patient can exert on the inflated balloon when it is inserted. This procedure requires hospitalization for one week for treatment that is administered 2 times a day.

A less invasive procedure attaches electrodes to the exterior of the anus to measure pressure. These devices are connected to transducers that are connected to a computer. The computerized equipment is used to present visual images designed to teach patients to easily learn how to voluntarily squeeze their anal sphincter and recognize associated physiological sensations. The child may be required to contract or relax the sphincter muscle to control a visual image on the computer's monitor screen. For example, he or she might be asked to catch an egg and then drop it into a basket that is moving along the bottom of a computer monitor screen by contracting and relaxing his sphincter muscles.

In order to teach the patient how to generalize this skill to controlling his or her sphincter muscle, he or she might be shown a circle that expands and contracts with the relaxation and contraction of the patient's anal sphincter. The visual images on the computer are combined with auditory instructions from the clinician who conducts the training. Children can improve voluntary sphincter function and rectal sensation using similar procedures and can learn to master the process within 15 to 20 minutes.

Studies of children with fecal incontinence treated with biofeedback therapy have shown variable results. The role of biofeedback therapy remains unclear. However, this may be an option for children with a rectal evacuation disorder and persistent symptoms despite optimal conventional treatment. Also, this is only performed on older children who can cooperate due to the intensive training that is required. Biofeedback used alone is not considered to be an effective adjunctive therapy for treating functional encopresis. Prognosis for successful treatment using behavioral interventions or biofeedback is worse for those children who have a long history of fecal incontinence or suffer from severe constipation. The longer a child has been incontinent or constipated, the longer it will take for him or her to respond to treatment and maintain therapeutic gains (i.e., no fecal staining, fecal incontinence or constipation). Treatment is considered effective when the child has been "clean" for 6 months.

Additional considerations

For refractory constipation, antegrade continence enemas administered via cecostomy is an option (31). This also treats fecal overflow incontinence associated with constipation. A retrospective study found that normal colonic and anorectal manometry were associated with good outcome; also, obesity and abdominal pain tend to be associated with poor outcomes after cecostomy for refractory constipation (31).

A prospective observational study evaluated the long-term efficacy of sacral nerve stimulation (SNS) in children with constipation and describe patient benefit and parent satisfaction (32). The investigators concluded that sacral nerve stimulation is a promising treatment for children with refractory constipation and appears particularly effective in decreasing fecal incontinence. Although a quarter of patients experienced complications requiring additional surgery, nearly all parents reported health-related benefit.

Another study evaluated parental perception of current treatments, incontinence burden, and attitudes toward novel and alternative therapies in a single pediatric institution (33). Sacral neuromodulation (SNM) and transcutaneous nerve stimulation (TENS) are alternative therapies to refractory incontinence and constipation. The investigators concluded that pediatric refractory fecal incontinence has a large impact on patients' as well as caregivers' quality of life and alternative therapies with the potential to quality of life of patients and caregivers should be further investigated as a substitute for surgery (33).

In recent years, internet interventions have become more common as a tool to educate and provide health intervention to parents (34, 35). A particular program called U-CAN-POOP-TOO used animations and graphics to provide tutorials for children aged 5 to 12 years that could engage them in this program (35). Along with this and other sources of internet interventions, most parents reported favorable outcomes with significant reduction in episodes of fecal incontinence. These researchers found that subjects had a higher success rate when they participated in the internet intervention than subjects who were treated with traditional methods (35).

Conclusion

Encopresis is a common condition seen in children. It can be effectively treated in most cases; however, relapses are not uncommon during the treatment process. The most common reason for relapse is premature discontinuation of the maintenance regimen. In children, long-term use of a laxative regimen has been shown to cause no significant side effects or result in habit formation. Various studies show that 50%-60% of children will achieve acceptable bowel control free of incontinence within 12 months, and up to 80% will do so by 2 years of treatment. A few children will require continued treatment for more than 2 years.

Acknowledgment

This chapter is modified and updated with permission from Patel DR, Pratt HD: Encopresis. In: Greydanus DE, Patel DR, Pratt HD, Calles JL Jr, Nazeer A, Merrick J, eds. Behavioral pediatrics, 4th edition, New York: Nova Biomedical, 2015:399-409.

References

[1] Abi-Hanna A, Lake AM. Constipation and encopresis in childhood. Pediatr Rev 1998;19(1):23-30.

[2] Loening-Baucke V. Encopresis. Curr Opin Pediatr 2002;14(5):570-5.

[3] Har AF, Croffie JM. Encopresis. Pediatr Rev 2010;31;368-374.

[4] Yilanli M, Gokarakonda SB. Encopresis. In: StatPearls. Treasure Island, FL: StatPearls Publishing, 2020 Jan-.

[5] LeLeiko NS, Mayer-Brown S, Cerezo C, Plante W. Constipation. Pediatr Rev 2020; 41(8):379-92.
[6] Lu PL, Mousa HM. Constipation: beyond the old paradigms. Gastroenterol Clin North Am 2018;47(4):845-62.
[7] Patel DR, Pratt HD. Encopresis. Ind J Pediatr 1999;66:439-46.
[8] Loening-Boucke V. Encopresis and soiling. Pediatr Clin N Amer 1996;43(1):279–98.
[9] Benninga MA, Faure C, Hyman PE, St James Roberts I, Schechter NL, Nurko S. Childhood functional gastrointestinal disorders: Neonate/toddler. Gastroenterology 2016;150:1443-55.
[10] Hyams JS, Di Lorenzo C, Saps M, Shulman RJ, Staiano A, van Tilburg M. Functional disorders: Children and adolescents. Gastroenterology 2016 Feb 15:S0016-5085(16)00181-5.
[11] American Psychiatric Association: Elimination disorders: Encopresis. Diagnostic and statistical manual of mental disorders 5th edition Arlington, VA: American Psyciatric Association, 2013:357-58.
[12] Nevéus T, von Gontard A, Hoebeke P, Hjälmås K, Bauer S, Bower W, et al. The standardization of terminology of lower urinary tract function in children and adolescents: report from the Standardisation Committee of the International Children's Continence Society. J Urol 2006;176(1):314-24.
[13] von Gontard A. Ausscheidungsstörungen – Klassifikation und Definition nach ICD-11 [Elimination disorders - ICD-11 classification and definitions]. Z Kinder Jugendpsychiatr Psychother 2020 Sep 21:1-8. doi: 10.1024/1422-4917/a000751. [German]
[14] Mellon MW, Natchev BE, Katusic SK, Colligan RC, Weaver AL, Voigt RG, et al. Incidence of enuresis and encopresis among children with attention-deficit/hyperactivity disorder in a population-based birth cohort. Acad Pediatr 2013;13(4):322-7.
[15] Gizli Çoban Ö, Önder A, Sürer Adanır A. Psychiatric comorbidities of children with elimination disorders. Arch Pediatr 2020 Nov 19:S0929-693X(20)30222-0.
[16] Tabbers MM, DiLorenzo C, Berger MY, Faure C, Langendam MW, Nurkos S, et al. Evaluation and treatment of functional constipation in infants and children: Evidence-based recommendations from ESPGHAN and NASPGHAN. J Ped Gastro Nutrit 2014;58(2):258-74.
[17] Nurko S, Zimmerman LA. Evaluation and treatment of constipation in children and adolescents. Am Fam Physician 2014;90(2):82-90.
[18] Baird DC, Bybel M, Kowalski AW. Toilet training: common questions and answers. Am Fam Physician 2019;100(8):468-74.
[19] Reiner WG. Pharmacotherapy in the management of voiding and storage disorders, including enuresis and encopresis. J Am Acad Child Adolesc Psychiatry 2008;47;5:491-7.
[20] Hansen SE, Whitehill JL, Goto CS, Quintero CA, Darling BE, Davis J. Safety and efficacy of milk and molasses enemas compared with sodium phosphate enemas for the treatment of constipation in a pediatric emergency department. Pediatr Emerg Care 2011;27(12):1118-20.
[21] Koppen IJ, von Gontard A, Chase J, Cooper CS, Rittig CS, Bauer SB, et al. Management of functional nonretentive fecal incontinence in children: Recommendations from the International Children's Continence Society. J Pediatr Urol 2016;12(1):56-64.
[22] Rowan-Legg A, Canadian Paediatric Society Community Paediatrics Committee. Managing functional constipation in children. Paediatr Child Health 2011;16(10):661–70.
[23] von Gontard A, Neveus T. The management of disorders of bladder and bowel control in childhood. Cambridge, UK: Cambridge University Press, 2006.
[24] Van der Plas RN, Benninga MA, Taminiau JA, Büller HA. Treatment of defaecation problems in children: the role of education, demystification and toilet training. Eur J Pediatr 1997;156(9):689-92.
[25] Shepard JA, Poler JE Jr, Grabman JH. Evidence-based psychosocial treatments for pediatric elimination disorders. J Clin Child Adolesc Psychol 2017;46(6):767-97.
[26] Beaudry-Bellefeuille I, Booth D, Lane SJ. Defecation-specific behavior in children with functional defecation issues: a systematic review. Perm J 2017;21:17-47.
[27] Brazzelli M, Griffiths P. Behavioural and cognitive interventions with or without other treatments for the management of faecal incontinence in children. Cochrane Database Syst Rev 2006;12:CD002240.
[28] Culbert TP, Banez GA. Integrative approaches to childhood constipation and encopresis. Pediatr Clin North Am 2007;54(6):927-47.
[29] Goodman G. Encopresis happens: theoretical and treatment considerations from an attachment perspective. Psychoanalytic Psychology 2013;30(3):438–55.

[30] Cox DJ, Sutphen J, Ling W, Quillian W, Borowitz S. Additive benefits of laxative, toilet training, and biofeedback therapies in the treatment of pediatric encopresis. J Pediatr Psychol 1996;21(5):659-70.

[31] Gomez-Suarez RA, Gomez-Mendez M, Petty JK, Fortunato JE. Associated factors for antegrade continence enemas for refractory constipation and fecal incontinence. J Pediatr Gastroenterol Nutr 2016;63(4):e63-8.

[32] Lu PL, Koppen IJN, Orsagh-Yentis DK, Leonhart K, Ambeba EJ, Deans KJ, et al. Sacral nerve stimulation for constipation and fecal incontinence in children: Long-term outcomes, patient benefit, and parent satisfaction. Neurogastroenterol Motil 2018;30(2). doi: 10.1111/nmo.13184.

[33] Dos Santos J, Marcon E, Pokarowski M, Vali R, Raveendran L, O'Kelly F, et al. Assessment of needs in children suffering from refractory non-neurogenic urinary and fecal incontinence and their caregivers' needs and attitudes toward alternative therapies (SNM, TENS). Front Pediatr 2020;8:558.

[34] Ritterband LM, Ardalan K, Thorndike FP, Magee JC, Saylor DK, Cox DJ, et al. Real world use of an Internet intervention for pediatric encopresis. J Med Internet Res 2008; 10(2):e16. doi: 10.2196/jmir.1081.

[35] Ritterband LM, Thorndike FP, Lord HR, Borowitz SM, Walker LS, Ingersoll KS, et al. An RCT of an internet intervention for pediatric encopresis with one-year follow up. Clin Pract Ped Psychol 2013;1(1):68–80.

Section two: Sexuality (editor: Donald E. Greydanus)

Chapter 6

Pediatric and adolescent sexuality: An overview

Donald E. Greydanus[1,*], MD, DrHC(Athens), Cheryl A. Dickson[1,2], MD, MPH and Hatim A. Omar[3], MD

[1]Department of Pediatric and Adolescent Medicine
[2]Health and Community Affairs, Western Michigan University Homer Stryker MD School of Medicine, Kalamazoo, Michigan, United States of America
[3]Section of Adolescent Medicine, Lehigh Valley Reilly Children's Hospital, Allentown, Pennsylvania, Lehigh Valley Health Network, LVPG, Pennsylvania and Department of Medical Education and Department of Pediatrics, University of South Florida Morsani College of Medicine, Tampa, Florida, United States of America

Abstract

Human sexuality is a complex phenomenon involving the interaction of one's biologic sex, core gender identity, and gender role behavior. Successful completion of normal stages of sexuality development is important for children and adolescents to enhance optimal life as an adult. Controversies arise for clinicians as they work with their pediatric patients regarding health care sexuality issues. It is important that clinicians help these patients in an unbiased and neutral manner. As adults, these children and adolescents will function in a number of sexuality roles, whether heterosexual, homosexual, pansexual, or other. This discussion considers many of these complex and critical issues that involve the fascinating development of human sexuality in pediatric patients.

Introduction

Sexuality education is the knowledge that we are all sexual human beings, that our sexuality is part of our lives and can be an enhancement or enrichment of our total personality (1). Sexuality is a complex phenomenon involving interaction between one's a) biologic sex; b) core gender identity (sense of maleness, femaleness, or neither); c) gender role behavior (nonsexual as well as sexual) (see Tables 1 and 2) (1-4). Sexuality is also a basic yet profound recognition that humans need other humans and that this human capacity to give and receive love represents a

[*] ***Correspondence:*** Professor Donald E Greydanus, MD, DrHC(Athens), Founding Chair, Department of Pediatric and Adolescent Medicine, Western Michigan University Homer Stryker M.D. School of Medicine, 1000 Oakland Drive, D48G, Kalamazoo, MI 49008-1284, USA. Email: Donald.greydanus@med.wmich.edu.

In: Behavioral Pediatrics II
Editors: Donald E. Greydanus, Dilip R. Patel, Ahsan Nazeer et al.
ISBN: 979-8-88697-019-7

continuum from birth to death (1, 2, 5, 6). Human sexuality involves the process of the individual at any age interacting with others and how one learns to get others to interact with oneself. As sexuality develops, the success or failure experienced by the child and teenager has much to do with eventual success or failure as an adult.

Table 1. Components of sexuality

Biologic sex: The biologic sex (XX or XY) is determined at conception, but postnatal sex hormones also have influence on the developing fetus. Between the sixth and twelfth fetal week, androgens program the XY fetus to develop biologically, and to some extent, behaviorally into a male. The presence of female hormones along with the absence of a critical level of fetal androgens allows the XX fetus to develop into a normal female. Rare situations involving an excess or deficiency of sex hormones can alter the normal male or female outcome; likewise, chromosomal abnormality can cause intersex conditions. However, in nearly all cases, the XX or XY fetus is normally programmed in a poorly understood manner; and the biologic sex is clearly assigned at birth.
Core gender identity: During early childhood, individuals learn various behaviors associated with masculinity or femininity and then establish what can be called non-sexual gender role behavior. Thus, girls play with dolls and wear dresses; boys do not and normally will not even consider such activities.
Gender role behavior: Gender role behavior from a sexual viewpoint refers to behavior influenced or precipitated by a personal desire for some type of sexual pleasure. This desire for physical sex resulting in orgasm is mainly explored during adolescence and frequently modified during adulthood. However, many experts emphasize that the sexual orientation (heterosexual or homosexual) of an individual develops in childhood by age 6 – 8, and not in adolescence.

Table 2. Definitions of terms in sexuality*

Definitions of Terminology
Anatomic sex Phenotypic appearance (male, female, intersex, includes variations such as the congenital adrenal hyperplasia (adrenogenital syndrome) and the incomplete masculinization syndrome).
Antihomosexualism The pervasive and often institutionalized attitudes denigrating homosexuality. Experienced as self-negating and precipitating significant insecurity, ambivalence, and self-loathing by persons who are homosexually oriented during childhood and adolescent development.
Asexuality The absence of erotic response or motivation.
Biologic sex The biologic sex (XX or XY) is determined at conception, but postnatal sex hormones also have influence on the developing fetus. Between the sixth and twelfth fetal week, androgens program the XY fetus to develop biologically, and to some extent, behaviorally into a male. The presence of female hormones along with the absence of a critical level of fetal androgens allows the XX fetus to develop into a normal female. Rare situations involving an excess or deficiency of sex hormones can alter the normal male or female outcome; likewise, chromosomal abnormality can cause intersex conditions. However, in nearly all cases, the XX or XY fetus is normally programmed in a poorly understood manner; and the biologic sex is clearly assigned at birth.
Bisexuality The capacity to respond to both sexes to a significant but not necessarily equal degree.

Definitions of Terminology
Casual relationship Physical and emotional relationship between two people who may have a sexual relationship or a near-sexual relationship without necessarily demanding or expecting a more formal relationship as a goal. It is different from a one-night stand or more than just casual sex. *Cisgender* Cis; gender identify is the same as the sex assigned at birth; versus transgender *Core gender identity* Self-identification as either male or female typically occurs by age 3 years. *Cross dressing* Dressing in clothing of the opposite sex with the intention of expressing identification with or caricaturing the opposite sex role identity; does not generally involve erotic stimulation. *Friends with benefits (FWB)* Two friends with a very casual dating relationship. The benefits can be really good, long, flirty conversations, make-out sessions, and sex with no other commitments. *Gender role identity* The summation of actions that indicate to self and society the degree to which one is male, female, or ambivalent. It is influenced by familial, cultural, and social role expectations, and includes but is not limited to sexual arousal and response. It may also be referred to as one's "sex role." *Gender role behavior* Gender role behavior from a sexual viewpoint refers to behavior influenced or precipitated by a personal desire for some type of sexual pleasure. This desire for physical sex resulting in orgasm is mainly explored during adolescence and frequently modified during adulthood. However, many experts emphasize that the sexual orientation (heterosexual or homosexual) of an individual develops in childhood by ages 6 – 8, and not in adolescence. *Genetic sex* Chromosomally determined sex (XX, XY, XXY, XYY, XO, others). *Heterosexuality* An erotic preference, including fantasies and experiences, for persons of the opposite sex, with minimal erotic interest in the same sex. *Homosexuality* An erotic preference, including fantasies and experiences, for persons of the same sex, with minimal erotic interest in the opposite sex. *Homophobia* The condition in which those whose love and lust are attached to others of the same sex are dreaded or feared. During early childhood, individuals learn various behaviors associated with masculinity or femininity and then establish what can be called non-sexual gender role behavior. Thus, girls play with dolls and wear dresses; boys do not and normally will not even consider such activities. *Hyposexuality* The paucity of erotic response or motivation. *LGBTQ* Lesbian, Gay, Bisexual, Transgendered, Questioning *LGBTIA+* Lesbian, gay, bisexual, transgender, intersexed, agender, asexual, pansexual, genderqueer, queer, others)

Table 2. (Continued)

Definitions of Terminology
Oral sex Fellatio (stimulating the penis with the lips, tongue, throat, teeth); Cunnilingus (stimulating the clitoris, vulva, labia with the lips, tongue, throat, teeth)
Pansexuality (Omnisexuality) Sexual or romantic attraction not dependent on specific sex or gender of others.
Sex buddy (F... buddy; FB) Sexual partner (male or female) with whom there is no danger of attachment, commitment or other complications. A person with whom you have sexual relations, on the mutual understanding that you both want sex and nothing more.
Sexual (erotic) orientation Defined by one's prevailing, unrepressed sexual longings and fantasies.
Sexual dimorphism The structural, physiologic, and behavioral differences between the sexes.
Transgender (Transsexualism) The expression or belief that one's gender identity does not match one's anatomic sex ("woman trapped in a man's body, or the reverse)
Transvestism Dressing in clothing of the opposite sex, predominantly by males, for the purpose of erotic stimulation.

* Adapted with permission: Greydanus DE, Patel DR, Pratt HD, eds. Behavioral pediatrics, 2nd ed. New York: iUniverse, 2006:331-3.

Adapted with permission: DE Greydanus, DR Patel, HD Pratt, Calles JL Jr, Nazeer J, Merrick J, eds. Behavioral pediatrics, 4th edition. New York: Nova Science, 2015:430-1.

Childhood sexuality is often viewed in terms of how concepts of human sexuality progress throughout stages of childhood – infancy, toddlerhood, preschool period, school age period, and adolescence (see appendix A). A key component to the healthy development of the teenager is how he/she proceeds with the stages of adolescent sexuality. While puberty is the word commonly used to describe the physical changes of adolescence, adolescence should be thought of altogether as a critical period of physical as well as psychosocial and cognitive growth in the progression of childhood to maturation. During the adolescent years, the individual must develop a healthy self-esteem and also sexual comfort – learning to deal with those in his/her "sexual" universe. As one looks at adolescent sexuality, it is important to reflect beyond the traditional research just focusing on consequences of coitus with resultant sexually transmitted diseases (STDs) and adolescent pregnancy. Childhood sexuality leads to adolescent sexuality and this leads to adult sexuality with its complicated aspects involving sexual desire (craving or passion), arousal (excitation, awakening), behaviors and sexual functioning (6).

This discussion considers various aspects of pediatric and adolescent sexuality: psychosocial development, attitudes regarding sexuality with emphasis on masturbation, the role of central nervous system (CNS) maturation, normal adolescent sexuality stages, adolescent coital experiences, modern changes in pediatric sexual developments, adolescent pregnancy, hypersexuality, sexual abuse, dating violence, adolescent sexual offenders, responsible teen sexuality, and perspectives on LGBTIA+ (6). In the summary, it is concluded that appropriate and comprehensive sexuality education should be provided to our children and adolescents to prepare them for life as sexual human beings in the 21st century.

Psychosexual development

The process of sexuality development begins at birth and perhaps during the process of gestation. At age 8-10 months, infants become aware of their genitalia (penis or vagina) and by the age of three, they usually have developed a fixed gender identity. By the time of their fourth birthday, the majority perceive themselves as being either boys or girls for life. The psychoanalytic view of adolescent sexual development by Sigmund Freud (1856-1939) offers health care professionals a framework for assessing adolescent sexuality and reflects some of the major importance of Freud's development of the major concept of psychoanalysis (6-8).

Freud contended that adults develop as sexual beings from birth through adulthood (see Table 3) (9). Though various scholars disagree on the exact meaning of these stages, there is agreement that by the time a child enters puberty, he/she should have developed a healthy self-image, a sense of security, a willingness to trust others, and a conscience with a normal sense of right versus wrong. It is the parents that must first accept their children's gender and then communicate to them that they are intact, beautiful, and normal. If this is not the case, major problems in adolescence and adulthood are likely to unfold.

Table 3. Freud's psychosexual states of development

1. Oral: Feeding; pleasure derived through the mouth; ages birth-1½ years; security and optimism develop, while conflicts at this stage may lead to distrust of one's environment and a sense of generalized hostility.
2. Anal: Toilet training and control over self and environment through elimination functions; ages 1-6 years.
3. Phallic phase: Discovery of genitals, pleasure derived through the genitals. Boys experience castration anxiety, fearing genital damage or loss. Oedipus Complex in males as a result of competitive feelings with the father is resolved when the boy develops normal identification with the father. Girls develop penis envy—similar concept for girls is called Electra Complex. This stage is considered ended when temporary resolution of the Complex occurs; ages 3-6 years.
NOTE: Freud's controversial theories of psychosocial development provide a framework for understanding human psychopathology as a failure to resolve the Oedipus or Electra Complex.
4. Latency phase: Child expands intellectual and social skills while repressing childhood sexuality development. End of this stage signaled by the onset of puberty; ages 6 to 9 years.
5. Genital phase: Oedipus or Electra Complex is once again raised; the development of normal sexual health dictates successful resolution of this complex. Healthy adult sexuality begins to occur with puberty; ages 6-15 years.

A review of normal childhood behavior reveals that physiologic components to sexuality are evident at an early age (see Tables 1, 2 and appendix A). During the first year of life (infancy), exploration is through mouthing and sucking while trust in the caretaker (especially the mother) develops; aggression may develop in the form of biting. Infants learn to be sexual by touching and being touched; how they are held, soothed, and nurtured impacts their emerging sexuality and sets the stage for their sexuality throughout life. Sexual exploration may involve the skin as an erotic organ and some genital touching. Male erections are noted even in utero; orgasm as a neurophysiological phenomenon can occur as early as the fourth month of life and is common in males 6 to 8 years of age. Female newborns often have leukorrhea or vaginal discharge as a result of maternal hormones suddenly cut off during the process of birth.

During the toddler period (ages 2-3 years), children develop mobility and language skills; the process of autonomy is noted and parents learn to deal with the word "no!" The toddler also learns what boys and girls do, how sex roles are different, and the names of body parts. Masturbation or self-genital manipulation for pleasure is very common between ages 2-6 years. Children during the pre-school period (ages 3-5 years) continue with an interest in masturbation, but also learn more of the differences in males versus females. During this process, a natural curiosity develops about sex play experimentation and exhibitionism. Primary care clinicians and other caring for pediatric patients must learn to distinguish between experimentation and sexual exploitation (6, 10-13). The reaction of parents to their child's growing interest in sexuality sets the tone for the incorporation of human sexuality into the child's sense of self-esteem.

Children first learn about their personal boundaries from their parents (e.g., that not all exploratory behaviors are appropriate in every place and time); thus, trusting relationships and open communication between parent and child are very significant. Parents should also communicate the rights for privacy and hygiene, as well as the necessity to share fears and concerns with trusted adults (e.g., nobody is to touch their body inappropriately or have them keep secrets from either parent). The establishment of core gender identity develops as the child enters the school-age period (5 years of age to the beginning of puberty). The latency age child has same-sex friends and sexuality is often expressed with an intense interest in prurient or salacious stories, jokes, riddles, and songs; interest in masturbation may recede until puberty develops. However, latency stage children are naturally curious about the anatomy of the opposite sex.

These are normal developmental phenomena, and parental attitudes are a major influence on attitudes that children develop about sexual behavior and feelings. As noted by Mary Calderone (1904-1998) (1):

> Whatever happens, it is clear that by the time the child arrives at school, it has already received, for good or ill, the most profound as well as the most unchangeable sex education it will ever receive in its life.

If a parent finds a 4-year-old masturbating and aggressively reacts to inform the child it is "unclean" and not "respectable," the child clearly learns to associate normal sexuality with negativism – a lesson carried throughout his/her life. If the natural curiosity of the latency age child is totally repressed, the child receives the wrong message about human sexuality.

Misinformation on the part of parents and failure to teach the child normal sexual concepts result in numerous psychosexual difficulties in adolescence and adulthood. It is curious to see 5-year-olds who can name the most common body parts, but not their own genitals. It is even more curious to see health care professionals contribute to this by not exploring such ideas with parents and by not even including the genitals as part of the normal physical examination. Health care professionals must teach normal concepts of human sexuality and encourage parents to do so also. Proper naming of their infant's genitalia (e.g., vagina or penis) is a step towards this goal. Other groups, such as religious and educational institutions, profoundly affect children and must actively join parents in the area of appropriate sexuality education of children and adolescents.

As the grade school child transitions into adolescence, their interests and actions regarding their sexuality expands. The manner in which the adolescent deals with his/her/their sexuality is far more influenced by what he/she/they experienced as a child at home, viewing and interacting with parents, rather than from what they may learn during adolescence. Unfortunately, the negative mixed messages they receive about human sexuality contribute to the many sexuality-related problems seen in many youth and adults: a) depression, b) serious rebellion against society, c) sexually transmitted diseases/infections (STDs/STIs), d) unwanted pregnancy, e) incest, f) runaway behavior, g) adolescent prostitution, h) marital dysfunction, and i) sexual dysfunction (1-4). It is important to remember that sexuality is simply a very important, normal, and crucial part of life and that failure to deal with its normal concepts contributes to the development of major problems in adolescence and adulthood.

Attitudes and sexuality: Masturbation

An excellent example of the potential detrimental effect that negative societal attitudes can have on sexuality is offered by looking at historical views on masturbation (1, 6, 14). For countless centuries, this persistent aspect of sexuality has been condemned as sinful and/or harmful to human health. Some incorrectly attributed this conclusion to Genesis 38:9 (*Pentateuch; Old Testament*), when Onan was condemned for not impregnating his brother's wife after the brother died. This was actually part of the *Levirate Marriage Concept* that was intended to assure survival of human civilization at a time of very high infant mortality rates and relatively short human life spans. Onan performed coitus interruptus, but his action was incorrectly called masturbation or onanism by later generations. Galen of Pergamum (129-200/217 AD), the famous Roman physician, wrote that masturbation was a very harmful habit and when encountering a male who engaged in this practice, he warned:

> Watch carefully over this young man, leave him alone neither day nor night; at least sleep in his chamber. When he has contracted this fatal habit (masturbation), the most fatal to which a young man can be subject, he will carry its painful effects to the tomb – his mind and body will always be enervated. (1, 8)

In 1716, Bekker wrote a book called "Onania. The heinous sin of self population", which strongly advocated the view that masturbation was immoral and caused many health problems. In 1766, an influential Swiss physician, Samuel Auguste Tissot (1728-1797), wrote what was to become a well-known book called "A treatise on the diseases produced by onanism" (15). His book offered this same thesis and such a conclusion, became the dominant medical view for the next 150 years or more; it was taught in medical schools that most of human medical and mental illnesses were the result of masturbation.

Various treatments were devised to stop masturbation including prayer, diverse dermatological agents, opium, diet, genital cautery, electrodesiccation of rectum or genitals, devices to prevent penile tumescence (including the spermatorrhea ring with spikes in its middle), circumcision, clitorectomy, castration and others. From 1890 to 1925 there was an

American group of surgeons (called the *Orificial Surgery Society*) who taught and practiced genital surgery as treatment measures for masturbation. The roots of such ideas are deeply imbedded in religious bias and fear that masturbation injures sperm – thus possibly interfering with the survival of civilization.

A gradual change in such attitudes was observed in the past century. During the early part of the 20th century, authors stressed that masturbation as such may not be harmful, but guilt over such worry certainly can be injurious to mental health. By the middle of the 20th century, many physicians accepted this concept and numerous researchers began to study masturbation as a very common aspect of normal human sexuality. It was noticed that genital self-stimulation for pleasure is practiced by most adults in some manner or other without deleterious effects on human physiology.

Pediatricians now teach that "excessive" masturbation in infants may result from such problems as pinworm infestation, diaper dermatitis, tight clothes, non-specific genital pruritus, phimosis, and other medical conditions. Sigmund Freud's view that masturbation drained energy from children is not accepted now. However, it is known that certain masturbation variations can be harmful; an example is the adolescent sexual asphyxia syndrome – in which the young person attempts to partially hang himself/herself by the neck ("partial hanging"), while masturbating in order to achieve an orgasm (16).

Current teaching among academic medical or psychological groups is that masturbation is not harmful by itself and can be useful as part of a therapeutic approach to correct various sexual dysfunctions (17, 18). Some youth, encouraged by their "peer" journals, are encouraged to masturbate in order to relieve sexual tension. However, there still exists considerable worry by parents about the "perceived" effects of masturbation on their children. Thus, anxiety about masturbation and other important aspects of human sexuality remains today, especially because comprehensive sexuality education is rarely granted to children and youth in the United States – despite its positive effects on youth (19-25).

Young children reflect this ignorance and uneasiness about their own sexuality with resultant negative effects. As parents have the greatest influence on sexual decision-making of youth, a partial solution for this complex issue is to encourage them to acquire a broad knowledge of human sexuality, which is consistent with their own moral philosophy as well as culture, and then to share this with their offspring. Health care professionals can assist in this goal as well due to close interactions with children and youth (6, 26, 27).

The role of CNS maturation

Prior to discussing puberty, this discussion considers the role of central nervous system (CNS) maturation in this process of ascension from childhood to adolescence and adulthood. Brain cells consist of neurons and glia; the latter support, nourish, and clean the neurons in addition to dynamic roles of modulating metabolic features of neurons and being alert to metabolic alterations (28, 29). After the billions of central nervous system (CNS) cells are developed by late fetal life, CNS pruning and differentiation occurs in an aggressive fashion in the young child and young adolescent (30, 31). While approximately three-fourths of the brain growth in weight occurs by age 2 years, CNS maturation continues throughout childhood and adolescence. One process this occurs through is axon myelination, a process aimed at increasing the efficiency and speed of nerve conduction (32). The ability of CNS cells to adapt to challenges is called plasticity; another process of CNS maturation is the pruning or sculpting of these cells starting in late fetal life with acceleration in the young child and young adolescent (32-37).

The excessive number of CNS cells that develops in fetal life is reduced by the process of apoptosis (programmed cell death) in which cells are destroyed and in contrast to necrosis or uncontrolled cell death as well as effects on various systems including those in gynecology (38, 39). As the hormones of puberty are increasing, apoptosis accelerates leading to massive death of neurons and the removal of half of the exuberant cortical synaptic connections. This pruning allows for the refinement of the particular balance of excitatory and inhibitory neurons in the prefrontal cortex (an area of higher order cognitive function) which is crucial for the normal development of adult executive function (40). Puberty is a very significant neurobiological event that has profound effects on the growth and development of the adolescent. This process, also discussed elsewhere in this symposium, is briefly considered now.

Puberty

The hallmark of adolescence is the process of puberty (see Table 4), a profound neurobiological/psychological event in the life of each child that prepares the way for eventual adulthood (6, 32, 41-45). The exact trigger for puberty is not yet clear, but it involves central nervous system (CNS) maturation with reduced hypothalamic sensitivity to gonadal steroids by changes in the GnRH pulse generator; there is also adrenal gland maturation (42). The progression (see Table 5) through puberty is predictable, but there is considerable variation in its onset, timing, tempo, and magnitude of changes (see Table 6). There are five stages of pubertal development due to hypothalamic-pituitary-gonadal maturation, called Sexual Maturity Ratings (SMR) or Tanner Stages (see Tables 7 and 8) (6, 46-48).

Eventually there is a rise in gonadotropins (follicle stimulating hormone [FSH], luteinizing hormone [LH]), sex hormones (i.e., estrogen, testosterone), adrenal gland steroids, growth hormone, insulin-like growth factors (IGFs or somatomedins) and other hormones. Thelarche (breast budding or SMR 2) is the first clinical evidence of puberty in females, developing between 6 and 13 years of age, typically between 10 and 12 years of age. A decreased mean of nearly 3 months per decade in thelarche has been observed from 1977 to 2013 with various implications, including the exact definition of precocious puberty in some areas of the globe (49).

Table 4. Major physical changes of puberty

Major increase in genital system (primary and secondary sex characteristics)
Gaining of 25% of final height (distal growth, e.g., of feet, may precede that of proximal parts, e.g., the tibia, by 3 to 4 months)
Doubling of lean and nonlean body mass (gaining by 50% of the ideal body weight)
Doubling of the weight of the major organs
Central nervous system maturation (without increase in size)
Maturation of facial bones
Marked decrease in lymphoid tissue

Table 5. The sequential changes of puberty

Adolescent female [a]
Breast bud (thelarche)
Pubic hair development (pubarche)
Height velocity peak
Menarche (onset of menstruation)
Axillary hair
Final pubertal changes, e.g., full breast, pubic hair, and completed height development
Adolescent male [a]
Early testicular growth
Pubarche
Testicular and penile growth
Nocturnal emissions
Height velocity peak
Marked voice changes
Facial hair growth and final pubertal changes, e.g., full genital, height, and muscle development

[a] Normally over a 2 to 4 year period.

Reprinted with permission: Greydanus DE, Patel DR, Pratt HD, eds. Behavioral pediatrics, 2nd ed. New York: iUniverse, 2006:331-3.

Table 6. Variations in pubertal changes

Pubertal changes	**Age Range of Appearance (yrs)**
Thelarche	6-15
Pubarche	9-14
Menarche	10-17
Testicular enlargement	9-15
Peak height velocity (male)	10-17
Peak height velocity (female)	10-14
Adult breast stage (V)	12-19
Adult genitalia (male V)	13-18

Table 7. Sexual maturity rating or Tanner staging in females

Stage	**Breasts**	**Pubic hair**	**Range**
I	None	None	Birth to 15 yr
II[a]	Breast bud (thelarche): areolar hyperplasia with small amount of breast tissue	Long downy pubic hair near the labia; may occur with breast budding or several weeks to months later (pubarche)	6 to 15 yr
III[b]	Further enlargement of breast tissue and areola	Increase in amount of hair with more pigmentation	10 to 15 yr
IV[c]	Double contour form: areola and nipple form secondary mound on top of breast tissue	Adult type but not distribution	10 to 17 yr
V[d]	Larger breast with single contour form	Adult distribution	12 ½ to 18 yr

Reprinted with permission: Greydanus DE, Patel DR, Pratt HD, eds. Behavioral pediatrics, 2nd ed. New York: iUniverse, 2006:306.

[a] Peak height velocity often occurs soon after stage II.

[b] 25% develop menarche in late III.

[c] Most develop menarche in stage IV 1 to 3 yr after thelarche.

[d] 10% develop menarche in stage V.

Table 8. Sexual maturity rating or Tanner staging in males

Stage	Testes	Penis	Pubic hair	Range
I	No change, testes 2.5 cm or less	Prepubertal	None	Birth to 15 yr
II	Enlargement of testes, increased stippling and pigmentation of scrotal sac	Minimal or no enlargement	Long downy hair often occurring several months after testicular growth; variable pattern noted with pubarche	10 to 15 yr
III[a]	Further enlargement	Significant penile enlargement, especially in length	Increase in amount, now curling	10 ½ to 16 ½ yr
IV[b]	Further enlargement	Further enlargement, especially in diameter	Adult type but not distribution	Variable; 12 to 17 yr
V[c]	Adult size	Adult size	Adult distribution (medial aspects of thighs, linea alba)	13 to 18 yr

Reprinted with permission: Greydanus DE, Patel DR, Pratt HD, eds. Behavioral pediatrics, 2nd ed. New York: iUniverse, 2006:307.

[a] Peak height spurt usually between III and IV.

[b] Axillary hair develops, as well as some facial hair.

[c] 20% have peak height velocity now. Body hair and increase in musculature, others, continues for several months to years.

Menarche (onset of menstruation) usually follows in 1 to 3 years in SMR 4, often between 12 and 13 years of age (range of 10 -17 years). Research has suggested that the increased percent of breast density in young females may be associated with increased time in months from thelarche to menarche (called a slower pubertal tempo) that may increase risks for breast cancer in later life (50).

The first clinical event of puberty (SMR 2) in the male is enlarged testicles (over 3 mL or 2.5 cm in diameter) and scrotal thinning; ejaculation is seen at SMR 3 and fertility at SMR 4 (46-48). The growth spurt results in the final 25% of the adult height and is an early pubertal event in females (SMR 2) often at age 11.5 years and a late pubertal event in males (SMR-4), typically at age 13.5 years of age - the average growth spurt lasts 24 to 36 months. Those who have early (precocious) or late (delayed) puberty can have considerable psychosocial consequences that include mood issues, behavior dysfunction, weight problems and other repercussions (51). For example, the female and male who develop much earlier than peers may be subjected to sexual behavior (including adolescent dating abuse) much earlier than peers who develop puberty over a normal chronological period (52).

Puberty stimulates more interest in sexuality in the growing and rapidly changing adolescent. Young teen males may be concerned about spontaneous erections, nocturnal emissions, and same-sex sexual experimentations. Males may also be concerned about the development of gynecomastia otherwise known as the usually transient development of breasts noted in as many as two-thirds of SMR 2-3 males (53-55). Though usually resolved in 12 to 18 months, gynecomastia may cause confusion about male identity and intense anxiety while undressing in front of peers in physical education classes.

Reassurance from the trusted clinician about the benign nature of this phenomenon is very helpful to the male. Though typically temporary, release from situations of being undressed in front of peers may be necessary to alleviate anxiety associated with transient male breast enlargement; surgery may also be necessary in some situations of persistent gynecomastia, large breasts, or severe psychosocial stress (54, 55). Education about important aspects of puberty is an important and needed task for primary care clinicians (43).

Females may be worried about vaginal discharge (estrogen-stimulated "physiologic leukorrhea"), nocturnal sexually oriented sex dreams, homosexual interests (including sexual experimentation) and pressure from peers as well as society to be sexually active (also seen in the male as well). Both males and females may be concerned with the effects of acne vulgaris, body odor, seborrheic dermatitis, and other dermatologic effects of puberty. Crushes on non-parent figures are common in both sexes, and include interest in teachers, youth leaders, coaches, and others. If adults misinterpret these "crushes," sexual abuse may result with severe negative consequences for this adolescent. The influence of parents' reactions to these changes, the youth's emerging sexuality and that of the family's religious beliefs have profound effects on how adolescents deal with these emerging concepts of human sexuality (56-58).

Normal adolescent sexuality stages

Adolescent psychosocial and cognitive development is traditionally divided in three classic periods: early, middle, and late adolescence (see Table 9) (2, 6, 14). Complications of self- and/or family-isolation due to societal stresses, such as the 2020-2022 COVID-19 pandemic, remain to be identified by research studies.

Early Adolescence

The young adolescent resumes previously acquired interest in the development of interpersonal relationships. Typically, the youth approaches this from a narcissistic viewpoint in which the individual's interest comes first and concerns of others are not considered. This "selfish" attitude starts with those of the same sex and extends to those of the opposite sex during mid-adolescence. First, there is exploration of one's own body linked with concerns of normality; then comes the comparison with peers of the same gender. When interest towards the opposite sex finally occurs, it is basically platonic during early adolescence and it is gradually expressed through sexual experimentation during middle adolescence. In both early and middle adolescence, crushes on and friendships with peers as well as others can be dramatic and influential in overall stability in adolescence and adulthood (59-61).

Considerable energy is spent acquiring social skills and friendships with same-sex individuals. Thus, boys tend to develop "gangs" of males who engage in various behaviors, as each member tests the others in diverse aspects of adolescence. Definitions of masculinity are tested and confirmed within such groups. Homosexual experimentation and considerable false braggadocio about sexuality are quite common.

Girls tend to associate with a few very close girlfriends and then, to a lesser extent, deal with a larger group of females. The extent of female masturbation and homosexual experiences is unknown. This early adolescent phase of development has been referred to as the homosexual phase and is considered normal. Also, classic Freudian theory teaches that early adolescence is the time for reemergence of the Oedipus complex and, if normal sexual health is to occur, it must be finally resolved (see Table 3) (1, 9).

Table 9. Adolescent psychosocial development

	Early adolescence (11-14 yr)	**Middle adolescence (15-17 yr)**	**Late adolescence (18-25 yr)**
Cognitive thinking	Concrete thinking: here and now. Appreciate immediate reactions to behavior but no sense of later consequences	Early abstract thinking: Inductive/deductive reasoning. Able to connect separate events, understand later consequences. Very self-absorbed, introspective, lots of daydreaming and rich fantasies	Abstract Thinking: Adult ability to think abstractly. Philosophical. Intense idealism about love, religion, social problems
Task areas			
1. Family –Independence	– Transition from obedient to rebellious – Rejection of parental guidelines – Ambivalence about wishes (dependence/independence) – Underlying need to please adults – Hero worship (“crushes”)	– Insistence on independence, privacy – May have overt rebellion or sulky withdrawal – Much testing of limits – Roleplaying of adult roles (but not felt to be “real” – easily abandoned)	– Emancipation (leave home) – Reestablishment of family ties – Assume true adult roles with commitment
2. Peers – social/sexual	– Same-sex “best friend” – “Am I normal?” concerns – Giggling boy-girl fantasies – Sexual experimentation not normal at this age.– counteract fears of worthlessness – Obtain “friends” – Humiliate parents	– Dating, intense interest in “boys” – Sexual experimentation begins – Risk-taking actions – Unrealistic concept of partner’s role – Need to please significant peers (of either sex)	– Partner selection – Realistic concept of partner’s role – Mature friendships – True intimacy possible only after own identity is established – Need to please self too (“enlightened self-interest”)
3. School – Vocation	– Still in a structured school setting – Goals unrealistic, changing – Want to copy favorite role models	– More class choices in school setting – Beginning to identify skills, interests – Start part-time jobs – Begin to react to system’s expectations: may decide to beat the establishment at its own game (super achievers) or to reject the game (dropouts)	– Full-time work or college – Identify realistic career goals – Watch for apathy (no future plans) or alienation, since lack of goal-orientation is correlated with unplanned pregnancy, juvenile crime, etc.
4. Self-perception	– Incapable of self-awareness while still concrete thinkers	– Confusion about self-image	– Realistic, positive self-image
Identity	– Losing child’s role but do not have adult role, hence low self-esteem	– Seek group identity – Very narcissistic	– Able to consider others’ needs, less narcissistic
Social Responsibility	– Tend to use denial (it can’t happen to me)	– Impulsive, impatient	– Able to reject group pressure if not in self-interest

Table 9. (Continued)

	Early adolescence (11-14 yr)	**Middle adolescence (15-17 yr)**	**Late adolescence (18-25 yr)**
Values	– Stage II values (back-scratching) (good behavior in exchange for rewards)	– Stage III values (conformity) (behavior that peer group values)	– Stage IV values (social responsibility) (behavior consistent with laws and duty)
Chief health issues (other than acute illness)	– Psychosomatic symptoms – Fatigue and "growing pains" – Concerns about normalcy – Screening for growth and development problems	– Outcomes of sexual experimentation – Prevention of pregnancy, STD – HIV/AIDs – Health-risk behaviors (drugs, alcohol, driving) – Crisis counseling (run-aways, acting-out, family, etc.)	– Health promotion/healthy lifestyles – Contraception and STD – HIV/AIDs prevention – Self-responsibility for health and health care
Professional approach To retain sanity, you and your staff should: -Like teenagers -Understand development -Be flexible -Be patient	– Firm, direct support – Convey limits-simple, concrete choices – Do not align with parents, but do be an objective caring adult – Encourage transference (heroworship) – Sexual decisions-directly encourage to wait, to say "NO" – Encourage parental presence in clinic, but interview teen alone	– Be an objective sounding board (but let them solve own problems) – Negotiate choices – Be a role model – Don't get too much history ("grandiose stories") – Confront (gently) about consequences, responsibilities – Consider: what will give them status in eyes of peers? – Use peer-group sessions – Adapt system to crises, walk-ins, impulsiveness, "testing" – Ensure confidentiality – Allow teens to seek care independently	– Allow mature participation in decisions – Act as a resource – Idealistic stage, so convey "professional" image – Can expect patient to examine underlying wishes, motives (e.g., pregnancy wish if poor compliance with contraception) – Older adolescents able to adapt to policies/needs of clinic system

Reproduced with permission from Dr. Roberta K. Beach, MD, Emeritus Director, of Adolescent Ambulatory Services, Denver Department of Health and Hospitals, Denver, CO.
Reprinted with permission: Greydanus DE, Patel DR, Pratt HD, eds. Behavioral pediatrics, 2nd ed. New York: iUniverse, 2006:308-10.

Middle adolescence

Middle adolescence is traditionally called the heterosexual stage, as youth acquire diverse experiences with the opposite sex (even those who may later identify as homosexual [gay, lesbian, bisexual, pansexual, transgender, other]); these experiences can be quite short (even one or two days) and intensive (see Table 9). This mainly occurs during this "selfish" period as a result of partner idealization which is followed by disappointment and moving on to the next partner (e.g., serial monogamy phenomenon). During middle adolescence – depending on the youth's self-image, opportunity, and parental influence – there is a normal sequencing of this heterosexual development with a long historical influence of serial monogamy in *Homo sapiens* (62).

It begins with interest in the opposite gender, and is followed by group dating, individual dating, and eventually sexual intimacy. Such intimacy runs an individual course including hand-holding, superficial versus "serious" kissing, petting, oral sex, anal sex, and/or vaginal coitus. This relationship is also described as narcissistic (generated from self-interest) and deeply embedded in resolution of the Oedipus or Electra complex (see Table 3) (63-67).

Late adolescence

Late adolescence is normally the time to begin consideration of available adult lifestyles. The ability of having functional non-selfish relationships finally develops and stability in adulthood in various areas has links to developments in early to late adolescence (see Table 9) (68-70).

Adolescent coital experience

Sexual behavior of *Homo sapiens* has been studied over the eons of human history (6, 71). Over the decades there have been changes in the adolescent coital experience resulting in an earlier age onset of first intercourse as time progresses. Alfred C Kinsey (1894-1956) published his ground-breaking, controversial reports on sexual behavior in the male (1948) and female (1953); he reported that 20% of American females aged 16-20 years were coitally experienced (72, 73). The search was on for understanding sexual behavior of humans, including adolescents.

Kantner and Zelnik published several well-known survey reports in the 1970s; they noted that 30% of females 15-19 years were coitally experienced in 1971, 43% in 1976 and 50% in 1979; males aged 17-21 years were at 70% (74). The average age of sexarche was 16.2 years for females and 15.7 for males (75). The average age of sexual "debut" (first sexual intercourse; sexarche) is approximately the same (16 years) in Canada and Western (United Kingdom, France) and Eastern Europe (Ukraine, Russia) (76). Early age at first intercourse can be influenced by many factors, such as socio-economical that involves such issues as personal or family income or level of education (77).

By the mid-1990s, surveys showed 66% of females and 70% of males had coitus before their 18th birthday; 9% of 12 year olds and 38% of 14 year olds were sexually active—this increased to 47% by age 16 and 68% by age 18 years (75, 76). This data also noted that 13%

of those 14-17 years of age and 41% of those 18-21 years of age had 4 or more sexual partners; 79% of African Americans were sexually active vs. 48% of Caucasians, and 56% of Hispanic students (75, 78).

The 1999 U.S. Centers for Disease Control (CDC) Youth Risk Behavior Surveillance (YRBS) noted that 49.9% of high school students (12-18 years of age) were coitally experienced; this was broken down as 45.1% for Caucasians, 54.1% for Hispanics, and 71.2% for African Americans (79). Also, 8% were coitally active before age 13 (12.2% for males, 4.4% for females) and 16% had 4 or more partners (19.3% in males and 13.1% in females). Adolescents are noted to practice serial monogamy, having one partner at a time, though often for a short time. Studies noted that 31% of sexually active female adolescents reported two to three sex partners, 9% had four or five partners, and 10% reported over five sex partners (79).

Data from the 2002 National Survey of Family Growth notes that 47% of never-married female youth (ages 15-19 years of age-4.6 million) have had coitus and 46% of never-married male youth (ages 15-19 years-4.7 million) ever had coitus (80). Among sexually active females in the 2002 survey, 83% said they used contraception the last time having sex, in contrast with 71% in 1995 (80). The 2017 YRBSS reported that youth ever having sex dropped from 48% in 2007 to 40% in 2017 while the contrast for those noting four or more sexual partners was 15% in 2007 versus 10% in 2017 (81). This data shows that as time progressed from the last decades of the 20th century to the first two decades of the 21st century, there had been an improvement in rates of contraception use perhaps due to increased education and availability of contraception.

Concepts of chronic illness and disability

Adolescents with chronic illnesses and deformities (i.e., cerebral palsy, spina bifida, others) are also invested in the development of their sexuality, even if society and parents are not focused on these issues (6, 82-91). Growing youth worry over their changing bodies, and disabled adolescents need to learn to accept actual abnormalities and tolerate deviations from an idealized body image.

Table 10. Psychosexual development problems in youth with chronic illness/deformities

Concerns about ability to reproduce and parent
Difficulties finding peer friends
Doubts about future self-sufficiency
Increased risk for abuse (physical and sexual)
Increased risk for bulling and harassment
Limited social skills
Poor body image
Reduced self-esteem

Table 10 lists potential complications in the psychosexual development of youth with chronic deformities/illnesses. For example, youth with colostomies become anxious about being accepted because of odor, while those with arthritis become concerned about problems with pain as well as limitations. Some chronically ill teens are stimulated to coital activity to prove normalcy, while others are slow to develop healthy sexuality; the clinician can be of considerable help to both groups to encourage normal sexual development. Parents and clinicians should seek to help adolescent females develop a positive self-esteem and body image despite impaired fertility noted with various genetic and endocrine disorders (6, 92, 93).

Second decade of the 21st century

Based off of US Centers for Disease and Prevention (CDC) data from 2011-2015, it is noted that 42.4% of teenage females and 44.2% of teenage males have had sex at least once which is consistent with the 2002 survey (94). This indicates that overall rates of adolescent coital experiences have remained relatively stable over 10 years. However, this is a dynamic and ever-changing process; for example, it was noted that the demographics changed with a decrease in rates of non-Hispanic black female teenagers and an increase in rates of non-Hispanic white males (94). Youth risk behavior surveillance system (YRBSS) data from 2017 notes that 39.5% of high school students ever had coital experience, 9.7% had four or more sexual partners, and condom use during last coital experience was limited—53.8% (81). Rates of sexual behavior in males under age 13 can vary based on multiple factors race/ethnicity, maternal level of education, living location and others (95). Research also notes that teen pregnancy and sexually transmitted diseases are well-known consequences of teen sexual behavior (6, 96-98).

Modern changes in pediatric sexual developments

In the 21st century, pediatric sexuality develops in a society characterized by a rapidly changing environment, intense migration, and expanding opportunities to communicate with others through a global online network that has become a widely used resource for sexual health information among adolescents around the world (99-103). Major problems for childhood and adolescent sexuality that are emerging in today's global society including a progression from previous expectations of heterosexual relationships as the norm to acceptance of LGBTQIA+ relationships (lesbian, gay, bisexual, pansexual, transgender, genderqueer, queer, intersexed, agender, asexual and others), the development of casual relationships, and changes in what is termed the love ideology (104-109). The love ideology notes that following the sexual revolution of the 1960's, the concepts of marriage and sex have been increasingly separated as pre-marital sex has become increasingly accepted.

There is a noticeable cultural difference in the acceptance of and breadth of the casual relationships in youth. Examples of visible changes in the love ideology among young people throughout the world include the increase in the number of sexual partners, a rise in casual sex episodes, more openness to group sex relationships, and open discussion among youth as well as popularity of such relationships as a sex buddy (f*** buddy or FB), friends with benefits (FWB), and sexualized friendships (see Table 2) (110-112).

There is enormous influence from the mass media on adolescents around the world in which sex is often presented as a casual pastime that is normative behavior without negative consequences (113-115). The media (television, movies) presents the message that "everyone is doing it and having fun." Some youth view oral sex as not "real sex" and use it to maintain a state of "technical" virginity, not realizing that sexually transmitted diseases are acquired with this form of sexual behavior including gonorrhea, syphilis, herpes, human papillomavirus (HPV) infection and AIDS/HIV (116). One study of 9th graders in San Francisco noted that nearly 30% were engaged in oral sex and 13.5% intended to have oral sex in the next six months (117); another study of 10th graders in New England noted that nearly 48% of the males and 42% of the girls reported experience with oral sex (118).

Adolescent pregnancy

Approximately 750,000 adolescent pregnancies occur each year in the United States; delivery of a live baby occurs in 51%, while 35% end in abortion (400,000) and 14% in a miscarriage (6, 119). Birth rates for American females aged 15-19 years of age dropped from 66/1000 in 1970 to 43.0 in 2002; studies note a 21st century decrease in adolescent pregnancy and adolescent birth rates that includes a 57% decline of birth rates from 2000 to 2016 for females 15- to 19-year-old (80, 81, 118-126). US teen birth rates had a low of 22.3 per 1000 15–19-year-old females in 2015 and in 2017---18.8 births per 1,000 15–19-year-old females (194,377 babies) (80, 81, 119-121). Ethnic variations in teen pregnancy are considered elsewhere is this overall publication (122, 123).

Issues involved in teen pregnancy declines include a change in behavior of sexually active youth, increase in use of contraception by sexually active teens, and the availability of more effective contraceptive methods (127-135). A number of contraceptive methods, as considered elsewhere, have become available over the past few decades that allow effective contraception without the need for consumption of a daily pill or use of a patch; these include long-acting reversible contraceptive (LARC) methods (133).

Various factors increase the risk of teen pregnancy; these include teen pregnancies that may develop within 6 months of sexarche (coital initiation) along with effects of early puberty, early sexual behavior, sexual abuse (i.e., incest, child abuse), compulsive adolescent sexual behavior, teen sexting, illicit substance use, limited school performance with school dropout, limited career goals, poverty, parental neglect and other factors (2, 81, 95, 136-146).

The negative psychosocial risks to the adolescent mother and offspring are well described in the literature (6, 124-126, 136). Marriage is often not seen as a consequence of adolescent pregnancy in contemporary American society; 11% of teens are married before age 18 and percentage of teen births taking place out of marriage has risen from 15% in 1960 to 80% in 1999 (47). The divorce rate among adults is 50% and 70% among teens (68).

Hypersexuality

The term, hypersexuality, has been used in various ways to refer to adolescent sexual behavior. However, it should be used to refer to inappropriate or ill-regulated behavior and can be a cause of disruption among children as well as adolescents who are hospitalized for psychiatric disorders. It refers to "inappropriate" sexual behavior that involves sexual fantasies that increase abruptly in frequency and become of sufficient severity to disrupt expected or usual functioning. Though not a common cause of hypersexuality, virilization should be considered in its differential diagnosis (147). Hypersexuality can also be seen in the overall context of compulsive sexual behavior (148).

Sexual abuse

Although most data on sexual abuse is focused on females, recent research is acknowledging that males are also sexually abused. Surveys of adults note 27% of adult females were sexually abused, with a peak at 16-19 years of age and 25% of college females report sexual assault at some point in their lives (6, 78, 149, 150). The child and adolescent must survive in a world with many dangers of unwanted sexual and physical abuse (see chapter on child abuse). There are three million reported annual cases of abuse in those under 18 years in the United States; these are classified as neglect (53%), physical abuse (26%), sexual abuse (14%), and emotional abuse (5%) (151). The abuse is more commonly from known close family/personal contacts (such as father, step-father, uncle, teachers, boyfriends) rather than complete strangers as was previously believed, except in 10% to 33% of the cases (152). Finkelhor noted that 5 of every 1,000 college female reported being victims of incest from their fathers (153). Pregnancy and sexually transmitted diseases (STDs) may be signs of sexual abuse in young teens (138-142).

Between 50,000 and 70,000 cases of rape are reported each year, while the estimated number of actual cases exceeds 400,000 to 700,000 each year (47, 154). Adolescents have the highest rates of rape and other sexual assaults (152). The United States Department of Justice notes there are 3.5 assaults per 1,000 ages 12-15 years, 5.0 for 16-19 years, 4.6 for those 20-24, and 1.7 for those 24-29 years; half of these rapes and other sexual assaults are to those under age 25 and the female-male ratio is 13.5 to 1 (155).

Sexual abuse is reported in 13% of females aged 13-14 years in the United States; forced coital behavior occurs in over 70% of sexually active females under 14 years of age and 60% in sexually active females under age 15 (156, 157). Forced sex among sexually active teens occurs in 74% at 13 years of age, 60% at 14 year of age, 40% at 15 year of age, and 15% at 19 years of age (78). In the 1999 YRBS, sexual assault was noted in 12.5% of high school females and 5.2% of males (79).

The 2001 Youth Risk Behavior Surveillance reports 10% of high school girls with forced coitus in contrast to 5% of the males (158). In the 2017 YRBSS, 9.7% of high school students had been forced to do "sexual things" once or more during the 12 months prior to the survey; sexual violence was reported by 15.2% of the females versus 4.3% of the males (81).

However, sexual abuse against males have previously been understudied; thus, its incidence may be higher than previously reported. There were 272,350 victims of sexual assaults (including rapes and attempted rapes) reported in 2006 (versus 191,670 in 2005) with over 40% being under age 18 years and an estimated one-sixth being under age 12 (159, 60). Factors increasing chances of being sexually assaulted include hitchhiking, living on the streets (i.e., being homeless), and prior assault. Unwanted sexual overtures and harassment can even occur over the internet (161). Issues of sexual abuse in the pediatric population is also considered elsewhere in this publication.

Dating violence

Dating violence is a serious issue for many adolescent females and is linked to sexual risk behaviors with negative implications for overall sexual health (6, 75, 81, 162, 163). Up to 87% of high school students receive unwanted sexual comments or actions at school-lewd comments, jokes, being touched or grabbed by others (78). Studies suggest that the majority of female youth eventually become victims of some violence while dating. This may be physical, verbal, and/or sexual in nature (164, 165). As many as 60% of adolescents experience dating violence and this involves youth from all ethnic groups and socioeconomic strata (166). Studies with college students note dating violence in 36% of the males and 59% of the females (166). Acquaintance or date rape may be the cause in 60-70% of adolescent assaults (47).

Adolescents need to learn potential signs that their dating partner may be too aggressive and may resort to violent means to control the relationship. Concerns in this regard should be raised under these circumstances as noted in Table 11 (162-167). Youth and their parents need to be educated that these are warning signs and to avoid dating or stop dating such individuals (55). Adolescents should also know that violent dating partners become violent spouses and that witnessing violence in childhood raises this risk as well (168).

Table 11. Signs warning of a potential violent dating partner (162-167)

1.	Partner prevents the teen from associating with friends
2.	Becomes jealous with minimal (if any) reason
3.	Becomes upset with the teen for little or no reason
4.	Uses any means of violence in the relationship
5.	Always apologizes for being mean or violent
6.	Induces sadness in the teen when with him/her
7.	Uses drugs, including Rohypnol or other date rape drugs when dating

Adolescent sexual offenders

Adolescents as well as adults (males and females) can also be sexual perpetrators as various result studies have revealed (10, 169, 170). Teens under age 18 years of age account for 20% of arrests for all sexual offenses (not including prostitution), 20-30% of rape cases, 14% of aggravated sexual assault offenses, and 27% of child sexual homicides (10, 47). Adolescent sexual offenders represent a serious problem in the American society. These offenders commit multiple offenses, usually have more than one victim, and may not limit their offenses to one type of victim (10). These adolescents represent all races, social classes, and regions throughout the United States.

This supports the need for comprehensive service delivery and the importance of having a continuum of treatment services that are available in all communities for this disorder. Within the context of anticipatory guidance, child health clinicians can incorporate office-screening questions regarding sexually deviant behaviors to detect aberrant or deviant sexual behavior, allowing for early referral and intervention.

They can play an important role in the education of parents about the importance of appropriate professional help for deviant sexual behavior in children and adolescents that include paraphilic disorders (171). Once these identified individuals are connected with professional mental health resources, treatment may occur in the form of cognitive behavioral therapy or multisystem therapy with involvement of the core family; indeed, this approach is the treatment of choice with additional pharmacotherapy medications incorporated according to the Risk Need Responsivity Model where the number of medications is proportional to the severity of impulsivity (171).

Other adverse consequences in youth

There are an estimated one million runaway youths, and an estimated one million adolescent prostitutes (male and female), who exist in the United States (6, 172-177). Some youth run away from home while others are thrown out by parents or guardians ("throwaways"), leading to a harsh life on the street as homeless youth. Many will turn to prostitution, using survivor sex as a way to remain alive. Children and adolescents living on the streets of the world are the product of war, poverty, domestic violence, and abuse (physical, sexual, mental) (178-185).

Homeless youth are subject to many dangers of the street—as physical/sexual abuse, substance abuse, sexually transmitted diseases, various medical disorders, and others (167, 178-185). Their main medical treatment is usually through the hospital emergency department, if they receive any care at all. Estimates of the number of children and adolescents who live on the world's streets range from 30 million to 170 million. Children and youth are sold into slavery and prostitution in various parts of the world. There are an estimated one million children abducted or coerced into the global sex trade industry each year. Estimates suggest there are 300,000 child soldiers around the world—some as young as 10 years of age; their duties are varied, from overt soldiers to providing sexual services for the older solders (47, 68, 174).

Responsible teen sexuality

Researchers and educators in sexuality often note considerable differences in how both sexes view sexuality (6, 68, 177). The male development of sexuality is termed prosocial, which is in comparison to females who learn their early concepts of sexuality in the context of social relationships. American society conditions males early in their development to define masculinity as synonymous with such destructive concepts as dominance, competition, performance, and achievement.

The American media is often indicted in this regard for teaching males that masculinity implies that one is aggressive, has a "duty" to perform (whether scoring in basketball or coitus), and has an out-of-control sex drive that can only be controlled by one's partner. This same philosophy implies that if a girl becomes pregnant (by not saying "no" or not using contraceptives), it is her fault, not his. Males are taught that "shared contraceptive" responsibility is not an important concept that applies to them. Even the media censors may remove the topic of contraception when coitus is demonstrated or implied. Insurance plans in the United States often cover prescriptions for erection dysfunction medications but not oral contraceptives!

Males lacking extended contact with their fathers for appropriate role model patterns are especially vulnerable to such misogynic cues from the media. Males are taught from early life and throughout life to be more distrustful and insecure than females. Males are taught to control their sexual thoughts in regard to other males and to use homophobia as a guiding principle. Males are more likely to carry negative attitudes about their bodies from their childhood throughout adolescence and adulthood.

The adolescent male is generally exposed to very limited sexuality education and receives little contraceptive information/services. Sexuality education programs are often geared toward females, and birth control clinics often provide inadequate services to males or exclude males altogether. A common reason given by males for not using contraception is their limited knowledge base, and studies also suggest that the male exerts more influence than the female regarding the use (or non-use) of contraception.

Others conclude that the changes in sexual values in America over this past century have allowed males to be raised with much conflict and confusion in regard to their sexuality as well as in methods of sexual expression. This confusion and lack of control contribute to the high morbidity and mortality currently described in adolescent males (166, 167, 186, 187). The current adolescent male is exposed to a hostile environment that promotes violence (suicide and homicide), homophobia, limited sexuality education, limited exposure to medical services, and limited knowledge of disease prevention (such as use of condoms or self-testicular examinations) (2, 3, 177, 188).

Such a dangerous risky environment continues throughout adulthood. Health care professionals should be trained in techniques helping to talk with males and females about their specific concerns as well as needs (189). While females are expected to control their sexuality, males are not by society. Males use the internet more for sexual purposes, though both sexes also use the internet for social contact (99, 111-115, 190). Certainly more open communication between sex partners is important to increase effective contraceptive use for improved responsible sexual decision-making that can be encouraged by health care providers.

Perspectives on LGBTIA+

As puberty progresses, attraction to and sexual experimentation with the opposite sex is a classic feature of youth. Also, during early puberty, transient attraction to and sexual experimentation with members of the same sex may occur (6, 191-193). Some adolescents go through a phase of same-sex (homosexual) behavior and proceed toward a heterosexual behavior pattern; other adolescents learn to perceive homosexuality as a life pattern (191-200). Clinicians may not only care for heterosexual adolescents, but also gay, lesbian, bisexual, transgender, queer (GLBTQ) or pansexual youth (200, 201). Current terminology in this evolving area can be LGBTQIA+ relationships (lesbian, gay, bisexual, pansexual, transgender, genderqueer, queer, intersexed, agender, asexual and others) (see Table 2) (201-204).

Sexual behavior, whether heterosexual/homosexual or other, places adolescents at risk for sexually transmitted diseases or infections (STDs or STIs) (6, 194-199). However, adolescents with persistent homosexual attraction and sexual behavior additionally have to cope with social pressures associated with LGBTQIA+ that may place them at risk for various psychosocial problems as well as diverse medical complications (191-204). Table 2 provides definitions of terms used in this discussion and others related to the discussion of sexual orientation (191, 194, 200-204). Cisgender (cis; cisgender) refers to those whose gender identify is the same as the sex assigned at birth in contrast to transgender persons (205).

Perspectives on homosexuality

Though there has been considerable research about the etiology of homosexuality, controversy remains. Some maintain that homosexuality results from *in utero* sex hormone-controlled "programming" of the brain (hypothalamus) in combination with complex social learning factors in childhood (191-193). It has been observed that if a female (XX) fetus is exposed to excessive male hormones (as noted with some forms of congenital adrenal hyperplasia), the resultant female child may exhibit some "masculine" traits (such as seeking male aggressive play or ignoring doll playing) (191-193).

Genetic studies have shown a higher incidence of homosexual concordance among monozygotic twins than among dizygotic twins (191-193). Studies in epigenetics seek to provide etiologic factors for homosexuality; these results suggest a genetic predisposition, but chromosome studies have been unable to differentiate homosexual persons from heterosexual persons (206-209). Most homosexual individuals have the same sex hormone levels as their heterosexual counterparts. Though some data suggest that homosexuals respond differently to certain hormone injections (as opposed to heterosexuals), more research clearly is necessary in this area (206, 207). Some researchers point out differences in hypothalamic size and structure, anterior commissure size, or cerebral asymmetry (191-193, 210-214). However, there is no agreement on these biologic theories at this time and further research in the 21st century in this regard continues (210-214).

Psychological perspective

Psychological studies and theories abound regarding homosexuality, but so do the disagreements (6, 191-193, 212, 215, 216). Sigmund Freud wrote that individuals began human life with bipotentiality - that is they could become homosexual or heterosexual; in his view, usually the heterosexual aspect dominated (191). Freud did not consider homosexuality a mental illness, as noted by his famous 1935 response to an American mother of a homosexual:

> "Homosexuality assuredly is no advantage, but nothing to be ashamed of, no vice, no degradation; it cannot be classified as an illness; we consider it to be a variation of sexual functioning produced by a certain arrest of sexual development (47)."

Diagnostic perspectives

It was in 1973 when homosexuality as a diagnostic category of mental illness was eliminated by the American Psychiatric Association and the American Psychological Association officially accepted this same concept in 1975 (191-193). In 1980, it was removed from its Diagnostic and Statistical Manual (DSM-III); it was not present in the DSM-IV-TR edition nor the 2013 DSM 5 (191-193, 217, 218). The 10th revision of the International Statistical Classification of Diseases and Related Health Problems (ICD-10) states "Sexual orientation alone is not to be regarded as a disorder (219)." The 11th edition of the World Health Organization's International Statistical Classification of Diseases and Related Health Problems) (ICD-11) continues this theme and notes that issue of transgender is placed in a category apart from mental disorders that are identified as "conditions related to sexual health (220, 221)." This view reflects a change in the perception of homosexuality and others (i.e., transgender) on the part of most researchers from a pathological disorder to a variant form of human sexuality and eventually a normal aspect of sexuality (205, 217-226).

Homosexual identity perspectives

A variety of sexual orientations have been described since the ground-breaking work of Kinsey et al, who surveyed over 5,000 adult males and 6, 000 adult females in the 1930s and 1940s in the United States (227, 228). This research concluded that 4% of adult males and 2% of adult females are exclusively homosexual in their sexual fantasy and sexual behavior; also, these researchers concluded that 50% of these adult males had a homosexual experience before puberty, 37% had at least one such experience leading to orgasm, and 10% were homosexual for at least 3 years after puberty (227, 228). Table 12 lists the Kinsey scale used to rate sexual orientation in adults (191, 192, 227, 228).

Bell and Weinberg noted that 25% of those identifying themselves as homosexual also reported having heterosexual inclinations (229). McConaghy surveyed 138 male and 58 medical students in Australia, concluding that 60% of these students were aware of homosexual feelings as teenagers, with 40% still retaining these feelings at different levels (230). Further ratings of the male group (using the Kinsey scale) revealed: 55%-0, 37%-1, 4%: 2-4; 1%-5, and 3%-6.; the McConaghy female group rated themselves as: 52%-0, 33%-1, 7%-2-4%, 5%-5, and 3%-6 (230).

Table 12. Kinsey scale of sexual orientation (227, 228)

Rating	Description
0	Exclusive heterosexual (in sexual behavior and fantasy)
1	Essentially heterosexual with incidental or limited homosexual history
2	Largely heterosexual with distinct homosexual history
3	Equal heterosexual and homosexual orientation ("ambisexuality")
4	Largely homosexual with distinct heterosexual history
5	Essentially homosexual with limited heterosexual history
6	Exclusive homosexual in sexual behavior and fantasy

Remafedi et al. (1992) sampled 34,706 students in Minnesota, grades 7 through 12; 10.7% were unsure of their sexual orientation, 88.2% were predominately heterosexual, and 1.1% were bisexual or predominately homosexual (231). Other researchers conclude that 2% of adult males are exclusively homosexual while 3% are bisexual, that 3% of adult females are sexually active with other females since their teen years (126), and nearly 7% of adult females in the United States are involved in same-sex sexual activity after age 15 years (232-234). Studies noted that there are 25 million transgender persons in the world (205). Such prevalence and epidemiologic features of sexual orientation have been essentially consistent across the research data of the 20th and 21st centuries (205, 235).

Same-sex sexual orientation identity acquisition

The process of acceptance of a homosexual identity has been described by different researchers (191-195). Green identifies three stages in this process: a) first feeling "different," b) then developing a crush on a same sex person, and finally, c) becoming aware of his/her homosexual orientation (236). There may be a subsequent "coming out" phase in which the teenager seeks to reveal this "secret" to others, as family, peers or a health care professional. Troiden (1979) has outlined four stages in the development of a gay identity (see Table 13) (237,238).

Table 13. Troiden's stages of gay identity development (237, 238)

1. Stage One: Sensitization
2. Gains homosexual experiences in childhood and adolescence while learning of general society's negative view on homosexuality
3. Stage Two: Dissociation and Signification
4. Struggles to reject the concept that society's negative views on homosexuality applies to oneself
5. Stage Three: Coming Out
6. Identifies oneself as homosexual and reaches out to become involved in some aspect of the same-sex society culture; begins to consider homosexuality as a viable lifestyle option
7. Stage Four: Acceptance
8. Fuses one's concepts of sexuality and emotionality as an adult; some are "arrested" at stage 3 while others will eventually progress to Stage Four

Parents' reactions

The process of "coming out" for a homosexual youth can be very difficult, not just for the teenager, but also for the parents, who may feel they cannot talk to others and feel isolated (239). Parents may say it is "just a phase my child is going through" and may not take seriously the young person's exploration. They may feel that their adolescent's sexual orientation can be changed, or blame themselves for having a gay or lesbian teen. One can also see some parents who become so angry and threatened by this declaration that they physically abuse their teens or throw them out of the house ("throwaway teens"), forbid them from talking about this to anybody, and/or forbid them from contact with other siblings in the family. Parents may also worry about increased risks of violence their children may face and fear that their teen may not become a happy, adjusted adult. They mourn the loss of never becoming traditional grandparents and never having their child married in a heterosexual relationship having children (239).

Social perspectives

Past societal attitudes generally have been intolerant of same sex orientation or gender nonconformity, especially for males; indeed, various religions have often condemned such lifestyles as being immoral (191-193, 240-242). Homophobia (see Table 2) is a negative attitude toward or fear of homosexuality or homosexuals, while heterosexism is the belief that a heterosexual relationship is preferable to all others; it implies discrimination against those practicing homosexuality (240-245). Some adults prefer to identify sexual orientation by using terms like "lesbians" and "gay men" rather than homosexual which may imply pathology.

In the United States, following the civil rights movement were the first few gay rights movements in 1965 with the Stonewall Riots of June, 1969 serving as a turning point in the gay pride movement (246, 247). Over the course of the late 20th century into the 21st century, there was continued community and organizational social activism with greater media attention on the gay rights movement fostered by famous celebrity performers in the U.S. media heralding same sex equality (248-250). Despite significant barriers such as the HIV/AIDS epidemic and the infamous "Don't ask, don't tell" policy of the military, gay men and lesbian women continued to win legal battles and eventually won their rights for same sex marriage equality in the Supreme Court decision of Obergefell v. Hodge in June 2015 (251).

Changing attitudes on same sex marriage in the United States is evident by Pew Research Center polling that showed an opposition of same-sex marriage by 60% to 31% in 2004 compared to an opposition by a margin of 31% to 61% in 2019 (252). Despite this improvement in American approval statistics on same sex marriage, homosexual individuals continue to face lingering intolerance and significant discrimination.

Evaluation and management

Part of the process of being a competent clinician is being aware of personal issues that may influence clinical evaluation and management. The clinician should be able to review personal attitudes and feelings related to sexuality, sexual behaviors, and homosexuality. The primary care practitioner ideally is comfortable in eliciting information regarding sexual fantasies, sexual history, and sexual behaviors when obtaining a comprehensive sexual history in adolescent and young adult patients (6). Though GLBTQ+ (gay, lesbian, bisexual, transgender, questioning, pansexual, others) youth often wish their clinician would ask them about their sexual orientation and provide information in this regard, most primary care clinicians fail in this regard, tending to ignore this important aspect of their adolescent patients' lives (223).

Clinicians should understand that GLBTQ+ youth have increased risks for depression, suicide attempts/completions, alcohol and drug abuse (including club or date-rape drugs), eating disorders, sexually transmitted diseases (including HIV), violence-related injuries (including homicides), homeless lifestyles, and other psychological as well as medical problems (6, 167, 172-176, 182, 183, 191-193, 198, 199, 205, 225, 245, 253-259). Clinicians must also understand that LGBTQ+ youth often have limited access to health care and variations in comfortability with their physician (199, 259, 260). Table 14 provides a sexuality evaluation checklist for clinicians when dealing with youth having issues related to sexual identity, gender, sexual orientation and/or behavior.

Table 14. Sexuality evaluation checklist for clinicians

Factor	Evaluation	Issues	Recommendations
1. Sexual Identity	Complete Physical Examination	1. Ambiguous Genitalia 2. Genital abnormalities	Genetic Testing Gynecological Evaluation Urological Evaluation
2. Gender Identity	Observation of gender behaviors Interview	1. History of persistent cross-dressing 2. Persistent feelings of being "trapped in the body of the opposite sex" 3. Persistent desire to be the opposite sex 4. Persistent repulsion towards genitals 5. Persistent gender behaviors of the opposite sex	Psychiatric Evaluation
3. Sexual Orientation	Interview	1. Predominant sexual fantasy and attraction towards the: Opposite sex Same sex Both sexes 2. Knowledge and awareness of variations of sexual orientations 3. Psychological Adjustment Depression Suicidal ideation and plan Substance abuse 4. Familial knowledge and support Family unaware Family unsupportive 5. Social knowledge and support School Friends Sexual relationships 6. Religious conflicts 7. Legal problems 7.1 Prostitution 8. Special problems Bullying Violence	Reassurance Advise on Gay and Lesbian resources (See Resources) Referral to Mental Health Professional
4. Sexual Behavior	Interview	1. Pattern of Sexual relationships Sexual Behaviors Masturbation Oral sex 2. Sexual intercourse Anal sex 3. Related behaviors Drugs Sex toys Pornography	Advise on options for Safe Sex and condom use Advise on Family Planning Advise on risk for STDs/STIs Hepatitis B immunization Medical Testing (See Tables 6 and 8)

Initiating the evaluation

Table 15 outlines various reasons why a LGBTQ+ adolescent may seek advice or an evaluation by the primary care clinician (6, 191-193). Table 16 provides an outline to the medical evaluation of this patient (82). The clinician should introduce himself or herself to the adolescent and explain that a complete medical evaluation includes both an interview and a physical examination.

Table 15. Reasons that GLBTQ+ youth seek medical attention (205)

- Information about homosexuality or other aspects of human sexuality
- Sexually transmitted disease(s), including fears of STDs and information
- Psychosocial difficulties
  - Family
  - School
  - Significant other(s)
  - Personal problems
  - Vocational concerns
  - Religious conflicts
- Infection with human immunodeficiency virus (HIV) or concerns about HIV or acquired immunodeficiency syndrome
- Other medical disorders
- Substance abuse
- Legal problems (including prostitution)

Table 16. Medical evaluation of GLBTQ+ adolescents (205)

- History (ensure confidentiality, privacy)
  - Social
  - School
  - Family
  - Employment
  - Substance use
  - Assessment of psychosocial problems, including suicidal ideations
- Review of systems
- Sexual history
- Physical examination
  - General
  - Close inspection for sexually transmitted diseases or infections (STDs/STIs)
  - Other procedures as indicated (pelvic examination, anoscopy)
- Laboratory evaluation (see table 20)
  - Neisseria gonorrhoeae
  - Chlamydia trachomatis
  - Treponema pallidum
  - Human immumodeficiency virus (HIV)
  - Others (herpes simplex virus [HSV], human papillomavirus [HPV], others)
- Hepatitis B immunization
- Human Papillomavirus Vaccine (and others as they become available)
- Appropriate treatment of STDs (including partners) and any medical problems
- Discussion of risk reduction, abstinence, contraception, condoms
- Referral to support groups as necessary
- Follow-up visit(s) with primary care physician (including family)

The clinician should also reassure the patient that whatever is discussed in the interview remains confidential except in situations that the safety of the patient may be compromised (47, 82, 154, 261-264). While evaluating an adolescent, the practitioner should not make assumptions about the youth's sexual orientation.

Sexuality is influenced by four interrelated psychosexual factors: sexual identity, gender identity, sexual orientation and sexual behavior (see Table 2) (191-193). The clinician should evaluate sexuality in all adolescents, asking questions in these different domains; these factors affect personality growth, development, and functioning.

Evaluation and management process

In evaluating the sexual identity of the adolescent, a general examination can help in addressing this concept. Table 14 provides a checklist for clinicians when evaluating concepts of sexuality in their adolescent patients. Should there be any genital anomaly, the adolescent should be further evaluated by the appropriate specialist whether by an endocrinologist, urologist, or gynecologist. In evaluating the gender identity of the adolescent, the clinician should determine any history of cross-dressing or the sense of feeling "trapped in the body of the opposite sex" (gender dysphoria or gender incongruence) (205, 256). These symptoms should be further evaluated by a psychiatrist or other appropriate mental health professional to determine the possibility of transvestic fetishism or gender dysphoria as well as to assess and treat any comorbid mental health concerns (see Tables 1 and 2) (205, 218, 265).

The mental health professional can then connect the individual and their family with community resources for various needs as well as refer the individual with a diagnosis of gender dysphoria to the proper medical professionals to discuss options for physical interventions (205, 265, 266). According to the World Professional Association for Transgender Health, physical interventions are based on three categories which include 1) fully reversible interventions such as GnRH agonists designed to suppress estrogen/testosterone production and delay the onset of pubertal physical changes 2) partially reversible interventions such as hormone therapy and 3) irreversible interventions such as surgeries (205, 266). Table 17 discusses the criteria for various physical interventions as suggested by the World Professional Association for Transgender Health (205, 266).

Sexual orientation is a very complex but poorly understood phenomenon which is established by middle childhood (ages 7-9 years) (191-193). In evaluating for sexual orientation, the clinician should identify whether the sexual attraction of the adolescent is directed towards the opposite sex, the same sex, or both sexes. Adolescents who have homosexual attraction and sexual behavior can be advised to wait until late adolescence or early adulthood before concluding their sexual orientation as gay, lesbian, bisexual, or asexual; by that time most are aware of their real sexual orientation. Early and mid-adolescence stimulate various stages of experimentation while late adolescence may allow some resolution in the area of acceptance of one's sexual orientation (191-193, 205).

Some youth enter adulthood committed to a homosexual lifestyle; they state that their sexual orientation as well as commitment began even in early adolescence. Variations on such timing certainly do occur. Part of the management of adolescents with homosexual attraction or gender dysphoria and sexual behavior includes evaluation of their knowledge and misconceptions regarding GLBTQ+.

Table 17. Criteria for physical interventions in gender sysphoria and gender non congruent individuals (205)

Criteria for puberty surpressing hormones

In order for adolescents to receive puberty-suppressing hormones, the following minimum criteria must be met:

1. The adolescent has demonstrated a long-lasting and intense pattern of gender nonconformity or gender dysphoria (whether suppressed or expressed);
2. Gender dysphoria emerged or worsened with the onset of puberty;
3. Any coexisting psychological, medical, or social problems that could interfere with treatment (e.g., that may compromise treatment adherence) have been addressed, such that the adolescent's situation and functioning are stable enough to start treatment;
4. The adolescent has given informed consent and, particularly when the adolescent has not reached the age of medical consent, the parents or other caretakers or guardians have consented to the treatment and are involved in supporting the adolescent throughout the treatment process.

Criteria for hormone therapy

1. Persistent, well-documented gender dysphoria;
2. Capacity to make a fully informed decision and to consent for treatment;
3. Age of majority in a given country
4. If significant medical or mental health concerns are present, they must be reasonably well controlled. The presence of coexisting mental health concerns does not necessarily preclude access to feminizing/masculinizing hormones; rather, these concerns need to be managed prior to, or concurrent with, treatment of gender dysphoria.

Criteria for surgical therapy

Criteria for breast/chest surgery (one referral)

Criteria for mastectomy and creation of a male chest in FtM patients:

1. Persistent, well-documented gender dysphoria
2. Capacity to make a fully informed decision and to consent for treatment
3. Age of majority in a given country (if younger, follow the SOC for children and adolescents)
4. If significant medical or mental health concerns are present, they must be reasonably well controlled. Hormone therapy is not a prerequisite.

Criteria for breast augmentation (implants/lipofilling) in MtF patients:

1. Persistent, well-documented gender dysphoria
2. Capacity to make a fully informed decision and to consent for treatment
3. Age of majority in a given country
4. If significant medical or mental health concerns are present, they must be reasonably well controlled. Although not an explicit criterion, it is recommended that MtF patients undergo feminizing hormone therapy (minimum 12 months) prior to breast augmentation surgery. The purpose is to maximize breast growth in order to obtain better surgical (aesthetic) results.

Criteria for genital surgery (two referrals) The criteria for genital surgery are specific to the type of surgery being requested.

Criteria for hysterectomy and salpingo-oophorectomy in FtM patients and for orchiectomy in MtF patients:

1. Persistent, well-documented gender dysphoria
2. Capacity to make a fully informed decision and to consent for treatment
3. Age of majority in a given countr
4. If significant medical or mental health concerns are present, they must be well controlled.
5. 12 continuous months of hormone therapy as appropriate to the patient's gender goals (unless hormones are not clinically indicated for the individual).

Criteria for metoidioplasty or phalloplasty in FtM patients and for vaginoplasty in MtF patients

6. Persistent, well-documented gender dysphoria
7. Capacity to make a fully informed decision and to consent for treatment
8. Age of majority in a given country
9. If significant medical or mental health concerns are present, they must be well controlled
10. 12 continuous months of hormone therapy as appropriate to the patient's gender goals (unless hormones are not clinically indicated for the individual).
11. 12 continuous months of living in a gender role that is congruent with their gender identity.

Also, the perceived need for secrecy and their often limited sexuality education result in various potential psychological and physiological difficulties (6, 191-193, 198, 199, 205, 245, 253-259). In this regard, the Internet, as noted previously, can be a dangerous place for youth seeking accurate information about sexuality, including homosexuality; the result may be sexual abuse and sexual grooming instead of appropriate sexuality information (161, 180, 267-270).

Evaluating support systems

Part of the evaluation of adolescents with homosexual attraction and sexual behavior includes a review of family and social supports. Youth who are going through various stages of homosexual and gender nonconforming identity (see Table 14) need as much support as possible (191-193, 198, 199). They have to deal with society's prejudicial (homophobic) attitude, peers' ridicule, and parents' potential rejection (205, 240-245). Perceived rejection of one's religious upbringing and even of one's culture can be very difficult with resultant depression and suicidality (255-259, 271). Some end up on the street as homeless youth. Hate crimes and violence are also a major risk factor for LGBTQ+ teens; this may take the form of murder, rape, assault, and other crimes (205, 272).

The clinician can provide information regarding gay-straight alliances at some schools for all adolescents receiving support from others who are interested in them. The growth of organizations like Parents and Friends of Lesbians and Gays (PFLAG) has been very important in helping both parents and teenagers understand these issues. The clinician can address the lack of information by providing resources available on the Internet or through libraries (see resources section).

Evaluating social relationships

Evaluating adolescents with homosexual or bisexual attraction and sexual behavior includes assessing self-esteem and social integration. Reaction to Troiden's Stage Two (see Table 13) may include denial, despair, avoidance of social as well as sexual relationships, and perhaps, eventual acceptance or rejection of having a homosexual or bisexual orientation. They may develop poor social skills and suffer due to a lack of appropriate adult role models.

It is not surprising that many such youth struggle intensely to develop an acceptable self-identity. Health care professionals can help such individuals by a) providing non-prejudicial counseling (or referring to someone who can provide this), b) teaching improved social skills, c) arranging family counseling, and d) reminding youth to keep their sexual orientation options open while being safe (191-193, 205).

If the individual does seem disturbed by a homosexual orientation or gender dysphoria, referral to appropriate mental health or counseling facilities may be helpful. However, there is no scientific evidence to support the process of "reparative therapy" ("conversion therapy") or trying to force sexual orientation change on a youth who seems content with his/her/their LGBTQ+ lifestyle (216, 273-275). The 1980 DSM-III contained the term, "ego dystonic homosexuality" in reference to those who were homosexual but in conflict with this orientation or wished to change their orientation; the 1987 revision of the DSM-III deleted this term, noting that most individuals who are homosexual normally go through a phase of conflict over this orientation in current society (217, 218).

Depression and suicide

Part of the evaluation of adolescents with homosexual attraction and sexual behavior includes assessment of depression and suicide risk (253-260, 265, 266). Data suggest that gay youth account for approximately 30% of completed suicides in adolescents, while 30% of a surveyed group of gay and bisexual males have attempted suicide at least once (253-255).

One study of 137 gay and bisexual males (ages 14-21 years) noted nearly 30% had a suicide attempt, and almost half of this group had multiple suicide attempts (254). The clinician can help those with overt depression and suicide risks by referral to an appropriate mental health professional (205, 265, 266).

Sexually transmitted diseases (STDs)

In evaluating for sexual behavior, the clinician should ask about the different aspects of the adolescent's sexual behavior and risk factors---as considered elsewhere in this publication. Youth may unknowingly be exposed to various sexually transmitted diseases (STDs) (see Table 18) (6, 47, 95-98, 104, 117, 118, 158, 196, 197, 199, 205, 225). Young adolescents may only find gay contact at public places where problems with sexually transmitted diseases (including HIV infection) often exist. Lesbian teens may have sex with males as part of their adolescent sexual experimentation and some are at increased risk of HIV infection because of coitus with infected males; pregnancy risks also occur in this situation if unprotected sex occurs. About 25% of those with HIV/AIDS in the United States contracted their infection by the age of 21; for those in their twenties with HIV, many, if not most of them, were infected while they were still teenagers or in their early twenties (276). Even if the adolescent engages in same-sex behavior for economic reasons and not because of being homosexual, risks for STDs remain (220, 222, 254).

Advice regarding testing for sexually transmitted diseases includes explaining possible risk factors, treatment options, and discussion regarding confidentiality as well as information for the adolescent's parents (2, 3, 6, 47, 154, 260-266). Advice regarding options for self-protection includes safe sex awareness and practice, such as sexual abstinence and use of latex condoms (127-135, 196). In addition, the adolescent can be taught techniques to handle peer pressure regarding sexual behavior. Part of the evaluation of sexual behavior includes inquiry about the use of alcohol or substances (including other illicit drugs, sildenafil citrate, others; "chem-sex") before or during sexual activity (137, 167, 277-281). Violence is a serious reality for many LGBTQ+ youth in America and the clinician should provide anticipatory guidance on what can be done if violence has become a threat to the life and well-being of this young individual; such violence can include assaults, homicides, and even suicides (158, 253-255, 265, 266). Also, as noted with heterosexuals, adolescents involved in non-heterosexual relationships may experience dating violence (160-166).

Table 18. Sexually transmitted diseases in GLBTQ+ adolescents (194-199)

Urethritis
Neisseria gonorrhoeae
Chlamydia trachomatis
Mycoplasma hominis/genitalium
Ureaplasma urealyticum
Acquired immunodeficiency syndrome or AIDS
(persons with HIV infection may acquire various other opportunistic infections not listed)
Genital warts (infection with human papillomavirus [HPV])
Ectoparasites.
Pediculosis pubis (Phthirus pubis)
Scabies (Sarcoptes scabiei)
Hepatitis A, B, C, D, and/or E virus
Cytomegalovirus
Epstein-Barr virus
Ulcerative lesions
Syphilis (Treponema pallidum)
Herpes simplex virus (HSV)
Chancroid (Haemophilus ducreyi)
Lymphogranuloma venereum (Chlamydia trachomatis)
Granuloma inguinale (Calymmatobacterium granulomatis)
Enteritis/proctocolitis
Giardia lamblia
Salmonella enteritidis
Entamoeba histolytica
Cryptosporidium species
Campylobacter species
Shigella species

RESOURCES

National Federation of Parents and Friends of Lesbians and Gays (PFLAG)
1726 M Street NW-Suite 400
Washington, DC 20036
Phone: 202-467-8180
www.pflag.org

Gay and Lesbian Medical Association
459 Fulton Street, Suite 107
San Francisco, CA 94102
Phone: 415-255-4547
FAX: 415-225-4784
www.glma.org

National Youth Advocacy Coalition
1638 R Street., NW, Suite 300
Washington, DC 20009
Phone: 202-319-7596
FAX: 202-319-7365
E-mail: nyac@nyacyouth.org
http://www.nyacyouth.org
(Referral information for youth-serving agencies and services

Summary: LGBTQ+

The clinician (i.e., primary care clinician, others) should be able to summarize findings with the adolescent and discuss options that do not emotionally threaten the young person (2, 6, 68). It is important to establish a trusting relationship based on respect and honesty using a professional demeanor. Explanation for a laboratory work-up should be provided and issues regarding confidentiality clearly addressed. Additionally, information on how the clinician or others may be reached in case of crisis should be provided.

The clinician should be aware of personal issues regarding sexuality and homosexuality which may affect clinical evaluation of the adolescent. The clinician should be comfortable in asking questions regarding sexuality in their adolescent patients. The primary care provider should evaluate the different dimensions of sexuality for all adolescents, including the current changes in love ideology of youth and their potential preference for casual relationships. Clinicians should also be sensitive to unique issues of adolescents with LBGTQ+ questions/behavior (99, 192, 215-218, 205, 282).

Additionally, the clinician should also appreciate the possible need for other medical specialties, school as well as community resources, and internet sites that may be helpful for the adolescent with sexuality concerns (see resources). The LGBTQ+ youth lives in a very difficult and potentially dangerous environment and the clinician may serve as an important lifeline in stabilizing this youth---allowing successful transitioning from adolescence to adulthood. Both heterosexual and homosexual youth are resilient and can learn to lead stable and productive lives with the help of supportive family members, friends, and their clinicians.

Primary care clinicians should understand and appreciate the importance of sexuality in the lives of the children and adolescents they care for in their practices (1-4, 6). Normal sexuality is a critical part of normal growth and development. Children and adolescents need knowledgeable health care professionals who can supplement the parents' teaching about human sexuality in a confidential and sensitive manner. Clinicians can also learn of potential problems with sexuality development, including unwanted pregnancy, sexually transmitted diseases, sexual assault, dating violence, GLBTQ+ questions/behavior and others. Adolescents who are not sexually active, can be encouraged to continue in this lifestyle. Those who choose to be sexually active, need information about STDs/STIs (safe sex) and pregnancy prevention. Counselling about fertility, sexual dysfunction, and other aspects of sexuality is an important role for clinicians caring for adolescents (see appendix A) (6). Many of these issues are discussed elsewhere in this publication.

Conclusion: Appropriate sexuality education

Various aspects of childhood and adolescent sexuality have been considered including psychosexual development, issues of masturbation and attitudes regarding pediatric sexuality, central nervous system maturation, normal adolescent sexuality stages (early, middle and late adolescence), adolescent coital experiences, concepts of chronic illness and disability, adolescent pregnancy, hypersexuality, sexual abuse, dating violence, adolescent sexual offenders, and perspectives on LGBTQ+ youth (LGBTIA+) (1, 2, 6, 10, 14, 32, 47, 68, 78, 82, 93, 104, 120, 127-129, 134, 154, 166, 167, 186, 187, 192, 193, 205, 260, 264).

Limited sex education can be invoked as a partial explanation for current adolescent sexuality statistics (2, 6, 68, 81, 94-96). Youth are naturally curious about sexuality and often experiment widely, especially starting during mid-adolescence. The twenty-first century society stresses the enjoyment of human sexuality but often, paradoxically, ignores the responsibility and potentially negative consequences of unwise sexual experimentation. Part of this is the "normal" narcissistic stage of adolescent sexuality, while part of it results from a society that exposes young people to sexual advertisements and promiscuous lifestyles that do not show the consequences of irresponsibility. As noted, the modern media (cable TV, movies, You-tube, others in modern media technology) has a profound effect on America's youth, without parents really being aware of what is being taught (190, 267-270). Pornography ("porno") websites are also used by adolescents (especially males) for sexual education needs. Sex is presented on these websites in a non-realistic way, in order to please the experienced and not by any means to educate the non-experienced.

As previously noted, most youth begin to overcome their narcissistic heterosexual experimentation in late adolescence; at this stage youth begin to prepare for adulthood by serious consideration of a job investment as well as an adult lifestyle. Relationships in late adolescence should switch from "selfish" concerns to overt caring about the other individual (s), which should be the goal of adult sexual relationships. Unfortunately, the high rate of divorce and sexual dysfunction reported in current adult populations indicates that this is not always the case (283-285).

The result of fewer teens being sexually active and more of the sexually-active teens using contraception has resulted in a decline in adolescent pregnancy from the early 1990s to the early part of the 21st century (68, 120-125). However, despite access to effective contraception and use of condoms, pregnancy rates in the United States, Western Europe, Eastern Europe and Russia remain high (76, 77, 36).

Primary care clinicians can encourage those who are abstinent to continue with this choice until they really feel mature and ready to become involved in a sexual relationship. Abstinence is the best way to prevent unwanted pregnancy and sexually transmitted diseases (STDs). Primary care clinicians should be prepared to ask basic questions about their teenage patients' sexuality, including if they are sexually active, what type of sex are they doing, when was the last time, how many partners, are they using condoms, and are they interested in using contraception (1-4, 6)?

Clinicians should be aware of factors that place youth at increased risk for early coital activity such as poor school attendance, early menarche, behavioral problems, drug use (including tobacco, cannabis, alcohol, methamphetamine, heroin, cocaine, others), limited training in refusal of unwanted sex, survival sex, and others (167). Those who choose to be sexually active should have appropriate information about contraception and STD protection (6, 68, 82, 95, 129-133, 188, 196). Role plays on refusal of unwanted sex or convincing one's partner to use effective contraceptive methods if sexual activity is about to take place, are very helpful in this education.

Sexuality education is important for all adolescents that is offered and encouraged from various segments of society, including parents, clinicians, and schools (6, 20-23). Advice about sexuality should be provided in a friendly, confidential, and safe manner. The attitudes and beliefs of clinicians can influence their ability and willingness to provide counsel for teens regarding sexual orientation, pregnancy, abortion, contraception, and STDs. Clinicians can introduce the subject of sexuality into the doctor-patient communication on a regular basis and set the youth at ease while talking about sexuality. Youth may have a hidden agenda regarding various aspects of sexuality, and clinicians should be attuned to this agenda. A number of factors can compromise sexual health and careful screening will often uncover these issues. Sexuality involves various family, legal, ethical, moral, and religious issues; also, clinicians need training to be able to help these youth as these various factors influence their young patients (6).

Anticipatory guidance by clinicians is important to promote healthy sexuality development in children as well as adolescents and prevent complications (as unwanted pregnancy, STDs, abuse) (**6**). Youth involved in abusive relationships need the guidance of trusted clinicians to steer them toward healthy adulthood. Counseling can encourage the growth of various resiliency factors that promote healthy sexuality and healthy living, enabling these youth to deal with adversities and lead a productive adolescent as well as adult life. These factors include a sense of belonging with other peers, acquiring a healthy value system, receiving appropriate education (including sexuality education), and learning to enjoy the fascinating phenomenon of life itself.

Youth need an adviser and a guide in life, one who can provide support and accurate education in important facets of life, such as human sexuality. One should follow local laws for confidentiality and provision of reproductive rights (1-4, 6, 82, 261-264). Also, the potentially devastating impact of the 2020-2022 global COVID-19 (SARS-CoV-2) pandemic on human sexuality remains under observation and research as the third decade of the 21st century proceeds (286-290). Finally, research continues on sexuality including sexual violence in the lives of children and adolescents as this century continues into its third decade (291-300).

Acknowledgments

Consultation over the years with Lyubov Matytsina MD, PhD and Helen D Pratt PhD (1948-2020) in the preparation of this manuscript is gratefully acknowledged.

Appendix A. Anticipatory guidance: Sex education

Age	Child's needs or interests	Anticipatory guidance
Newborn	– Cuddling, sucking, loving touch (foundations for security, trust and later ability to give physical affection are established now)	– Teach parents the importance of touch, of warm, loving cuddling – Encourage breastfeeding, front packs, rocking chairs – "You can't spoil a baby at this age – it's okay to pick her up when she cries" – Observe parents' interactions with newborn – demonstrate behaviors if parents seem uncomfortable – Comment on role expectations – by choosing "pink or blue" we are already sending sex role messages to the infant
6 months	– Infant discovers body – Self-stimulation and touching of genitals	– Tell parents to expect this behavior and that it's normal – Ask parents about their own attitudes toward infant self-stimulation – Remind them, "Don't slap his hands", as this sets up negative messages (i.e., that part of your body is "bad") – Show the parents the parts of genitalia – teach them the vocabulary to use – Encourage questions – let them know sexually related topics are appropriate to discuss during health care visits
1 year	– Curiosity as to what daddy and mommy look like without clothes on	– Guidelines for household nudity. Explore parents' own attitudes – what's best is what they are comfortable with – Children begin to establish gender identity by observing differences in male and female bodies – Use picture books if nudity is uncomfortable – Parents should avoid messages that convey nudity as "dirty" or "pornographic"

Age	Child's needs or interests	Anticipatory guidance
11/2 – 3 years	– Self-respect and self-esteem develop. Feelings form about being a boy or a girl – Effectiveness of toddler discipline at this age determines later ability to handle frustration and have self-control – Exploration of body parts is common – Bathroom activities are of great interest (toilet training) – Sense of privacy develops	– Teach parents how self-esteem is developed. Need for lots of positive feedback ("catch them being good"). Give praise and positive messages about being either a girl or a boy. Let children seek own preferences for sex role behavior (okay for boys to play with dolls or girls to play with trucks) – Discuss plans for discipline. Teach parents methods (e.g., time out). Emphasize how to give positive reinforcement ("I like it when you__") – Encourage parents to help children learn correct words for genitals and body functions (penis, vulva, BM) – Discuss toilet training – using rewards and reinforcing positive attitudes about genitals
3 - 5 years	– Child needs answers to "sexual questions" appropriate to cognitive level of development – Grasping genitals is clearly pleasurable, may occur when child is upset – Children become very seductive toward opposite sex parent – Role-modeling (assimilation of characteristics of same-sex role model) takes place – Children begin learning what is socially acceptable, what behaviors are public or private, and how to show respect for others	– Tell parents to expect sexual questions ("where do babies come from") and give examples of how to answer them – Give techniques for determining level of understanding ("where do you think they come from") – Child needs to learn it's okay to talk about sex – Give booklets or suggest additional educational materials – Prepare parent for child's seductive behavior – Encourage parents to support each other and put their needs as a couple first (bad time to get divorced) – Remind them to role model the kind of male-female relationship they want their children to imitate (because the kids will) – This is the time to begin demonstrating that women have rights and men are equally responsible for outcomes
5 – 7 years	– "Playing doctor" is universal – Kids have learned parents' discomforts, starting "keeping secrets" about sex – Peer discussions provide many ideas about sex – dirty jokes among playmates common – Four-letter words (for exhibitionist behavior) used for shock value – Starting school – so stranger awareness is important	– Let parents know that childhood genital exploration is typical – it satisfies curiosity about opposite sex – Ask parents about their own childhood experiences "playing doctor" – Discuss ways to handle the situation ("It's normal to be curious – we consider other people's bodies private – I'd like you to get dressed and play other games") – Same with four-letter words ("be cool") – Encourage parents to bring up sexual questions, rather than waiting to be asked, utilize "teachable moments" to reinforce that it's okay to talk about sex. Need ample family discussion to balance what is learned from playmates – Discuss sexual molestation as a risk – discuss prevention techniques to teach children
7 – 9 years	– Child needs answers to more advanced sexual questions (often scientific) e.g., "How does the baby get into the womb" – Needs preview of changes in sexual development that will be associated with puberty – Values are instilled now that will last a lifetime (e.g., self-responsibility, kindness)	– Ask if parents have been getting any sexual questions (if not, child may feel it's not okay to ask). Dispel myth that information leads to sexual experimentation or that child is "too innocent" to hear about sex – Encourage them to use experiences such as TV shows, mating animals, new babies in neighborhood, as opportunities to bring up questions – Assure parents it's okay not to know all the answers. Guide them to resources (books) for information – Give parents an understanding of wide range of pubertal development (e.g., breast budding at age 8-9 is normal) – Encourage parents to teach difference between facts and opinions, e.g., that nearly all young men masturbate is a fact; that masturbation is bad (or good) is an opinion (with which others may not agree) – Important to teach child the family values and beliefs, as well as facts

Appendix A. (Continued)

Age	Child's needs or interests	Anticipatory guidance
10 – 12 years	– Pubertal changes are of great importance – hormone levels rise – Both sexes need to know about body changes, menarche, wet dreams, and sexual fantasies – Sex behavior "rehearsal" is common (looking through Playboy, spin-the-bottle games) – Questions about homosexuality arise – Need for privacy intensifies – Self-esteem is very fragile	– By now, caregivers should start giving anticipatory guidance directly to young teens as well as to parents – Parents need to understand the normalcy of preadolescent sexual concerns and be willing to discuss them in a nonjudgmental way (last chance to be an important source of information – later it will be peers) – Empathize with parental discomfort ("sometimes we feel uneasy talking about sex, but-") – Model nonjudgmental ways of asking questions ("some parents don't mind their children looking at Playboy, and some parents disapprove. What are your feelings about that?") – Parents must set aside time to talk with children about puberty and sexual changes – School and community groups (Scouts, Church) should be encouraged to provide sex education for young adolescents – Build self-esteem – preteens need lots of positive feedback
11 – 15 years (early adolescence)	– Obsessive concern with body and appearances (breast size, penile erections, acne, etc.) – Pubertal changes are completed – need for a solid understanding of reproductive physiology – Sexual behaviors emerge (masturbation, homosexual encounters, sex dreams) – "First dates" start – questions about "what is love" – Peer pressure become significant – Need for assertiveness skills, right say "NO" – Boys need to know they are equally responsible for consequences of sexual activity – Both sexes need to be prepared to use contraception when the time comes – Educations about STDs, AIDs prevention is a priority – Self-esteem still low	– At puberty, parents will reap the results of their past efforts – Parents need to learn how to "let go with love" and let the teen take responsibility for choices – Reflective listening is far more important than talking – Affirm wholesomeness of sexual feelings ("it's natural to want to have sex") while conveying own opinions ("it would be wiser to wait until you're sure") – Parent should be sure teens have access to educational resources (e.g., books) that will answer questions in detail – Many heterosexual young teens have some experimental homosexual encounters prior to dating. They may need reassurance and information – Parents need to prepare teens to use contraception – discuss realities, give permission, explain about resources. Dispel parental myths (e.g., that access to family planning promotes promiscuity) – Message should be "wait until you're sure you're ready, then use reliable birth control each and every time" – Do not give messages that "good girls" don't have sex – guilt induction leads to denial and inability to accept responsibilities for choices (e.g., unprotected sex) – Risks of STDs and AIDs should be discussed openly. Help teen realistically plan for self-protection (abstinence, monogamy, condoms) – Continue to discuss personal values (continue to separate facts from opinions) – Continue to reinforce positive self-esteem – Caregivers: The same anticipatory guidance should be given directly to teen in the office setting

Age	Child's needs or interests	Anticipatory guidance
15 – 17 years (middle adolescence)	– Sexual activity begins – Services for sexual issues (family planning, STD, pregnancy tests) are essential – Meaning of relationships is explored ("Does he really love me") – Life planning becomes serious (high-risk low-income teens needs to see options beyond pregnancy) – Increased independence can lead to risks (date-rape, sexual assault) – Sexual preference becomes apparent to self – homosexual teens may feel much confusion and self-doubt	– Ask parent, "What have you done to prepare your teen to use contraception when the time comes?" "How much have you discussed STD or AIDS with your teen?" – Encourage parents to give teens permission to obtain contraception, and acquaint them with resources and means – Allow confidentiality and independence for teens seeking health care – Parents can continue to raise questions ("What did you think of that TV scene that showed __?") and give teens a chance to look at choices and consequences. But be prepared for either unwillingness to talk or challenges to parental viewpoints – Most teens do not want to discuss their personal sexual activities with their parents – Suggest to parents that they discuss teen's plans for the future, and then ask how plans would be affected by pregnancy, or marriage, etc. – Teens need to know family, society expect them to prevent unplanned pregnancy, STDs if they choose to have sex – Discuss prevention techniques for sexual assault – Sexual orientation should be asked about (rather than presumed) – Referral to support resources may be helpful to gay teens or their parents if emotional or societal stress is present

Reproduced with permission from Dr. Roberta K. Beach, MD, Emeritus Director of Adolescent Ambulatory Services, Denver Department of Health and Hospitals, Denver, CO.

Reprinted with permission: Greydanus DE, Patel DR, Pratt HD, eds. Behavioral pediatrics, 2nd ed. New York: iUniverse, 2006:326-30.

Adapted with permission: Greydanus DE, Patel DR, Pratt HD, Calles JL Jr, eds. Behavioral pediatrics, 3rd Edition. New York: Nova Science, 2009:265-96.

References

[1] Greydanus DE. Adolescent sexuality: An overview and perspective for the 1980's. Pediatr Ann 1982;11:714-26.

[2] Fonseca F, Greydanus DE. Sexuality in the child, teen, and young adult: Concepts for the clinician. Prim Care Clin Off Pract 2007;34(2):275-92.

[3] Rosenthal SL, Blythe MJ. Adolescent sexuality. Adolesc Med State Art Rev 2007; 18:425-587.

[4] Alderman EM, Breuner CC, Committee on Adolescence. Unique needs of the adolescent. Pediatrics 2019;144(6). pii: e20193150. doi: 10.1542/peds.2019-3150.

[5] Burunat E. Love is a physiological motivation (like hunger, thirst, sleep or sex). Med Hypotheses 2019;129:109225. doi: 10.1016/j.mehy.2019.05.011.

[6] Omar HA, Greydanus DE, Patel DR, Merrick J, eds. Pediatric and adolescent sexuality and gynecology. Principles for the primary care clinician, Second edition. New York: Nova Science, 2021.

[7] Rudnytsky PL. Inventing Freud. Am J Psychoanal 2008;68(2):117-27.

[8] Pitman SR, Knauss DPC. Contemporary psychodynamic approaches to treating anxiety: theory, research, and practice. Adv Exp Med Biol 2020;1191:451-64.

[9] Freud S. Three essays on the theory of sexuality. Vol 7. London: Hogarth Press, 1953:125-243.

[10] Pratt HD, Greydanus DE, Patel DR. The adolescent sexual offender. Prim Care Clin Office Pract 2007;34:305-16.

[11] Mesman GR, Harper SL, Edge NA, Brandt TW, Pemberton JL. Problematic sexual behavior in children. J Pediatr Health Care 2019;33(3):323-31.

[12] De Jong AR. Sexual interactions among siblings and cousins: Experimentation or exploitation? Child Abuse Negl 1989;13:271-9.

[13] Miragoli S, Camisasca E, Di Blasio P. Child sexual behaviors in school context: Age and gender differences. J Child Sex Abus 2017;26(2):213-31.
[14] Greydanus DE, Geller B. Masturbation: Historic perspective. NY State J Med 1980; 80:1892-96.
[15] Tissot SA. Onanism or a treatice upon the disorders produced by masturbation; or the dangerous effects of secret and excessive venery. Translated by A Hume. London: M Chapins, 1776.
[16] Cowell DD. Autoerotic asphyxiation: secret pleasure—lethal outcome? Pediatrics 2009;124(5):1319-24.
[17] Herbenick D, Reece M, Schick V, Sanders SA, Dodge B, Fortenberry JD. Sexual behavior in the United States: results from a national probability sample of men and women ages 14-94. J Sex Med 2010;7(Suppl 5):255-65.
[18] Rowland D, Donarski A, Graves V, Caldwell C, Hevesi B, Hevesi K. The experience of orgasmic pleasure during partnered and masturbatory sex in women with and without orgasmic difficulty. J Sex Marital Ther 2019;45(6):550-61.
[19] Kohler PK, Manhart LE, Lafferty WE. Abstinence-only and comprehensive sex education and the initiation of sexual activity and teen pregnancy. J Adolesc Health 2008;42(4):344-51.
[20] Stanger-Hall KF, Hall DW. Abstinence-only education and teen pregnancy rates: why we need comprehensive sex education in the US. PLoS One 2011;6(10):e24658. doi: 10.1371/ journal.pone.0024658.
[21] Hall KS, McDermott Sales J, Komro KA, Santelli J. The state of sex education in the United States. J Adolesc Health 2016;58(6):595-7.
[22] Breuner CC, Mattson G. Committee on Adolescence; Committee on Psychosocial Aspects of Child and Family Health. Pediatrics 2016;138(2). pii: e20161348. doi:10.1542/peds.2016-1348.
[23] Rabbitte M, Enriquez M. The role of policy on sexual health education in schools: Review. J Sch Nurs 2019;35(1):27-38.
[24] Fox AM, Himmelstein G, Khalid H, Howell EA. Funding for abstinence-only education and adolescent pregnancy prevention: Does state ideology affect outcomes? Am J Public Health 2019;109(3):497-504.
[25] Santelli JS, Grilo SA, Choo TH, Diaz G, Walsh K, Wall M, et al. Does sex education before college protect students form sexual assault in college. PloS One 2018; 13(11):e0205951. doi: 10.1371/journal.pone.0205951.
[26] McGregor AJ, Chin EL, Rojek MK, Digre KB, Lopez AM, Jenkins K, et al. Sex and gender health education summit: advancing curricula through a multidisciplinary lens. J Womens Health (Larchmt) 2019;28(12):1728-36.
[27] Cahill SR, Geffen SR, Fontenot HB, Wang TM, Viox MH, Fordyce E, et al. Youth-serving professionals' perspectives on HIV prevention tools and strategies appropriate for adolescent gay and bisexual males and transgender youth. J Pediatr Health Care 2020;34(2):e1-11.
[28] Barros LF, Brown A, Swanson RA. Glia in brain energy metabolism: A perspective. Glia 2018;66(6):1134-7.
[29] Jha MK, Morrison BM. Glia-neuron energy metabolism in health and disease: New insights into the role of nervous system metabolic transporters. Exp Neurol 2018;309: 23-31.
[30] Mosser CA, Baptista S, Arnoux I, Audinat E. Microglia in CNS development: Shaping the brain for the future. Prog Neurobiol 2017;149-150:1-20.
[31] Bilimoria PM, Stevens B. Microglia function during brain development: New insights from animal moels. Brain Res 2015 Aug 18;1617:7-17. doi: 10.1016/j.brainres.2014.11.032.
[32] Greydanus DE, Pratt HD, Patel DR. The first three years of life and the early adolescent: Comparisons and differences. Lessons for child rearing. Int Pediatrics 2004;19:68-80.
[33] Johnston MV, Nishimura A, Harum K, et al. Sculpting the Brain. Adv Pediatrics 2001; 48:1-38.
[34] Chaudhury S, Sharma V, Kumar V, Nag TC, Wadhwa S. Activity-dependent synaptic plasticity modulates the critical phase of brain development. Brain Dev 2016;38(4): 355-63.
[35] Ismail FY, Fatemi A, Johnston MV. Cerebral plasticity: Windows of opportunity in the developing brain. Eur J Paediatr Neurol 2017;21(1):23-48.
[36] Birnie MT, Kooiker CL, Short AK, Bolton JL, Chen Y, Baram TZ. Plasticity of the reward circuitry: After early-life adversity: Mechanisms and significance. Biol Psychiatry 2019 Dec 24. pii: S0006-3223(19)31959-6. doi: 10.1016/j.biopsych.2019.12.018.

[37] Laube C, van den Bos W, Fandakova Y. The relationship between pubertal hormones and brain plasticity: Implications for cognitive training in adolescence. Dev Cogn Neurosci 2020;42:100753. doi: 10.1016/j.dcn.2020.100753.

[38] D'Arcy MS. Cell death: a review of the major forms of apoptosis, necrosis and autophagy. Cell Biol Int 2019;43(6):582-92.

[39] Taghavipour G, Sadoughi F, Mirzaei H, Yousefi B, Moazzami B, Chaichian S, et al. Apoptotic functions of microRNAs in pathogenesis, diagnosis, and treatment of endometriosis. Cell Biosci 2020;10:12. doi: 10.1186/s13578-020-0381-0.

[40] Selemon, L. A role for synaptic plasticity in the adolescent development of executive function. Transl Psychiatry 2013;3:e238. doi:10.1038/tp.2013.7.

[41] Siegel EJ. Adolescent growth and development. In: Greydanus DE, Patel DR, Pratt HD, eds. Essentials of Adolescent Medicine. New York: McGraw-Hill, 2006:1-16.

[42] Biro FM. Puberty. Adol Med State Art Rev 2007;18:425-34.

[43] Omar HA, Merrick J. Adolescents and puberty. In: Merrick J, Omar HA, eds. Adolescent behavior research: International perspectives. New York: Nova Science, 2007:109-14.

[44] Vijayakumar N, Op de Macks Z, Shirtcliff EA, Pfeifer JH. Puberty and the human brain: Insights into adolescent development. Neurosci Biobehav Rev 2018;92:417-436.

[45] Herting MM, Sowell ER. Puberty and structural brain development in humans. Front Neuroendocrinol 2017;44:122-37.

[46] Tanner JM. Growth at adolescence, 2nd ed. Oxford: Blackwell, 1962.

[47] Greydanus DE, Patel DR, Pratt HD, Bhave SY, eds. Course manual for adolescent health. Indian Acad Pediatr. Delhi, India: Cambridge Press, 2002.

[48] Lauffer P, Mooij CF, Zwaveling-Soonawala N, van Trotsenburg ASP. Reforming the male Tanner genital scale. J Pediatr Endocrinol Metab 2020 Feb 12. pii: /j/jpem.ahead-of-print/jpem-2019-0501/jpem-2019-0501.xml. doi: 10.1515/jpem-2019-0501.

[49] Eckert-Lind C, Busch AS, Petersen JH, Biro FM, Butler G, Bräuner EV, et al. Worldwide secular trends in age at pubertal onset assessed by brain development among girls: A systematic review and meta-analysis. JAMA Pediatr 2020 Feb 10:e195881. doi: 10.1001/jamapediatrics.2019.5881.

[50] Houghton LC, Jung S, Troisi R, LeBlanc ES, Snetselaar LG, Hylton NM, et al. Pubertal timing and breast density in young women: a prospective cohort study. Breast Cancer Res 2019;21(1):122. doi: 10.1186/s13058-019-1209-x.

[51] Cheng HL, Harris SR, Sritharan M, Behan MJ, Medlow SD, Steinbeck KS. The tempo of puberty and its relationship to adolescent health and well-being: A systematic review. Acta Paediatr 2019 Nov 15. doi: 10.1111/apa.15092.

[52] Chen FR, Rothman EF, Jaffee SR. Early puberty, friendship group characteristics, and dating abuse in US girls. Pediatrics 2017;139(6). pii: e20162847. doi: 10.1542/peds.2016-2847.

[53] Reinehr T, Kulle A, Barth A, Ackermann J, Lass N, Holterhus PM. Sex hormone profile in pubertal boys with gynecomastia and pseudogynecomastia. J Clin Endocrinol Metab 2020 Jan 30. pii: dgaa044. doi: 10.1210/clinem/dgaa044.

[54] Leung AKC, Leung AAC. Gynecomastia in infants, children, and adolescents. Recent Pat Endocr Metab Immune Drug Discov 2017;10(2):127-37.

[55] Soliman AT, De Sanctis V, Yassin M. Management of adolescent gynecomastia: An update. Acta Biomed 2017;88(2):204-13.

[56] Lantos JD. When deeply held personal beliefs conflict with collective societal norms. Pespect Biol Med 2019;62(3):503-8.

[57] Moore E, Berkley-Patton J, Bohn A, Hawes S, Bowe-Thompson C. Beliefs about sex and parent-child-church sex communication among church-based African American youth. J Relig Health 2015;54(5):1810-25.

[58] McCann E, Donohue G, Timmins F. An exploration of the relationship between spirituality, religion and mental health among youth who identify as LGBT+: A systematic literature review. J Relig Health 2020 Feb 12. doi: 10.1007/s10943-020-00989-7.

[59] Bowker JC, Etkin RG. Evaluating the psychological concomitants of other-sex crush experiences during early adolescence. J Youth Adolesc 2016;45(5):846-57.

[60] Bowker JC, Stotsky MT, White HI, Kamble SV. Being an other-sex crush during early adolescence in India: Investigating socio behavioral and psychological concomitants. J Adolesc 2020;80:115-24.
[61] Chow CM, Ruhl H, Burhmester D. Romantic relationships and psychological distress among adolescents: Moderating role of friendship closeness. Int J Soc Psychiatry 2015; 61(7):711-20.
[62] Brandon M. Monogamy and nonmonogamy: Evolutionary considerations and treatment challenges. Sex Med Rev 2016;4(4):343-52.
[63] Lebovici S. The origins and development of the Oedipus complex. Int J Psychoanal 1982;63(Pt 2):201-15.
[64] Borovecki-Jakovljev S, Matacić S. The Oedipus complex in the contemporary psychoanalysis. Coll Antropol 2005;29(1):351-60.
[65] Hartke R. The Oedipus complex: A confrontation at the central cross-roads of psychoanalysis. Int J Psychoanal 2016;97(3):893-913.
[66] Halberstadt-Freud HC. Electra versus Oedipus. Femininity reconsidered. Int J Psychoanal 1998;79(Pt 1):41-56.
[67] Buchberg L. Oedipus in Brooklyn: reading Freud on women, watching Lena Dunham's girls. Psychoanal Q 2014;83(1):121-50.
[68] Greydanus DE. Overview on adolescence. In: Greydanus DE, Patel DR, Omar HA, Feucht C, Merrick J (eds). Adolescent Medicine: Pharmacotherapeutics in General, Mental, and Sexual Health. Berlin, Germany: De Gruyter, 2012;ch 2: 9-37.
[69] Masselink M, Van Roekel E, Oldehinkel AJ. Self-esteem in early adolescence as predictor of depressive symptoms in late adolescence and early adulthood: The mediating role of motivational and social factors. J Youth Adolesc 2018;47(5):932-46.
[70] D'Amico EJ, Rodriquez A, Tucker JS, Dunbar MS, Pedersen ER, Shih RA, et al. Early and late adolescent factors that predict co-use of cannabis with alcohol and tobacco in young adulthood. Prev Sci 2020 Jan. doi: 10.1007/s11121-020-01086-7.
[71] Smith KL. Sexual science in ancient Greece. Pharos Alpha Omega Alpha Honor Med Soc 2002;65(1):12-7.
[72] Wallis WA. Statistics of the Kinsey report. J Am Stat Assoc 1949;44(248):463-84.
[73] Kinsey AC, Pomeroy WR, Martin CE. Sexual behavior in the human male. 1948. Am J Public Health 2003;93(6):894-8.
[74] Zelnik M, Kantner JF, Ford K. Sex and pregnancy in adolescence. Beverly Hills, CA: Sage, 1981.
[75] Kann L, Warren CW, Harris WA. Collins JL, Williams BI, Ross JG, et al. Youth risk behavior surveillance--United States, 1995. MMWR CDC Surveill Summ 1996;45 (4):1-84.
[76] Matytsina LA, Greydanus DE. Contraception in high school environment. Woman's Health 2006;3(27):115-20.
[77] Regushevskaya E, Dubikaytis T, Nikula M, Kuznetsova O, Hemminki E. The socioeconomic characteristics of risky behaviour among reproductive-age women in St. Petersburg. Scand J Public Health 2008;36(2):143-52.
[78] Stewart DC, Hofmann AD. Adolescent sexuality. In: Hofmann AD, Greydanus DE, eds. Adolescent medicine, 3rd ed. Stamford, CT: Appleton Lange, 1997:457-72.
[79] Kann L, Kinchen SA, Williams BI, Ross JG, Lowry R, Grunbaum JA, et al. Youth risk behavior surveillance system--United States, 1999. MMWR CDC Surveill Summ 2000;49(SS-5):1-32.
[80] Abma JC, Martinez GM, Mosher WD, Dawson BS. Teenagers in the United States: Sexual activity, contraceptive use, and childbearing: 2002. National Center for Health Statistics. Vital Health Stat 2004;23(24):1-2.
[81] Kann L, McManus T, Harris WA, Shanklin SL, Flint KH, Queen B, et al. Youth Risk Behavior Surveillance — United States, 2017. MMWR Surveill Summ 2018;67(SS-8):1–114.
[82] Greydanus DE, Omar HA. Sexuality issues and gynecologic care of adolescents with developmental disabilities. Pediatr Clin North Amer 2008;5(6):1315-35.
[83] Murphy N, Young PC: Sexuality in children and adolescents with disabilities. Dev Med 2005;47:640-4.
[84] Murphy NA, Elias ER. Council on children with disabilities. Pediatrics 2006;118:398-403.

[85] Hibbard RA, Desch LW. Committee on child abuse and neglect and council on children with disabilities. Pediatrics 2007;119(5):1018-21.
[86] Rew L. Sexual health of adolescents with chronic health conditions. Adol Med State Arts Rev 2007;18(3):519-29.
[87] Shandra CL. Research on adolescent sexuality should be inclusive of disability. J Adolesc Health 2018;62(3):253-4.
[88] Kahn NF, Halpern CT. Experiences of vaginal, oral, and anal sex from adolescence to early adulthood in populations with physical disabilities. J Adolesc Health 2018; 62(3): 294-302.
[89] Kahn NF, Suchindran CM, Halpern CT. Variations in the timing of first sexual experiences among populations with physical disabilities in the United States. Disabil Health J 2019;12(2):155-63.
[90] Spinoit AF, Waterschoot M, Sinatti C, Abbas T, Callens N, Cools M, et l. Fertility and sexuality in congenital lifelong urology patients: male aspects. World J Urol 2020 Feb 17. doi: 10.1007/s00345-020-03121-2.
[91] Holland-Hall C, Quint EH. Sexuality and disability in adolescents. Pediatr Clin North Am 2017;64(2):435-49.
[92] Covington SN, Martinex PE, Popat V, Nandagopal R, Ryan M, Nelson LM. The psychology of antecedents to adult reproductive disorders in adolescent girls. Ann NY Acad Sci 2008;1135:155-62.
[93] Greydanus DE, Patel DR. The female athlete: Before and beyond puberty. Pediatric Clin North Am 2002;49:553-80.
[94] Abma JC, Martinez GM. Sexual activity and contraceptive use among teenagers in the United States, 2011-2015. Nat Health Stat Rep 2017;104:1-22.
[95] Kann L, Lindberg LD, Maddow-Zimet I, Marcell AV. Prevalence of sexual initiation before age 13 years among male adolescents and young adults in the United States. JAMA Pediatr 2019;173(6):553-60.
[96] Sieving RE, Gewirtz O'Brien JR, Saftner MA, Argo TA. Sexually transmitted diseases among US adolescents and young adults: Patterns, clinical considerations, and prevention. Nurs Clin North Am 2019;54(2):207-25.
[97] Wangu Z, Burstein GR. Adolescent sexuality: Updates to the sexually transmitted infection guidelines. Pediatr Clin North Am 2017;64(2):389-411.
[98] Bonar EE, Walton MA, Caldwell MT, Whiteside LK, Barry KL, Cunningham RM. Sexually transmitted infection history among adolescents presenting to the emergency department. J Emerg Med 2015;49(5):613-22.
[99] Herlitz CA, Forsberg M. Sexual behaviour and risk assessment in different age cohorts in the general population of Sweden (1989-2007). Scand J Public Health 2010;38(1): 32-9.
[100] Pizzol D, Bertoldo A, Foresta C. Adolescents and web port: a new era of sexuality. Int J Adolesc Med Health 2016;28(2):169-73.
[101] Gesser-Edelsburg A, Abed Elhadi Arabia M. Discourse on exposure to pornography content online between Arab adolescents and parents: Qualitative study on its impact on sexual education and behavior. J Med Internet Res 2018;20(10):e11667. doi: 10.2196/11667.
[102] Overbeek G, van de Bongardt D, Baams L. Buffer or brake? The role of sexuality-specific parenting in adolescents' sexualized media consumption and sexual development. J Youth Adolesc 2018;47(7):1427-39.
[103] Herbenick D, Fu TC, Wright P, Paul B, Gradus R, Bauer J, et al. Diverse sexual behaviors and pornography use: Findings from a nationally representative probability survey of Americans aged 14 to 60 years. J Sex Med 2020 Feb 17. pii: S1743-6095(20)30047-3. doi: 10.1016/j.jsxm.2020.01.013.
[104] Matytsina LA, Greydanus DE, Danisson LL, Pratt HD. Strategies of youth reproductive health and sex educational programs. Woman's Health 2004;4(20):126-35.
[105] Ventriglio A, Bhugra D. Sexuality in the 21st century: Sexual fluidity. East Asian Arch Psychiatry 2019;29(1):30-4.
[106] Rushton A, Gray L, Canty J, Blanchard K. Beyond binary: (Re)Defining "gender" for 21st century disaster risk reduction research, policy, and practice. Int J Environ Res Public Health 2019 Oct 18;16(20). pii: E3984. doi: 10.3390/ijerph16203984.

[107] Ventriglio A, Kalra G, Ghugra D. Human rights and sexuality: sexual fluidity. Lancet Psychiatry 2018;5(2):109-10.

[108] Yang HC. Education first: Promoting LGBT+ friendly healthcare with a competency-based course and game-based teaching. Int J Environ Res Public Health 2019 Dec 22;17(1). pii: E107. doi: 10.3390/ijerph17010107.

[109] Ufomata E, Eckstrand KL, Spagnoletti C, Veet C, Walk TJ, Webb C, et al. Comprehensive curriculum for internal medicine residents on primary care of patients identifying as lesbian, gay, bisexual, or transgender. MedEDPORTAL 2020;16:10875. doi: 10.15766/mep_2374-8265.10875.

[110] Auslander BA, Rosenthal SL, Fortenberry JD, Biro FM, Bernstein DI, Zimet GD. Predictors of sexual satisfaction in an adolescent and college population. J Pediatr Adolesc Gynecol 2007;20(1):25-8.

[111] Baranowski T. Sexual health in the 21st century. Games Health J 2015;4(2):67-8.

[112] Fortenberry JD. Adolescent sexual well-being in the 21st century. J Adolesc Health 2016;58(1):1-2.

[113] Strasburger VC, Donnerstein E. Children, adolescents, and the media in the 21st century. Adolesc Med 2000;11(1):51-68.

[114] Brown JD, Strasburger VC. From Calvin Klein to Paris Hilton and MySpace: Adolescents, sex, and the media. Adolesc Med State Art Rev 2007;18(3):484-507.

[115] Strasburger VC. Adolescents, sex, and the media. Adolesc Med State Art Rev 2012; 23(1):15-33.

[116] Habel MA, Leichliter JS, Dittus PJ, Spicknall IH, Aral SO. Heterosexual anal and oral sex in adolescents and adults in the United States, 2011-2015. Sex Trans Dis 2018; 45(12):775-82.

[117] Halpern-Felsher BL, Cornell JL, Kropp RY, Tschann JM. Oral sex versus vaginal sex among adolescents: perceptions, attitudes, and behavior. Pediatrics 2005;115(4):845-51.

[118] Prinstein MJ, Meade CS, Cohen GL. Adolescent oral sex, peer popularity, and perceptions of best friends' sexual behavior. J Pediatr Psychol 2003;28(4):243-9.

[119] Martin JA, Hamilton BE, Osterman MJK, Driscoll AK, Drake P. Births: final data for 2017. Natl Vital Stat Rep 2018;67(8):1-50.

[120] Greydanus DE. Adolescent pregnancy—a multifaceted problem. Peds Rev 2019. pedsinreview.org/pir40.https://pedsinreview.aappublications.org/sites/default/files/additional_assets/Files/GreydanusDE_AdolPreg1979_PIR.pdf.

[121] Hamilton BE, Rossen LM, Branum Am. Teen birth rates for urban and rural areas in the United States, 2007-2015. NCHS Data Brief 2016;(264):1-8.

[122] Charlton BM, Roberts AL, Rosario M, Katz-Wise SL, Calzo JP, Spiegelman D, et al. Teen pregnancy risk factors among young women of diverse sexual orientations. Pediatrics 2018;141(4). pii: e20172278. doi: 10.1542/peds.2017-2278.

[123] Charlton BM, Nava-Coulter B, Coles MS, Katz-Wise SL. Teen pregnancy experiences of sexual minority women. J Pediatr Adolesc Gynecol 2019;32(5):499-505.

[124] Leftwich HK, Alves MV. Adolescent pregnancy. Pediatr Clin North Am 2017;64(2): 381-8.

[125] McCracken KA, Loveless M. Teen pregnancy: an update. Curr Opin Obstet Gynecol 2014;26(5): 355-9.

[126] Holness N. A global perspective on adolescent pregnancy. Int J Nurs Pract 2015;21(5): 677-81.

[127] Bacopoulou F, Greydanus DE, Chrousos GP. Reproductive and contraceptive issues in chronically ill adolescents. Eur J Contracept Reprod Health Care 2010;15(6):389-404.

[128] Greydanus DE, Rimsza ME, Matytsina L. Contraception for college students. Pediatr Clin North Am 2005;52(1):135-61.

[129] Greydanus DE, Patel DR, Rimsza ME. Contraception in the adolescent: an update. Pediatrics 2001;107(3):562-73.

[130] Ngui EM, Greer DM, Bridgewater FD, Salm Ward TC, Cisler RA. Trends and progress in reducing teen birth rates and the persisting challenge of eliminating racial/ethnic disparities. J Racial Ethn Health Disparities 2017;4(4):615-22.

[131] Apter D. Contraception options: Aspects unique to adolescent and young adult. Best Pract Res Clin Obstet Gynaecol 2018;48:115-27.

[132] Robbins CL, Ott MA. Contraception options and provision to adolescents. Minerva Pediatr 2017;69(5):403-14.

[133] Bahamondes L, Fernandes A, Monteiro I, Bahamondes MV. Long-acting reversible contraceptive (LARCs) methods. Best Pract Res Clin Obstet Gynaecol 2020;66:28-40.

[134] Greydanus DE, Pratt HD, Patel DR. Concepts of contraception for adolescent and young adult women with chronic illness and disability. Dis Mon 2012;58(5):258-320.

[135] Raidoo S, Kaneshiro B. Contraception counseling for adolescents. Curr Opin Obstet Gynecol 2017;29(5):310-5.

[136] Klein JD; American Academy of Pediatrics Committee on Adolescence. Adolescent pregnancy: current trends and issues. Pediatrics 2005;116(1):281-6.

[137] Salas-Wright CP, Vaughn MG, Ugalde J, Todic J. Substance use and teen pregnancy in the United States: evidence from the NSDUH 2002-2012. Addict Behav 2015;45: 218-25.

[138] Noll JG, Guastaferro K, Beal SJ, Schreier HMC, Barnes J, Reader JM, et al. Is sexual abuse a unique predictor of sexual risk behaviors, pregnancy, and motherhood in adolescence? J Res Adoles 2019;29(4):967-83.

[139] Boyer D Fine D. Sexual abuse a factor in adolescent pregnancy and child maltreatment. Fam Plann Perspect 1992;24(1):4-11.

[140] Madigan S, Wade M, Tarabulsy G, Jenkins JM, Shouldice M. Association between abuse history and adolescent pregnancy: a meta-analysis. J Adolesc Health 2014;55(2): 151-9.

[141] Restrepo Martínez M, Trujillo Numa L, Restrepo Bernal D, Torres de Galvis Y, Sierra G. Sexual abuse and neglect situations as risk factors for adolescent pregnancy. Rev Colomb Psiquiatr 2017;46(2):74-81. [Spanish]

[142] Fortin-Langelier E, Daigneault I, Achim J, Vézina-Gagnon P, Guérin V, Frappier JY. A matched cohort study of association between childhood sexual abuse and teenage pregnancy. J Adolesc Health 2019;65(3):384-9.

[143] Soriano-Ayala E, Cala VC, Dalouh R. Adolescent profiles according to their beliefs and affinity to sexting. Int J Environ Res Public Health 2020 Feb 8;17(3). pii: E1087. doi: 10.3390/ijerph17031087.

[144] Ojeda M, Del Rey R, Hunter SC. Longitudinal relationships between sexting and involvement in both bullying and cyberbullying. J Adolesc 2019;77:81-9.

[145] Van Ouytsel J, Lu Y, Ponnet K, Walrave M, Temple JR. Longitudinal associations between sexting, cyberbullying, and bullying among adolescents: Cross-lagged panel analysis. J Adolesc 2019;73:36-41.

[146] Milton AC, Gill BA, Davenport TA Dowling M, Burns JM, Hickie IB. Sexting, web-based risks, and safety in two representative national samples of young Australians: Prevalence, perspectives, and predictors. JMIR Ment Health 2019;6(6):e13338. doi: 10.2196/13338.

[147] El-Gabalawi F, Johnson RA. Hypersexuality in inpatient children and adolescents: Recognition, differential diagnosis, and evaluation. CNS Spectrum 2007;12:821-7.

[148] Efrati Y, Gola M. Understanding and predicting profiles of compulsive sexual behavior among adolescents. J Behav Addict 2018;7(4):1004-14.

[149] Felitti VJ, Anda RF, Nordenberg D, Williamson DF, Spitz AM, Edwards V, et al. Relationship of childhood abuse and household dysfunction to many leading causes of death in adults: The Adverse Childhood Experience (ACE) Study. Am J Prev Med 1998;14(4):245-57.

[150] Felitti VJ, Anda RF, Nordenberg D, Williamson DF, Spitz AM, Edwards V, et al. Relationship of childhood abuse and household dysfunction to many leading causes of death in adults: The Adverse Childhood Experience (ACE) Study. Am J Prev Med 2019;56(6):774-86.

[151] United States Department of Health and Human Services, National Center on Child Abuse and Neglect. Child Maltreatment, 1994: Report from States to the National Center for Child Abuse and Neglect. Washington, DC: US Gov Printing Office, 1996.

[152] American Academy of Pediatrics. Care of the adolescent sexual assault victim. Committee on adolescence. Pediatrics 2001;107:1476-9.

[153] Finkelhor D. Child sexual abuse: New theory and research. New York: Free Press, 1984.

[154] Greydanus DE, Palusci VJ, Merrick J. Chronic disease and disability: Abuse and neglect in childhood and adolescence. NY: Nova Science, 2017.

[155] Rennison CM. Criminal victimization 1998: Changes 1997-1998 with trends 1993 to 1998. Washington DC: Bureau Justice Stat, 1997. Available at http://www.ojp.usdoj.gov/bjs/abstract/cv98.htm.

[156] Wilson M, Joffe A. Adolescent medicine. JAMA 1995;273:1657-9.

[157] Finkelhor V, Hotaling G, Lewis I. Sexual abuse in a national survey of adult men and women: Prevalence, characteristics, and risk factors. Child Abuse Negl 1990;14:9-11.

[158] Grunbaum A, Kann L, Williams B, Ross JG, Lowry R, Kolbe L. Youth risk behavior surveillance --- United States, 2001. CDC Surveill Summ 2002;51(SS:4):1-64.

[159] US Department of Justice. Crime victimization, 2006. Washington, DC: Bureau Justice Stat, 2007.

[160] Muram D. Sexual assault. In: Hillard PJA, ed. The 5-Minute obstetrics and gynecology consult. Philadelphia, PA: Wolters Kluwer/Lippincott Williams Wilkins, 2008:602-3.

[161] Mitchell KJ, Finkelhor D, Wolak J. Risk factors for and impact of online sexual solicitation of youth. JAMA 2001;285:3011-4.

[162] Joppa MC. Dating violence in adolescence: Implications for girls' sexual health. J Pediatr Adolec Gynecol 2020 Feb 19. pii: S1083-3188(20)30160-1. doi: 10.1016/j.jpag.2020.02.007.

[163] Basile KC, Clayton HB, Rostad WL, Leemis RW. Sexual violence victimization of youth and health risk behaviors. Am J Prev Med 2020 Feb 4. pii: S0749-3797(20)30010-6. doi: 10.1016/j.amepre.2019.11.020.

[164] Halpern CT, Oslak SG, Young ML, Martin SL, Kupper LL. Partner violence among adolescents in opposite-sex romantic relationships: Findings from the National Longitudinal Study of Adolescent Health. Am J Publ Health 2001;91(10):1679-85.

[165] Lin AJ, Raymond M, Catallozzi M, Ryan O, Rickert VI. Relationship of violence in adolescence. Adolesc Med State Art Rev 2007;18(3):530-43.

[166] Pratt HD, Greydanus DE: Adolescent violence: Concepts for a new millennium. Adolesc Med 2000;11:103-25.

[167] Greydanus DE, Kaplan G, Patel DR, Merrick J, eds) Substance use disorders in adolescents and young adults. A manual for pediatric and primary care clinicians. New York: Nova Science, 2019; 389 pages.

[168] Murshid NS, Murshid N. Intergenerational transmission of marital violence: Results from a nationally representative sample of men. J Interpers Violence 2018;33(2):211-27.

[169] Hornsveld RHJ, Zwets AJ, Leenaars EPEM, Kraaimaat FW, Bout R, Lagro-Janssen TALM, et al. Violent female offenders compared to violent male offenders on psychological determinants of aggressive behaviors. Int J Offender Ther Comp Criminol 2018;62(2):460-7.

[170] Seidl H, Nilsson T, Hofvander B, Billstedt E, Wallinius M. Personality and cognitive functions in violent offenders – Implications of character maturity? Front Psychol 2020 Jan 28;11:58. doi: 10.3389/fpsyg.2020.00058.

[171] Thibaut F, Bradford JM, Briken P, De La Barra F, Häßler F, Cosyns P; WFSBP Task Force on Sexual Disorders. The World Federation of Societies of Biological Psychiatry (WFSBP) guidelines for the treatment of adolescent sexual offenders with paraphilic disorders. World J Biol Psychiatry 2016;17(1):2-38.

[172] US General Accounting Office. Homeless children and youths. Washington, DC: US Gov Account Office, 1989.

[173] Finkelhor D, Hotaling G, Sedlak A. Missing, abducted, runaway, and throwaway children in America. First Report: Numbers and characteristics. Washington, DC: Department Justice, Office Juvenile Justice Delinquency Prev, 1990.

[174] Pratt HD. Homeless adolescents in the United States. Int Pediatr 2002;17:70-6.

[175] Abdalian SE. Street youth mortality. Leaning with intent to fall. JAMA 2004;292:624-6.

[176] Farrow JA, Deisher W, Brown R, Kulig JW, Kipke MD. Health and health needs of homeless and runaway youth: A position paper of the Society for Adolescent Medicine. J Adolesc Health 1992;13(8):717-26.

[177] Bell DL, Ginsburg KR. Connecting the adolescent male with health care. Adolesc Med 2003;14:555-64.

[178] Gerassi L. From exploitation to industry: Definitions, risks, and consequences of domestic sexual exploitation and sex work among women and girls. J Hum Behav Soc Environ 2015;25(6):591-605.

[179] Greenbaum VJ. Commercial sexual exploitation and sex trafficking of children in the United States. Curr Probl Pediatr Adolesc Health Care 2014;44(9):245-69.
[180] Moore JL, Kaplan DM, Barron CE. Sex trafficking of minors. Pediatr Clin North Am 2017;64(2):413-21.
[181] Franchino-Olsen H. Vulnerabilities relevant for commercial sexual exploitation of children/domestic minor sex trafficking: A systematic review of risk factors. Trauma Violence Abuse 2019 Feb 3:1524838018821956. doi: 10.1177/1524838018821956.
[182] Noh D. Psychological interventions for runaway and homeless youth. J Nurs Scholarsh 2018;50(5):465-72.
[183] Wang JZ, Mott S, Magwood O, Mathew C, Mclellan A, Kpade V, et al. The impact of interventions for youth experiencing homelessness on housing, mental health substance use, and family cohesion: a systematic review. BMC Public Health 2019;19(1):1528. doi: 10.1186/s12889-019-7856-0.
[184] Alessi EJ, Greenfield B, Manning D, Dank M. Victimization and resilience among sexual and gender minority homeless youth engaging in survival sex. J Interpers Violence 2020 Jan 10:886260519898434. doi: 10.1177/0886260519898434.
[185] Quintyne F, Harpin SB, How hospital practitioners can support sofa surfing adolescents to access community mental health services: An English perspective. Clin Child Psychol Psychiatry 2020 Feb 12:1359104520905072. doi: 10.1177/1359104520905072.
[186] Strasburger VC, Greydanus DE. The at-risk adolescent. Adolesc Med 1990;1:1-198.
[187] Strasburger VC, Greydanus DE. At-risk adolescents: An update for the new century. Adolesc Med 2000;11:1-210.
[188] Marcell AV, Monasterio EB. Providing anticipatory guidance and counseling to the adolescent male. Adolesc Med 2003;14:565-82.
[189] Rosen DS, Rich M. The adolescent male. Adolesc Med 2003;14:525-37.
[190] Kanuga M, Rosenfeld WD. Adolescent sexuality and the internet: the good, the bad, and the URL. J Pediatr Adolesc Gynecol 2004;17:117-24.
[191] Greydanus DE, Dewdney D. Homosexuality in adolescence. Sem Adol Med 1985;1: 117-30.
[192] Sison AC, Greydanus DE. Deconstructing adolescent same-sex attraction and sexual behavior in the twenty-first century: Perspectives for the clinician. Prim Care Clin Off Pract 2007;34:293-304.
[193] Rowlett JD, Greydanus DE. Homosexuality in adolescence. Adolesc Med 1994;5:509-26.
[194] Frankowski BL. Committee on Adolescence. American Academy of Pediatrics. Sexual orientation and adolescents. Pediatrics 2004;13:1827-32.
[195] American Academy of Pediatrics. Homosexuality and adolescence. Committee on Adolescence. Pediatrics 1993;92:631-4.
[196] Workowski KA, Bolan GA; Centers for Disease Control and Prevention. Sexually transmitted diseases treatment guidelines, 2015. MMWR Recomm Rep 2015;64(RR-03):1-137.
[197] Achterbergh RCA, Drückler S, van Rooijen MS, van Aar F, Slurink IAL, de Vries HJC, et al. Sex, drugs, and sexually transmitted infections: A latent class analysis among men who have sex with men in Amsterdam and surrounding urban regions, the Netherlands. Drug Alcohol Depend 2020;206:107526.
[198] Garofalo R, Harper GW. Not all adolescents are the same: addressing the unique needs of gay and bisexual male youth. Adolesc Med 2003;14:595-611.
[199] Catallozzi M, Rudy BJ. Lesbian, gay, bisexual, transgendered, and questioning youth: the importance of a sensitive and confidential sexual history in identifying the risk and implementing treatment for sexually transmitted infections. Adolesc Med 2004;15: 353-67.
[200] Grant R, Nash M, Hansen E. What does inclusive sexual and reproductive healthcare look like for bisexual, pansexual and queer women? Findings from an exploratory study from Tasmania, Australia. Cult Health Sex 2020;22(3):247-60.
[201] Morandini JS, Blaszczynski A, Dar-Nimrod I. Who adopts queer and pansexual identifies? J Sex Res 2017;54(7):911-22.
[202] Greaves LM, Barlow FK, Lee CHJ, Matika CM, Wang W, Lindsay CJ, et al. The diversity and prevalence of sexual orientation self-labels in a New Zealand national sample. Arch Sex Behav 2017;46(5):1325-36.

[203] Graham K, Treharne GJ, Ruzibiza C, Nicolson M. The importance of health(ism): A focus group of lesbian, gay, bisexual, pansexual, queer and transgender individuals' understandings of health. J Health Psychol 2017;22(2):237-47.

[204] Galupo MP, Lomash E, Mitchell RC. "All of my lovers fit into this scale": Sexual minority individuals' responses to two novel measures of sexual orientation. J Homosex 2017;64(2):145-65.

[205] Agana MG, Greydanus DE, Indyk JA, Calles JL Jr., Kushner J, Leibowitz S, Cabral MD. Caring for the transgender adolescent and young adult: Current concepts of an evolving process in the 21st century. Dis Mon 2019;65(9):303-56.

[206] Balter M. Behavioral genetics. Can epigenetics explain homosexuality puzzle? Science 2015;350(6257):148. doi: 10.1126/science.350.6257.148.

[207] Tu D, Xu R, Zhao G, Wang B, Feng T. Research progress on molecular genetics of male homosexuality. Zhonghua Yi Xue Yi Chuan Xue Za Zhi 2016;33(4):569-72. [Article in Chines]

[208] Jordan B. End of the road for the homosexuality gene. Med Sci (Paris) 2020;36(2): 181-4. [French]

[209] Haag ES. One gene is not enough to explain the evolution of homosexuality. Arch Sex Behav 2019 Nov 8. doi: 10.1007/s10508-019-01575-z.

[210] Allen L, Gorski R. Sexual orientation and the size of the anterior commissure in the human brain. Proc Natl Acad Sci USA 1992;89:7199-202.

[211] Savic I, Lindstrom P: PET and MRI show differences in cerebral asymmetry and functional connectivity beteen homo- and heterosexual subjects. PNAS Early Edition (National Academy of Sciences of the USA) 2009. URL: www.pnas org/cgi/doi.10.1073/pnas.0801566105.

[212] Friedman RC, Downey JI. Homosexuality. N Engl J Med 1994;331(14):923-30.

[213] Pillard RC, Bailey JM. A biologic perspective on sexual orientation. Psychiatr Clin North Am 1995;18:71-84.

[214] Wang Y, Wu H, Sun ZS. The biological basis of sexual orientation: How hormonal, genetic, and environmental factors influence to whom we are sexually attracted. Front Neuroendocrinol 2019;55:100798. doi: 10.1016/j.yfrne.2019.100798.

[215] Hubbard KA, Griffiths DA. Sexual offense, diagnosis, and activism: A British history of LGBTIQ psychology. Am Psychol 2019;74(8):940-53.

[216] Patra S. Conversion therapy for homosexuality: serious violation of ethics. Indian J Med Ethics 2016;1(3):194-5.

[217] American Psychiatric Association. Diagnostic and statistical manual of mental disorders, DSM-IV, 4th ed. (Text revision; DSM-IV-TR). Washington, DC: Am Psychiatric Association, 2000.

[218] American Psychiatric Association. Diagnostic and statistical manual of mental disorders, fifth edition (DSM-5). Arlington, VA: American Psychiatric Association, 2013.

[219] International classification of diseases and related health problems, 10th rev. Geneva: WHO, ICD-10, 2004.

[220] Wanta JW, Unger CA. Review of the transgender literature: Where do we go from here? Transgend Health 2017;2(1):119-28.

[221] Winter S. Gender trouble: The World Health Organization, the International Statistical Classification of Diseases and Related Health Problems (ICD-11) and the trans kids. Sex Health 2017;14(5):423-30.

[222] Drescher J. Queer diagnoses revisited: The past and future of homosexuality and gender diagnoses in DSM and ICD. Int Rev Psychiatry 2015;27(5):386-95.

[223] Allen LB, Glicken AD, Beach RK, Naylor KE. Adolescent health care experience of gay, lesbian, and bisexual young adults. J Adolesc Health 1998;23(4):212-20.

[224] East JA, El Rayess F. Pediatricians' approach to the health care of lesbian, gay, and bisexual youth. J Adolesc Health 1998;23:191-3.

[225] Ryan CR, Futterman D, eds. Gay and lesbian youth. Adolesc Med 1997;8(2):199-397.

[226] Alexander B, Schrauber S: Outside the margins: youth who are different and their special health care needs. Prim Care Clin Off Pract 2006;33(2):285-303.

[227] Kinsey A, Pomeroy W, Martin C. Sexual behavior in the human male. Philadelphia, PA: WB Saunders, 1948.

[228] Kinsey A, Pomeroy W, Martin C, Gebbard P. Sexual behavior in the human female. Philadelphia, PA: WB Saunders, 1953.

[229] Bell A, Weinberg M: Homosexuality: A study of diversity among men and women. New York: Simon Schuster, 1978.
[230] McConaghy N, Armstrong B, Birrell P, Buhrich N. The incidence of bisexual feelings and opposite sex behavior in medical students. J Nerv Ment Dis 1979;167(11):685-8.
[231] Remafedi G, Resnick M, Blum R, Harris L. Demography of sexual orientation in adolescents. Pediatrics 1992;89(4 Pt 2):714-21.
[232] Seidman SN, Rieder RO. A review of sexual behavior in the United States. Am J Psychiatr 1994;151:330-41.
[233] Diamond M. Homosexuality and bisexuality in different populations. Arch Sex Behav 1993;22:291-310.
[234] Sell RL, Wells JA, Wyrij D. The prevalence of homosexual behavior and attraction in the United States, the United Kingdom, and France: Results of national population-based samples. Arch Sex Behav 1995;24:235-48.
[235] Rahman Q, Xu Y, Lippa RA, Vasey PL. Prevalence of sexual orientation across 28 nations and its association with gender equality, economic development, and individualism. Arch Sex Behav 2020;49(2):595-606.
[236] Green R, ed. Sexual identity conflict in children and adults. New York: Basic Books, 1974.
[237] Troiden RT. Becoming homosexual: A model of gay identity acquisition. Psychiatry 1979;42:362-73.
[238] Troiden R. Homosexual identity development. J Adoles Health Care 1989;9(2):105-13.
[239] Dundas S. Family therapy in gay and lesbian-parented families. J Gay Les Med Assoc 1997;1:111-7.
[240] Moon D. Beyond the dichotomy: sex religious views of homosexuality. J Homosex 2014;61(9):1215-41.
[241] Mbote DK, Sandfort TGM, Waweru E, Zapfel A. Kenyan religious leaders' views on same-sex sexuality and gender nonconformity: religious freedom versus constitutional rights J Sex Res 2018;55(4-5):630-41.
[242] Darmansjah D, Kalra G, Ventriglio A. Religion, psychiatry, and alternative sexuality. East Asian Arch Psychiatry 2019;29(1):26-9.
[243] Lane J. Using queer phenomenology to disrupt heteronormativity and deconstruct homosexuality. J Homosex 2020 Mar 6:1-20. doi: 10.1080/00918369.2020.1733353.
[244] Calvo V, Cusinato M, Meneghet N, Miscioscia M. Perceived social support mediates the negative impact of insecure attachment orientations on internalized homophobia in gay men. J Homosex 2020 Mar 4:1-19. doi: 10.1080/00918369.2020.1734378.
[245] Lee H, Operario D, Yi H, Choo S, Kim SS. Internalized homophobia, depressive symptoms, and suicidal ideation among lesbian, bay, and bisexual adults in South Korea: An age-stratified analysis. LGBT Health 2019;6(8):393-9.
[246] Thorstad D. Homosexuality and the American left: the impact of Stonewall. J Homosex 1995;29(4):319-49.
[247] Thorstad D. Man/boy love and the American gay movement. J Homosex 1990;20(1-2):251-74.
[248] McNaught B. A disturbed peace: Selected writings of an Irish Catholic homosexual. Washington, DC: Dignity, 1981.
[249] Fisher K, Funke J. The age of attraction: age, gender and the history of modern male homosexuality. Gend Hist 2019;31(2)::266-83.
[250] Davies RD, Davies ME. The (slow) depathologizing of gender incongruence. J Nerv Ment Dis 2020;208(2):152-4.
[251] Morris B J. A brief history of lesbian, gay, bisexual and transgender social movements. URL: https://www.apa.org/pi/lgbt/resources/history.
[252] Pew Research Center. Changing attitudes on same-sex marriage. URL: https://www.pewforum.org/fact-sheet/changing-attitudes-on-gay-marriage/.
[253] Allen LB, Glicken AD. Depression and suicide in gay and lesbian adolescents. Phys Assist 1996;20:44-60.
[254] Remafedi G. Fundamental issues in the care of homosexual youth. Med Clin North Am 1990;74(5):1169-76.

[255] Remafedi G, Farrow JA, Deisher RW. Risk factors for attempted suicide in gay and lesbian youth. Pediatrics 1991;87:869-75.
[256] Fulginiti A, Goldbach JT, Mamey MR, Rusow J, Srivastava A, Rhoades H, et al. Integrating minority stress theory and the interpersonal theory of suicide among sexual minority youth who engage crisis services. Suicide Life Threat Behav 2020 Feb 12. doi: 10.1111/sltb.12623.
[257] Frimpong EY, Rowan GA, Williams D, Li M, Solano L, Chaudhry S, et al. Health disparities, inpatient stays, and emergency room visits among lesbian, gay, and bisexual people: Evidence from a mental health system. Psychiatr Serv 2020;71(2):128-35.
[258] Escobar-Viera CG, Whitfield DL, Wessel CB, Shensa A, Sidani JE, Brown AL, et al. For better or for worse? A systematic review of the evidence on social media use and depression among lesbian, gay, and bisexual minorities. JMIR Ment Health 2018;5(3): e10496. doi: 10.2196/10496.
[259] Lampalzer U, Behrendt P, Dekker A, Briken P, Nieder TO. The needs of LGBTI people regarding health care structures, prevention measures and diagnostic and treatment procedures: A qualitative study in a German metropolis. Int J Environ Res Public Health 2019 Sep 22;16(19). pii: E3547. doi: 10.3390/ijerph16193547.
[260] Greydanus DE, Codde JR. The transgender teen: Our duty to help! Int J Adolesc Med Health 2020; 32(2):1-3.
[261] Ford C, English A, Sigman G. Confidential health care for adolescents: Position paper of the Society for Adolescent Medicine. J Adolesc Health 2004;35:160-7.
[262] Lyren A, Silber TJ. Consent, confidentiality, and other related issues in the care of adolescents: medical, legal, ethical, and practical considerations. In: Greydanus DE, Patel DR, Pratt HD, eds. Essential Adolescent Medicine. New York: McGraw-Hill Med, 2005:444-54.
[263] English A. Sexual and reproductive health care for adolescents: Legal rights and policy challenges. Adolesc Med State Art Rev 2007; 18(3):571-81.
[264] Greydanus DE, Patel DR. Consent and confidentiality in adolescent health care. Pediatr Ann 1991;20:34-40.
[265] American Psychological Association. Guidelines for psychological practice with transgender and gender non-coforming people. Am Psychol 2015;70(9):832-64.
[266] Deutsch MB, ed. Guidelines for the primary and gender-affirming care of transgender and gender Nonbinary people, 2 edition. San Francisco, CA: : Center of Excellence for Transgender Health, Department of Family and Community Medicine, University of California San Francisco, 2016. URL: www.transhealth.ucsf.edu/guidelines.
[267] Döring N. Sexuality education on the internet: From Dr. Sommer to Dr. Google. Bundesgesundheitsblatt Gesundheitsforschung Gesundheitsschutz 2017;60(9):1016 1026. [German]
[268] de Santisteban P, Del Hoyo J, Alcázar-Córcoles MÁ, Gámex-Guadix M. Progression, maintenance, and feedback of online child sexual grooming: A qualitative analysis of online predators. Child Abuse Negl 2018;80:203-15.
[269] Kloess JA, Hamilton-Giachritsis CE, Beech AR. Offense processes of online sexual grooming and abuse of children via internet communication platforms. Sex Abuse 2019;31(1):73-96.
[270] Gámex-Guadix M, Almendros C, Calvete E, De Santisteban P. Persuasion strategies and sexual solicitations and interactions in online sexual grooming of adolescents: Modeling direct and indirect pathways. J Adolesc 2018;63:11-8.
[271] Thoma BC, Salk RH, Choukas-Bradley S, Goldstein TE, Levine MD, Marshal MP. Suicidality disparities between transgender and cisgender adolescents. Pediatrics 2019 Nov;144(5). pii: e20191183. doi: 10.1542/peds.2019-1183.
[272] Orr L, Shebl FM, Heimer R, Khoshnood K, Barbour R, Khouri D, et al. Violence and discrimination against men who have sex with men in Lebanon: The role of international displacement and migration. J Interpers Violence 2019 Oct 28:886260519884684. doi: 10.1177/0886260519884684.
[273] Salway T, Ferlatte O, Gesink D, Lachowsky NJ. Prevalence of exposure to sexual orientation change efforts and associated sociodemographic characteristics and psychosocial health outcomes among Canadian sexual minority men. Can J Psychiatry 2020 Jan 26:706743720902629. doi: 10.1177/0706743720902629.

[274] McGeorge CR, Carlson TS, Toomey RB. An exploration of family therapists' beliefs about the ethics of conversion therapy: the influence of negative beliefs and clinical competence with lesbian, gay, and bisexual clients. J Marital Fam Ther 2015;41(1):42-56.

[275] Streed CG Jr., Anderson JS, Babits C, Ferguson MA. Changing medical practice, not patients – putting an end to conversion therapy. N Engl J Med 2019;381(6):500-2.

[276] Hosek S, Henry-Reid L. PrEP and adolescents: The role of providers in ending the AIDS epidemic. Pediatrics 2020 Jan;145(1). pii: e20191743. doi: 10.1542/peds.2019 1743.

[277] Sullivan MC, Cruess DG, Huedo-Medina TB, Kalichman SC. Substance use, HIV serostatus disclosure, and sexual risk behavior in people living with HIV: An event-level analysis. Arch Sex Behav 2019 Dec 20. doi: 10.1007/s10508-019-01531-x.

[278] Dallelucci CC, Bragiato EC, Areco KCN, Fidalgo TM, da Silveira DX. Sexual risk behavior, cocaine and alcohol use among substance users in an outpatient facility: a cross section study. Subst Abuse Treat Prev Policy 2019;14(1):46. doi: 10.1186/s13011-019-0238-x.

[279] Bond KT, Yoon IS, Houang ST, Downing MJ Jr., Grov C, Hirshfield S. Transactional sex, substance use, and sexual risk: Comparing pay direction for an internet-based U.S. sample of men who have sex with men. Sex Res Social Policy 2019;16(3):255-67.

[280] Edmundson C, Heinsbroek E, Glass R, Hope V, Mohammed H, White M, et al. Sexualised drug use in the United Kingdon (UK): A review of the literature. Int J Drug Policy 2018;55:131-48.

[281] Hibbert MP, Brett CE, Porcellato LA, Hope VD. Psychosocial and sexual characteristics associated with sexualised drug use and chemsex among men who have sex with men (MSM) in the UK. Sex Transm Infect 2019;95(5):342-50.

[282] Mohammadi MR, Khaleghi A. Transsexualism: A different viewpoint to brain changes. Clin Psychopharmacol Neurosci 2018;16(2):136-43.

[283] Jackson KM, Rogers ML, Sartor CE. Parental divorce and initiation of alcohol use in early adolescence. Psychol Addict Behav 2016;30(4):450-61.

[284] Deighton S, Neville A, Pusch D, Dobson K. Biomarkers of adverse childhood experiences: A scoping review. Psychiatry Res 2018;269:719-32.

[285] Savoy M, O'Gurek D, Brown-James A. Sexual health history: Techniques and tips. Am Fam Physician 2020;101(5):286-93.

[286] Blanco JL, Ambrosioni J, Garcia F. COVID-19 in patients with HIV: Clinical case series. Lancet HIV 2020;7(5):e314-6.

[287] Hussein J. COVID-19: What implications for sexual and reproductive health and rights globally?. Sex Reprod Health Matters 2020;28(1):1746065. doi:10.1080/26410397.2020.1746065.

[288] Ghosh R, Dubey MJ, Chatterjee S, Dubey S. Impact of COVID -19 on children: special focus on the psychosocial aspect. Minerva Pediatr 2020;72(3):226-35. doi:10.23736/S0026-4946.20.05887-9.

[289] Jing Y, Run-Qian L, Hao-Ran W, Hao-Ran O, Ya-Bin L, Yang G, et al. Potential influence of COVID-19/ACE2 on the female reproductive system. Mol Hum Reprod 2020;26(6):367-73. doi:10.1093/molehr/gaaa030.

[290] Hough S. From the Editor of Sexuality and Disability: The impact of COVID-19 on sexuality and disability-are we closer or more isolated? Sex Disabil 2020;1-2. doi:10.1007/s11195-020-09634-3.

[291] Reddock R, Reid SD, Nickenig T. Child sexual abuse and the complexities of gender, power, and sexuality. J Interpers Violence 2022;37(1-2):NP176-NP208.

[292] Sansone A, Limoncin E, Colonnello E, Mollaioli D, Ciocca G, Corona G, et al. Harm reduction in sexual medicine. Sex Med Rev 2022;10(1):3-22.

[293] Toplu-Demirtaş E, Öztemür G, Fincham FD. Perceptions of dating violence: Assessment and antecedents. J Interpers Violence 2022;37(1-2):NP48-75.

[294] Enszer JR. Lesbian vitality: a provocation. J Lesbian Stud 2022;26(1):113-9.

[295] Fansher AK, Zedaker SB. The relationship between rape myth acceptance and sexual behaviors. J Interpers Violence 2022;37(1-2):NP903-NP924.

[296] Laursen L, Hebert L, Newton S, Norcott C, Gilliam M. Community violence exposure and adolescent pregnancy in Chicago. J Interpers Violence 2022;37(1-2):NP742-56.

[297] Ferguson CJ, Hartley RD. Pornography and sexual aggression: Can meta-analysis find a link? Trauma Violence Abuse 2022;23(1):278-87.

[298] Ferragut M, Rueda P, Cerezo MV, Ortiz-Tallo M. What do we know about child sexual abuse? Myths and truths in Spain. J Interpers Violence 2022;37(1-2):NP757-75.
[299] Chopin J, Beauregard E. Sexual sadism: Its role in the crime-commission process of sexual homicide of children. J Interpers Violence 2022;37(1-2):NP350-74.
[300] Finnie RKC, Okasako-Schmucker DL, Buchanan L, Carty D, Wethington H, Mercer SL, et al.; Community Preventive Services Task Force. Intimate partner and sexual violence prevention among youth: A community guide systematic review. Am J Prev Med 2022;62(1):e45-55.

Chapter 7

Child and adolescent gender identity, nonconformity, and dysphoria: An overview

Lydia Stetson*, **MA**
Outpatient Counseling, Rise Counseling Group and Holistic Wellness Center, Portage, Michigan, United States of America

Abstract

Gender nonconformity, gender identity, gender expression, and gender dysphoria are terms that, anecdotally, are gaining more traction in everyday culture. These terms may be lumped into the overall discussion about gender or even used interchangeably; however, it is important to have a solid understanding of each these concepts individually. Healthcare providers particularly are often in a position to educate and assist youth as well as families with navigating concerns that may come with a young person's developing gender identity. This discussion will begin to explore the many complexities of children's and adolescent's experiences of gender identity, gender nonconformity, and gender dysphoria within the framework of healthcare.

Introduction

It is essential for healthcare providers to refrain from pathologizing deviations from stereotypical gender constructs. As recently as in the Diagnostic and statistical manual, Fourth edition, Text Revision (DSM-IV-TR), gender identity that fell outside of traditional gender roles corresponding with biological sex could be labelled as gender identity disorder (1). In the most recent iteration of the DSM, the DSM-5, gender identity disorder has been replaced with gender dysphoria (2, 3). This new diagnosis of gender dysphoria is worded as such so as to emphasis the distress experienced by the individual, rather than stigmatizing the individual as disordered (3). Nonetheless, work must still be done to move away from the idea that cis-gender identities are the "norm" and that individuals with gender identities that do not correspond with natal sex are somehow abnormal (4).

---

* ***Correspondence:*** Email: Lydia.m.stetson@gmail.com.

In: Behavioral Pediatrics II
Editors: Donald E. Greydanus, Dilip R. Patel, Ahsan Nazeer et al.
ISBN: 979-8-88697-019-7

While healthcare providers should not pathologize nonconforming gender identities, providers should understand the impacts nonconformity has on an individual's wellbeing (5, 6). The Standards of Care put forth by the World Professional Association for Transgender Health (WPATH) cautions providers to be mindful of minority stress that may be faced by gender non-conforming individuals which may lead to the development of mental health and other concerns related to wellbeing (6). Indeed, a diagnosis of gender dysphoria requires that there is significant distress directly related to incongruence between an individual's experienced and/or expressed gender and the individual's assigned gender (3, 6).

Table 1. Basic terminology pertaining to gender identity (7)

Cisgender	Indicates congruence between one's experienced/expressed gender and sex assigned at birth.
Deadname/Deadnaming	Using a former/birth name for an individual when they have changed their name, socially and/or legally, as part of their gender transition.
Gender Binary	Viewing gender as a binary system, that is, only male or only female
Gender Expansive	Umbrella term referring to people who may or may not express or experience their gender within traditional social constructs.
Gender Dysphoria	Significant distress cause by incongruence between one's experienced/expressed gender and sex assigned at birth.
Gender Identity	One's internal experience of gender
Gender Nonconforming	Refers to an individual who eschews traditional gender roles, norms, experience, or expression associated with their sex assigned at birth.
Gender Variance	Refers to the full spectrum of gender rather than viewing gender as a binary construct.
LGBTQ+	Acronym used as an umbrella term to indicate persons who identify as Lesbian, Gay, Bisexual, Trans*, Queer/Questioning, Pansexual, Agender, Asexual, Gender Expansive/Nonconforming, or other identities associated with sexual orientation or identity and/or gender identity.
Natal Sex/Sex Assigned at Birth	Term referring to a person's sex assigned at birth due to physical characteristics which may or may not match a person's gender identity.
Nonbinary	Term referring to a person who identifies as neither or both male and female.
Sexual Identity	How one conceptualizes themselves in terms of who they are romantically or sexually attracted to.
Sexual Orientation	To whom a person is sexually attracted in terms of gender(s) or gender identity.
Transgender/Trans*	A person whose gender identity does not correspond with their natal sex.

It is imperative for healthcare providers to understand that not all gender nonconforming individuals will experience gender dysphoria and that individuals who do experience gender dysphoria will likely not experience it for the entirety of their lives (6). Long-term or chronic dysphoria may contribute to individuals seeking out of healthcare assessment or treatment; yet there remains a lack of education amongst the healthcare community as to effectively working with the gender nonconforming population or those experiencing gender dysphoria (7). In order to provide competent care, healthcare professionals should at the very least have an understanding of gender beyond the binary, i.e., beyond the limited framework of gender as only male or female, how gender nonconformity may influence healthcare needs, and the impact of gender dysphoria.

This discussion reviews basic terminology, differentiates gender dysphoria from gender nonconformity and gender identity, explores the role of healthcare professionals in navigating gender identity as well as expression, and considers the role of healthcare professionals in providing education to families of gender diverse youth. Finally, in the summary of this discussion, it is concluded that further steps towards gender affirming care and inclusivity are necessary within the field of healthcare.

Gender identity and gender nonconformity

As with gender as a whole, gender variance exists on a spectrum with various points on the spectrum. These include identifying with one's natal sex yet expressing their gender in ways outside of the sociocultural norms, identifying as nonbinary (i.e., identifying as neither or both male and female), or identifying and presenting as a gender other than their natal sex (7). Gender identity is commonly thought to develop in early childhood, specifically during the toddler years, with children as young as 18 to 24 months old able to identify their and others' genders (8). A child's gender identity may begin to show stability around three to four years of age (9). Moving into adolescence and puberty, youth place more focus on exploring their identity and who they are in the world in addition to undergoing physical changes (10). Children may also show more transient interest in play or activities not associated with their natal sex or that are more gender neutral than adolescents or adults. Transient interests should also be distinguished from children who show persistent or insistent interest in gender nonconforming play, activities, presentation, or identity (9).

Gender nonconforming children may choose to play with toys or games not typically associated with their natal sex and throughout childhood they may explore gender nonconforming play as well as roles. Gender nonconformity in childhood may lead to children experiencing pressure from peers, family, or others to engage in play or roles more typically associated with their natal sex, which may in turn lead to internalized concerns such as anxiety or low self-esteem (9). In the media, at school, and amongst peers, children may receive messages that some activities are "for boys" and are more masculine: these include rough-and-tumble play; playing with cars, trucks, or trains; or interest in contact sports. Other activities are more feminine and are "for girls:" these include playing with dolls, playing house, or interest in makeup or fashion. Research suggests that the importance placed on gender conformity in childhood varies and may be of higher import in kindergarten and adolescence versus lower import during middle childhood (11).

Research also suggests that gender nonconformity is linked to higher rates of victimization by peers in adolescence (11, 12). Furthermore, youths who are gender nonconforming and who experience same sex attraction to others face additional stressors from peers, families, and others (12). Although these risks and stressors do not negate a child's nonconforming gender identity development, they may be barriers to these children being able to express their experienced gender safely; this is discussed further in later sections.

Gender dysphoria

It is important to stress that gender identity is not a disorder and is not pathological even when it varies from generally accepted sociocultural norms. It is also important to reiterate that not all youth who identify as gender nonconforming will experience gender dysphoria. Gender dysphoria as a diagnosis also differentiates between gender dysphoria in childhood versus gender dysphoria in adolescence and adulthood; both, however, include significant incongruence between natal sex/sex assigned at birth and experienced/expressed gender and intense desire to be a different gender than what was assigned at birth.

Children who experience gender dysphoria may indicate strong preference or insistence on dressing in ways not stereotypically associated with their natal sex, preference for friends of the other gender, preference for toys or activities not stereotypically associated with their natal sex, and dislike of their anatomy. Conversely, adolescents who experience gender dysphoria may desire to be and/or be identified or treated as a gender other than which corresponds with their natal sex, desire to not have the primary and/or secondary sex characteristics associated with natal sex, to have the primary and/or secondary sex characteristic of another gender, or holding strong belief that their experiences or reactions are indicative of a gender other than that associated with their natal sex (13, 14).

A diagnosis of gender dysphoria in childhood often does not persist into adolescence or adulthood with some research suggesting that gender dysphoria desists for up to 80% of adolescents who experienced gender dysphoria prior in childhood (10, 15). Although, as of yet, there are no definitive indicators which identify whether gender dysphoria will persist beyond childhood, it is suggested that in cases in which gender dysphoria does persist, children will state more definitively that they are another gender rather than that they feel more like another gender (15). Typically, medical intervention such as puberty suppression are not suggested or completed unless gender dysphoria persists or intensifies during puberty, specifically for youth in Tanner stages II through III of puberty and interventions taken for younger children are typically reversible (9, 10).

Physical changes associated with puberty may be uncomfortable for even cis-gender adolescents. For adolescents experiencing gender dysphoria, the physical changes of puberty, if no medical intervention has been provided, are often even more uncomfortable and distressing. For adolescents experiencing gender dysphoria, the physical changes of puberty may serve to further accentuate the incongruence between their natal sex and their experienced or expressed gender. This contributes to mental health concerns, self-harm or suicidality, poor body image, and low self-esteem making timely, gender affirming care necessary and even life-saving (16).

It is noted that one particular line of research considers the prevalence of gender dysphoria alongside autism spectrum disorder (ASD) (17-19). This line of research suggests that younger children view gender more rigidly than older children and that children with ASD who show more general rigidity may then experience greater gender dysphoria (17). Nonetheless, treatment should be based on the level of distress and not on the clinician's hypothesis as to whether ASD or gender dysphoria are entirely separate or if one is an underlying concern (17). Further research exploring the relationship between ASD and gender dysphoria would be helpful to determine best practices for healthcare and mental health providers working with youth who may experience both ASD and gender dysphoria (17-19).

Healthcare roles regarding gender identity and expression

Just as gender is on a spectrum, so is the care and treatment healthcare professionals may provide to children regarding gender nonconformity and gender dysphoria (20). Healthcare providers may begin by asking youths about their gender identity, name, and pronouns, doing so discretely when indicated so as to not "out" the youth to others (21). Healthcare providers may consider sharing their own pronouns with the youth in an effort to model and normalize the discussion of gender identity rather than the assumption of gender based on natal sex (22). For example, stating, "Hi, my name is Jane and I use the pronouns she, her, and hers." For some youth, having a conversation about gender identity with their healthcare provider may be the first formal conversation or acknowledgment of gender nonconformity, or may occur while the youth is still developing or clarifying their own gender identity (23).

Electronic health record systems may not have a space to indicate differences between experienced/expressed gender and natal sex (21). In this case, the healthcare provider may need to explain that a person's natal or administrative sex, will be formally indicated in the record but that the youth's experienced/expressed gender, pronouns, or name may also be indicated within the provider's documentation with the youth's permission. This allows the healthcare provider to normalize non-cis-gender identities while beginning to acknowledge some of the challenges faced by gender nonconforming youth such as misgendering.

Challenges faced by gender nonconforming youth and youth who are experiencing gender dysphoria may include increased risk of victimization by peers, mental health concerns (such as anxiety or depression, increased risk of suicide or self-harm), and rejection or violence by family members or caregivers (5, 22, 24-26). Healthcare providers should take care to minimize the potential for victimization or harm to youth in their care. For instance, healthcare providers should not "out" the youth in situations in which the youth has not come out themselves in general social situations (i.e., in a clinic waiting room) or with family (i.e., when a parent is present in the exam room) such as by using the name or pronouns the youth has privately, but not socially identified as theirs.

It is also essential for health care providers to avoid misgendering or deadnaming the youth in their care such as by refusing to respect a youth's name change or using pronouns associated with natal sex rather than pronouns identified by the youth. Given the complexities of finding a balance between not misgendering a youth and not outing the youth inappropriately, healthcare providers should practice discretely asking a youth about their gender identity and pronouns and specifying if there are situations in which the youth does not wish the provider to use names or terms associated with their experienced gender (27).

Healthcare providers should also be able to identify appropriate places to where youth may be referred when care falls outside the scope of practice for that healthcare provider. For example, a healthcare provider may identify mental health professionals who are competent in concerns related to gender identity, crisis or legal resources available to youth, or other healthcare specialists. The section on educating families further explores how healthcare providers may intervene or provide support to families or to youth at risk of rejection or violence by their family or caregivers. Overall, it is the responsibility of the healthcare professional to provide affirming, individualized care to the youth they serve.

It is important to note that not all individuals who experience gender dysphoria seek surgical intervention and instead there is a range of gender affirming services that may be offered by the healthcare provider (20). The WPATH Standards of Care indicate criteria to help determine appropriate gender affirming medical intervention (6). This includes, for example, when it is appropriate and necessary to provide masculinizing or feminizing hormone therapy or to consider or perform surgery to change primary and/or secondary sex characteristics (6). Medical interventions such as hormone therapy and surgery are only a few types of intervention that may be provided.

There are other ways healthcare professionals may provide gender affirming services. These include participating in conversations with the youth about socially transitioning to their experienced gender (such as by living full or part time as the gender they experience), opening the doorway for youth to more fully explore their gender identity and expression, or engaging in honest but not fear-mongering discussions as to the stigma of gender dysphoria or nonconformity as well as the potential impacts on mental health (6). In the event that medical interventions such as hormone therapy or surgery are sought and identified as appropriate, it is advisable and necessary for a formal assessment regarding gender dysphoria to be completed (6, 20).

As noted in the section on gender dysphoria, gender dysphoria often does not persist past childhood, so what are healthcare providers to do when unsure if a child will continue to experience gender dysphoria (15)? One model, called the Dutch model or Dutch protocol, suggests that healthcare providers support the natural development of child's gender identity and engage in "watchful waiting" in regard to children (15). Watchful waiting or the wait and see approach does not disaffirm the child's developing gender identity prior to puberty but rather uses puberty as a guide to determine if gender dysphoria in childhood is likely to desist or persist (7, 15). As noted previously, to alleviate symptoms of gender dysphoria in childhood, healthcare providers may assist the child to express their experienced gender in a social and reversible sense (10).

Table 2. Healthcare providers' responsibilities for gender affirming care

- Privately or discretely inquire as to the youth's pronouns and name if other than those assigned at birth to avoid misgendering or deadnaming the youth.
  - Confirm in what situations and with whom the youth has transitioned to pronoun use or name other than those assigned at birth to avoid outing the youth which may pose risks to safety or wellbeing.
- Assess for gender dysphoria or collaborate other providers to assess for gender dysphoria.
- Educate youth and their parents or caregivers on gender affirming treatments available and appropriate.
  - When within the scope of practice, provide education and clarification on the reversibility and irreversibility of different available interventions, refer to appropriate providers able to provide this education when needed.
- Provide medically necessary gender affirming interventions, refer to providers with necessary scope of practice and expertise/specialization when needed.
- Maintain or improve understanding of mental health risks or impacts associated with gender dysphoria and socially or medically transitioning.
- Refer to mental health services as needed.
- Maintain understanding of and adherence to the WPATH Standards of Care.

Table 3. Resources for LGBTQ + youth, families, and allies

Crisis Intervention and Suicide Prevention **The Trevor Project** TrevorLifeline – 1-866-488-7362 TrevorChat - https://www.thetrevorproject.org/get-help-now/ TrevorText – text "START" to 678-678 **The GLBT National Youth Talkine (youth through 25 years old)** 800-246-7743 **Trans Lifeline** 877-565-8860 **National Suicide Prevention Hotline** 800-273-8255 https://suicidepreventionlifeline.org/chat/ **Crisis Text Line** Text "HOME" to 741-741 Additional Youth Resources **The National Runaway Safeline** 800-786-2929 https://www.1800runaway.org/youth-teens **Rape Abuse and Incest National Network (RAINN)** 800-656-4673 https://www.rainn.org/ **PFLAG** https://pflag.org/

Educating families regarding gender identity and expression

Healthcare providers working with children and adolescents face the challenge of providing care to the youth along with the youth's family members or caregivers. Gender nonconforming youth may experience pressure from family members to engage in more traditionally cis-gender activities or presentation and may therefore experience discomfort discussing concerns related to gender identity as well as expression with healthcare providers if their parents or caregivers are present or indirectly included in the encounter (9, 27). Providing education and support to family members of gender nonconforming youth is essential in promoting the safety and wellbeing of gender nonconforming youth as gender nonconforming youth whose family is gender affirming have better mental health outcomes than youth whose families are disaffirming (7, 28).

Healthcare providers may work with mental health providers in assisting youth to explore their gender identity and options for expressing their gender identity at home and socially (20, 29). Healthcare providers may also model gender affirming interactions to parents or caregivers such as by asking a child more open-ended questions about interests and gender expression rather than assuming stereotypical cis gender interests or expression. For example, healthcare providers may ask a child what toys or activities they enjoy rather than asking a child whose natal sex is female what dolls they like to play with or asking children whose natal sex is male what kind of sports they enjoy. Nonjudgmental questions asked of the child may communicate to both the child and caregivers that it is okay to like nontheoretically gendered activities (29). Healthcare providers may also need to educate parents or caregivers on the difference between sexual orientation and gender identity (25).

Conclusion: Directions for healthcare in the future

While not specific to gender nonconforming youth, many LGBTQ+ individuals are met with barriers in accessing healthcare services (22, 27, 30). Concerns such as not having a restroom available continue to be a concern for gender nonconforming and/or transgender individuals (28). Thus, having large scale conversations within healthcare facilities about restroom access, such as creating gender neutral restrooms or private restrooms is a necessary step in promoting overall health and wellbeing. As noted, medical records often only offer gender binary options (i.e., "are you male or female?") rather than allowing gender nonconforming individuals to indicate accurately how they identify on the gender spectrum (21). Healthcare providers and facilities should advocate for changes or make changes in routine documentation (such as intake forms, demographic information, others) to be more inclusive of individuals' gender identities.

When treating gender nonconforming or transgender individuals specifically, healthcare providers have reported a wide range of comfort levels in discussion reproductive concerns which is an important discussion to have particularly when providing gender affirming medical interventions for individuals of reproductive age (6, 22). Therefore, improving healthcare providers' knowledge and understanding of reproductive health for gender nonconforming individuals is also important. There are too many ways in which policies may be updated and other changes may be made to promote inclusivity as well as acceptance of all gender identities than are feasible to explore in this single article. Nonetheless, it is hoped that this brief discussion regarding gender identity may serve to begin or continue much needed conversations on the role of healthcare providers working alongside youth developing and understanding their gender identities.

References

[1] DSM-IV-TR Diagnostic criteria For gender identity disorder. Psychiatr News 2003; 38(14):32–32.

[2] Davy Z, Toze M. What is gender dysphoria? A critical systematic narrative review. Transgender Heal 2018;3(1):159–69.

[3] Byne W, Karasic DH, Coleman E, Eyler AE, Kidd JD, Meyer-Bahlburg HFL, et al. Gender dysphoria in adults: An overview and primer for psychiatrists. Transgender Heal 2018;3(1):57–70.

[4] Lev AI. Gender dysphoria: Two steps forward, one step back. Clin Soc Work J 2013; 41(3):288–96.

[5] Lagos D. Looking at population health beyond "male" and "female": Implications of transgender identity and gender nonconformity for population health. Demography 2018;55(6):2097–117.

[6] Coleman E, Bockting W, Botzer M, Cohen-Kettenis, DeCuypere G, Feldman J, et al. Standards of care for the health of transsexual, transgender, and gender-nonconforming people, version 7. Int J Transgend 2012;13(4):165-232.

[7] Kameg BN, Nativio DG. Gender dysphoria in youth: An overview for primary care providers. J Am Assoc Nurse Pract 2018;30(9):493–8.

[8] Steensma TD, Kreukels BP, de Vries AL, Cohen-Kettenis PT. Gender identity development in adolescence. Horm Behav 2013;64(2):288-97.

[9] Forcier MM, Haddad E. Health care for gender variant or gender non-conforming children. R I Med J 2013;96(4):17–21.

[10] Kaltiala-Heino R, Bergman H, Työläjärvi M, Frisen L. Gender dysphoria in adolescence: current perspectives. Adolesc Health Med Ther 2018;9:31–41.

[11] Toomey RB, Card NA, Casper DM. Peers' Perceptions of gender nonconformity: Associations with overt and relational peer victimization and aggression in early adolescence. J Early Adolesc 2014;34(4):463–85.

[12] Bos H, Sandfort T. Gender nonconformity, sexual orientation, and Dutch adolescents' relationship with peers. Arch Sex Behav 2015;44(5):1269–79.

[13] American Psychiatric Association. Diagnostic and statistical manual of mental disorders. 5th ed (DSM-5). Arlington, VA: American Psychiatric Publishing, 2013.

[14] Zucker KJ, Disorders GI. Management of gender dysphoria. Manag Gend Dysphoria 2015;(March):2008–13.

[15] Dora M, Grabski B, Dobroczyński B. Gender dysphoria, gender incongruence and gender nonconformity in adolescence – changes and challenges in diagnosis. Psychiatr Pol 2020; 2674 (162):1–15.

[16] Becker I, Auer M, Barkmann C, Fuss J, Möller B, Nieder TO, et al. A cross-sectional multicenter study of multidimensional body image in adolescents and adults with gender dysphoria before and after transition-related medical interventions. Arch Sex Behav 2018; 47(8):2335–47.

[17] Van Der Miesen AIR, Hurley H, De Vries ALC. Gender dysphoria and autism spectrum disorder: A narrative review. Int Rev Psychiatry 2016;28(1):70–80.

[18] Strang JF, Meagher H, Kenworthy L, de Vries ALC, Menvielle E, Leibowitz S, et al. Initial clinical guidelines for co-occurring autism spectrum disorder and gender dysphoria or incongruence in adolescents. J Clin Child Adolesc Psychol 2018;47(1):105–15.

[19] VanderLaan DP, Leef JH, Wood H, Hughes SK, Zucker KJ. Autism spectrum disorder risk factors and autistic traits in gender dysphoric children. J Autism Dev Disord 2015; 45(6):1742–50.

[20] Ahmad S, Barrett J, Beaini AY, Bouman WP, Davies A, Greener HM, et al. Gender dysphoria services: A guide for general practitioners and other healthcare staff. Sex Relatsh Ther 2013; 28(3):172–85.

[21] Knight RE, Shoveller JA, Carson AM, Contreras-Whitney JG. Examining clinicians' experiences providing sexual health services for LGBTQ youth: Considering social and structural determinants of health in clinical practice. Health Educ Res 2014;29(4):662–70.

[22] Gahagan J, Subirana-Malaret M. Improving pathways to primary health care among LGBTQ populations and health care providers: Key findings from Nova Scotia, Canada. Int J Equity Health 2018;17(1):1–9.

[23] Parmar DD, Alabaster A, Vance S, Ritterman Weintraub ML, Lau JS. Identification of sexual minority youth in pediatric primary care settings within a large integrated healthcare system using electronic health records. J Adolesc Heal 2019;66:255–7.

[24] Felner JK, Dudley TD, Ramirez-Valles J. "Anywhere but here": Querying spatial stigma as a social determinant of health among youth of color accessing LGBTQ services in Chicago's Boystown. Soc Sci Med 2018;213:181–9.

[25] Medicus J. Practice parameter on gay, lesbian, or bisexual sexual orientation, gender nonconformity, and gender discordance in children and adolescents. J Am Acad Child Adolesc Psychiatry 2012;51(9):957–74.

[26] Hailey J, Burton W, Arscott J. We Are family: Chosen and created families as a protective factor against racialized trauma and anti-LGBTQ oppression among African American sexual and gender minority youth. J GLBT Fam Stud 2020;16(2):176–91.

[27] Snyder BK, Burack GD, Petrova A. LGBTQ youth's perceptions of primary care. Clin Pediatr (Phila) 2017;56(5):443–50.

[28] Human Rights Campaign Foundation. Mental health and the LGBTQ community. 2017;(May):2013–6. URL: https://suicidepreventionlifeline.org/wp-content/uploads/2017/07/LGBTQ_MentalHealth_OnePager.pdf.

[29] MacMullin LN, Bokeloh LM, Nabbijohn AN, Santarossa A, van der Miesen AIR, Peragine DE, et al. Examining the relation between gender nonconformity and psychological well-being in children: The roles of peers and parents. Arch Sex Behav 2021;50(3):823-41.

[30] MacApagal K, Bhatia R, Greene GJ. Differences in healthcare access, use, and experiences within a community sample of racially diverse lesbian, gay, bisexual, transgender, and questioning emerging adults. LGBT Heal 2016;3(6):434–42.

Chapter 8

Sexually transmitted diseases/infections

Jocelyn Deleon, MD, Maria Demma Cabral*, MD, Selvy Kumaran, MD, Marine Bolliet and Nicole Coleman
Department of Pediatric and Adolescent Medicine, Western Michigan University Homer Stryker MD School of Medicine, Kalamazoo, Michigan, United States of America

Abstract

Sexually transmitted infections (STIs) continue to pose public health challenges to adolescents and young adults who continue to comprise half of all new infections diagnosed annually. Several factors have been implied to increase their risk of acquiring such infections. Understanding sexual practices in youth is important in recognizing spread of STIs. There are factors that increase their risk of acquiring STIs and research continues to focus on mitigating these factors to improve sexual health. All STIs are preventable, most are treatable, but not all are curable. In this discussion, we review the definition, clinical presentation, epidemiology, complications, diagnosis and treatment of diverse STIs and included the behavioral aspects to consider.

Introduction

Sexually transmitted infections (STIs) or venereal diseases, continue to pose challenges to the public health with an estimated 16 billion dollars in direct medical costs to the American healthcare system – particularly those infections requiring chronic treatment (1). According to the United States Centers for Disease Control and Prevention (CDC), adolescents and young adults aged 15-24 years particularly comprise half of all newly acquired STIs in the United States (2). These conditions are passed from one person to another when engaged in sexual activities, such as vaginal, oral and anal practices. Transmission can also occur in non-sexual methods such as sharing needles, breastfeeding, and though uncommon, through intimate physical contact such as heavy petting.

* ***Correspondence:*** Maria Demma Cabral, MD, Department of Pediatric and Adolescent Medicine, Western Michigan University Homer Stryker MD School of Medicine, 1000 Oakland Drive, Kalamazoo, MI 49008, United States. Email: mariademma.cabral@med.wmich.edu.

In: Behavioral Pediatrics II
Editors: Donald E. Greydanus, Dilip R. Patel, Ahsan Nazeer et al.
ISBN: 979-8-88697-019-7

A person who contracted an STI can remain asymptomatic or experience a range of symptoms from mild to severe presentations, some prompting hospitalization. Common presentations include:

- pain or discomfort during sex (dyspareunia)
- painful urination (dysuria)
- abnormal skin changes (i.e., ulcers, bumps, rashes) on or around the genitalia, buttocks, thighs, or mouth
- unusual penile or vaginal discharge
- genital bleeding
- testicular pain or swelling in males
- vaginal itching in females

Several factors have been implicated to increase risk of STI acquisition in young people; these include behavioral/developmental, biological, and sociocultural features. Adolescents in the early stages of development are concrete thinkers from their underdeveloped prefrontal cortex and possess the "I am invincible" attitude; such development makes them prone to high risk behavioral and sexual practices resulting in unintended pregnancies and STIs (3). There has been a steady decline in the number of sexually active youth based on the national Youth Risk Behavior Surveillance System (YRBSS) from 47.8% of high school student respondents in 2007 to 39.5% in 2017; however, 1 in 10 students still reported having at least 4 sexual partners in their lifetime and only half of currently sexually active students had used a condom in their last sexual encounter (4).

Young men are more likely to have sex compared to young women; however, the latter are more likely to acquire STIs and experience long-term health complications such as pelvic inflammatory disease (PID), ectopic pregnancies, and infertility. From a biological perspective, cervical ectopy in female adolescents is normal, but its presence makes the young woman susceptible to certain STIs such as infections caused by *Chlamydia trachomatis* and the human papillomavirus (HPV) affecting 25% of sexually active teen girls (2). Females were more likely to get tested than males, and a core reason for not getting tested was lack of perception that they were at risk for STIs (5).

Access to prevention, testing and treatment services continues to be problematic in this age group as well. Such barriers include payment issues, limited or absence of transportation, less readily available flexible clinic hours, and perceived lack of receiving confidential care (6). Males were less likely to seek testing due to confidentiality reasons (5). Ongoing research focuses on combatting these barriers to help improve the lives of affected youth and prevent further health and economic implications of STIs.

Adolescent sexuality has evolved over time and conducting clinical encounters should be confidential, respectful, non-biased and non-judgmental. The young person should be encouraged to discuss sexual and reproductive health concerns at any visit with a trusted health care professional (7-9). A thorough sexual history should be obtained followed by routine screening and treatment if indicated; such a history includes the number of sexual partners, sex practices, use of barrier methods as well as contraception, and past history of STIs (10). Promotion of healthy sexual choices and behaviors is key when counseling and educating adolescents as well as young adults to prevent infection that leads to diseases and potential exploitation.

STI caused by bacteria

Chlamydial infection caused by *chlamydia trachomatis* (CT) is the most commonly reported bacterial STI in the United States with high prevalence in individuals younger than age 25 years. Young age is a strong predictor. In 2018, 1.75 million cases were reported to the CDC from 50 states and the District of Columbia, yet an estimated 2.86 million chlamydial infections occur annually (2). Chlamydia is highly contagious with greater than 50% transmissibility. The incubation period is 1-3 weeks after exposure and most cases are asymptomatic. When symptomatic, females present with cervicitis manifested by vaginal discharge, intermenstrual bleeding, or dyspareunia; symptoms may mimic urinary tract infection.

The most common sequela is pelvic inflammatory disease (PID) characterized by abdominal or pelvic pain, cervical erythema and tenderness, and/or adnexal motion tenderness (11, 12). This occurs in up to 5% of women infected with chlamydia. If left untreated, it can result in infertility, ectopic pregnancy, and chronic pelvic pain.

Males with chlamydia commonly present with urethritis and up to two-thirds are symptomatic. They present with urethral discomfort, dysuria, and urethral discharge. An examination shows erythema of the urethral meatus and non-purulent mucoid discharge. A few present with orchitis or epididymitis where patients complain of testicular or scrotal pain seen with corresponding tenderness. CT and *neisseria gonorrhoeae* (NG) are the most common causes of acute epididymitis in sexually active men younger than age 25 years (11).

Rectal or oropharyngeal transmission can occur with CT. Rectal infection can be asymptomatic or may cause proctitis in those who have anal sex. Patients with oropharyngeal CT are usually asymptomatic but may also have pharyngitis or cervical lymphadenopathy. More than half of newborns will get the infection during passage through birth canal; the most common clinical manifestation in newborns is conjunctivitis (11).

Nucleic acid amplification testing (NAAT) is recommended for both screening and diagnosis of chlamydia with high specificity and sensitivity. Samples should be from first-catch urine in both men and women, as well as urethral swab in men and endocervical or vaginal swab in women (13). NAATs are also recommended for rectal and oropharyngeal chlamydial testing. NAATs are available in laboratories but standardization is recommended to ensure validity of results. Culture of chlamydia is only suggested in cases of sexual abuse in children (11, 12).

The CDC recommends that all sexually active females younger than age 25 years should be screened annually for CT, as should women 25 years and older who are at increased risk for infection. STI risk increases with new sexual partners, multiple sexual partners, and having a sexual partner with an STI (14, 15). Screening increases the chance of early diagnosis and has been shown to reduce rates of complications. In pregnant women, prenatal screening for both CT and NG is recommended. Appropriate treatment is given when diagnosed. Another retesting is performed at the third trimester of pregnancy due to risk of transmission during delivery (11).

In men, chlamydial testing, even if it not routinely recommended, may still be performed annually for populations at high risk. This includes patients in STI clinics or prisons, and men who have sex with men (MSM) (11). Co-infection with NG, syphilis, and human immunodeficiency virus (HIV) infection should be recognized. Testing must be considered and performed on all sexual partners during the last 60 days and they should be treated accordingly (11).

The recommended and alternative treatment regiments for chlamydial genitourinary infections is summarized in Table 1. The CDC favors treatment with azithromycin over doxycycline due to better patient compliance. Concern regarding not completing the 7 day-course of doxycycline causes partially treated infections. Doxycycline can be administered once daily using the single daily dose of a delayed-release doxycycline formulation (brand name Doryx) which can be administered as 200 mg orally once daily, but is more expensive (14). Both doxycycline regimens (the generic and Doryx) should be administered for 7 days. While both regimens are equally efficacious with similar microbial cure rates, treatment with azithromycin offers more adherence to treatment and may be better tolerated.

Rectal and oropharyngeal infections are treated similarly. However, some data has suggested reduced efficacy of single-doze azithromycin for treatment of rectal chlamydial infections (16). For pregnant patients, a single dose of azithromycin is proven safe with avoidance of use of doxycycline. Alternatives for pregnant women are erythromycin with similar dose for nonpregnant patients or amoxicillin 500 mg orally 3 times a day for 7 days.

Table 1. Recommended and alternative treatment regimens for chlamydia

Recommended	**Azithromycin** 1 g orally in a single dose, or **Doxycycline** 100 mg orally twice a day for 7 days
Alternative	**Erythromycin** base 500 mg orally four times a day for 7 days, or **Erythromycin** ethylsuccinate 800 mg orally four times a day for 7 days, or **Levofloxacin** 500 mg orally once daily for 7 days, or **Ofloxacin** 300 mg orally twice a day for 7 days

During treatment, patients should abstain from sexual activity for seven days after one dose regimen or until a 7-day regimen is completed and any symptoms resolve, as well as until all sexual partners have completed treatment (11). The patient and their partner should be counseled on safe sex practices including use of condoms or other barrier methods of contraception to minimize the risk of transmission as well as acquisition of chlamydia and other STIs.

Test of cure 3–4 weeks after therapy to detect treatment failures is not recommended unless adherence is in question, symptoms persist, or reinfection is suspected. Repeat NAAT is not recommended because it may lead to false positive results due to the presence of nonviable organisms (11). However, for pregnant woman, repeat testing at a minimum of 3 weeks following treatment is recommended to identify persisting or repeat infection so that retreatment can be instituted to reduce the risk for neonatal morbidity. For all other patients, retesting 3 months after treatment is recommended because re-infections are associated with higher risk for PID. Prevention of chlamydia lies on good implementation of screening programs to identify and treat asymptomatic individuals. Prompt treatment of patients and partners can reduce transmission.

Expedited partner therapy (EPT) may be an option in cases where sexual partners of a patient with chlamydia may not have access to care or do not wish to be seen (11). It is the clinical practice of treating the sexual partners of patients diagnosed with chlamydia by providing prescriptions or medications to the patient to take to their partner without the health care provider seeing the partner. Legality of EPT depends on state health department regulations, and is currently prohibited in South Carolina. EPT is currently permissible in 45 states. Under certain circumstances, EPT may be allowed in Alabama, Kansas, Oklahoma and

South Dakota. Due to the high risk of HIV or other STDs, EPT should not be offered to partners of MSM diagnosed with chlamydia (11).

Gonococcal infection

Gonorrhea is the most common cause of urethritis in men and cervicitis in women with risk of disseminated infection. It is caused by *Neisseria gonorrhoeae* and is the second most common bacterial cause of STI as well as implicated in most PID cases (2). Risk factors include young age, previous history of STI, new sexual partner, multiple sexual partners, sexual partner with STI, inconsistent condom use, incarcerated population and military recruits. It is more common in black and Hispanic groups (11). In 2018, more than half a million cases were reported to the CDC, yet an estimated 1.14 million new gonococcal infections occur annually (2).

Men with acute gonococcal urethritis, which is the most common presentation, usually presents with urethral discharge and dysuria; see Figure 1 (17). The incubation period is 2–5 days after exposure and few men remain asymptomatic (18-20). Acute, unilateral epididymitis can be a complication of urogenital gonorrhea. It commonly affects sexually active men between 15-35 years of age and older MSMs. Other less common presentations include periurethral abscess, penile lymphangitis, prostatitis and vesiculitis (18).

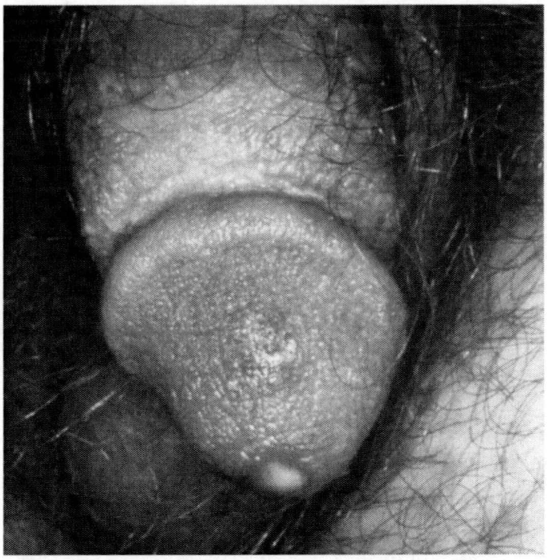

This image is in the public domain and thus free of any copyright restrictions. As a matter of courtesy we request that the content provider be credited and notified in any public or private usage of this image. URL: *https://phil.cdc.gov/Details.aspx?pid=16961.*

Figure 1. Mucopurulent penile discharge caused by *N gonorrhea.*

Gonococcal urogenital infections in women may be asymptomatic (19). The incubation period is 5–10 days following exposure and the most common symptoms are vaginal discharge, bleeding, discomfort and dysuria. Urethritis is the primary manifestation in women after hysterectomy. Symptoms of abdominal pain or dyspareunia suggests the presence of upper genital tract involvement. PID is the most common complication in women with increased risk of developing endometritis, salpingitis, tubo-ovarian abscess, peritoneal and pelvic adhesions; fifteen percent of women experience fallopian tube obstruction and infertility (18). Fitz-Hugh – Curtis syndrome is an infection of the liver capsule without involvement of the liver parenchyma due to retrograde spread of infection. It can be a complication of PID due to both NG and CT. It is mostly seen in women; but there are case reports of affected males. It usually presents with right upper quadrant pain and tenderness on examination (21).

Other extragenital manifestations can occur such as pharyngitis and conjunctivitis. Pharyngitis is due to receptive oral sex and often occurs in women as well as MSM; patients are usually asymptomatic (22). The most common presentation of gonococcal conjunctivitis is in neonates who acquire them from mothers who have the infection (18). Person-to-person nonsexual contact or fomites can also occur and cause conjunctivitis especially in outbreak settings; blindness may develop if left untreated. Anorectal infection can be asymptomatic and can occur in both women and MSM. Men acquire this through unprotected receptive anal intercourse. In women, contaminated cervical secretions can lead to this infection. MSM can develop acute proctitis and may present with rectal pain, anal pruritis and tenesmus; acute gonococcal proctitis is associated with an increased risk of human immunodeficiency virus (HIV) infection (22).

Disseminated gonococcal infection (DGI) can occur through hematogenous dissemination from any mucosal site. It occurs in 1% of patients with gonorrhea and occurs approximately 2 weeks after the primary infection (18). It is preceded by mucosal symptoms. Host factors play a role and patients with complement deficiencies are likely to experience this complication; thirteen percent of patients with this complication have a complement deficiency.

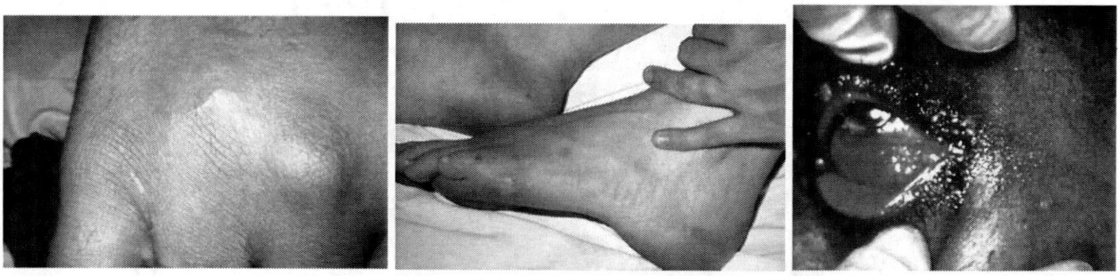

a b c

a) URL: https://phil.cdc.gov/Details.aspx?pid=22337;
b) URL: https://phil.cdc.gov/Details.aspx?pid=5326;
c) URL: https://phil.cdc.gov/Details.aspx?pid=5175

Figure 2. DGI: a) swelling and erythema of the fourth metacarpophalyngeal joint, b) characteristic skin lesions on the left foot, c) gonococcal ophthalmia.

DGI can be classified into stages. The first stage is a bacteremic stage, also known as arthritis-dermatitis stage, is characterized by presence of high fever, asymmetric polyarthralgias and tenosynovitis affecting the knees, elbows, and distal joints. Painless skin lesions develop in the majority of patients, and these lesions are most often petechial or maculopapular; however, it can progress to characteristic hemorrhagic pustules with central necrosis.

The second stage of DGI, also known as joint localized stage with septic arthritis, is characterized by the presence of localized gonococcal arthritis that is generally suppurative and monoarticular. Most patients do not develop polyarthralgia, tenosynovitis, or skin lesions associated with the bacteremic stage. Complications, though rare, may occur such as osteomyelitis, endocarditis, myopericarditis, meningitis, and epidural abscess (23).

The diagnosis of gonorrhea can be made with culture or by using the NAAT. Cultures can be obtained with endocervical or urethral swabs. NAAT has greater sensitivity compared to culture. Urine specimens or swabs from the endocervix and vagina in women, and urethra in men can be collected (24). NAAT urine specimens are 10% less sensitive compared to vaginal and endocervical swabs. NAAT is not approved by the US Food and Drug Administration (FDA) for diagnosis of rectal, oropharyngeal, or conjunctival infections (24). However, there are several Clinical Laboratory Improvement Amendments (CLIA)-approved tests that are able to use NAAT to diagnose rectal and oropharyngeal infection.

Despite the high specificity of NAAT, false positives can occur from the oropharynx tests. A culture should be considered if deemed necessary. If both NAAT and culture are being collected from the same site, the culture should be obtained first to increase the culture yield (24). In symptomatic men, a Gram stain from the urethral swab showing polymorphonuclear leukocytes with intracellular gram-negative diplococci can establish a highly sensitive and specific diagnosis; see Figure 3 This technique is less sensitive in asymptomatic men and other specimen sites (i.e., endocervical, pharyngeal, rectal) (24).

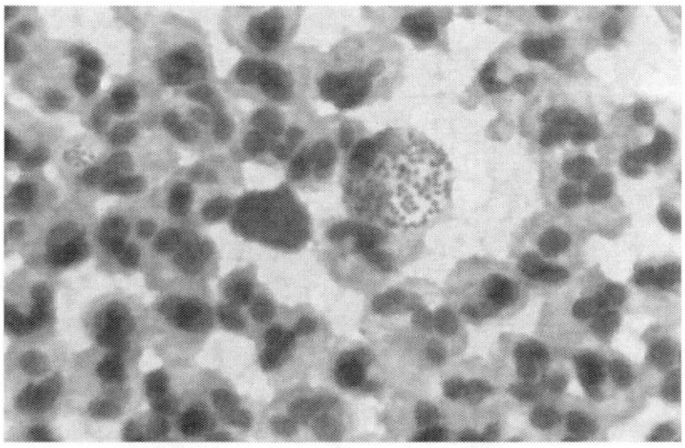

This image is in the public domain and thus free of any copyright restrictions. As a matter of courtesy we request that the content provider be credited and notified in any public or private usage of this image. URL: https://phil.cdc.gov/Details.aspx?pid=21365.

Figure 3. Gram-stained specimen showing *N. gonorrhea* with classic intracellular diplococcic.

Overt diagnosis of disseminated infection from gonorrhea can be difficult since blood cultures are not always positive. NAAT and culture of all mucosal surfaces should be obtained and up to 80% will have evidence of a mucosal infection (i.e., genital, anorectal, and oropharyngeal) (23). Moreover, if appropriate, NAAT and cultures can be performed on blood, synovial fluid, cerebral spinal fluid, and skin lesions. Sex partners should also be tested. Evaluation for complications such as meningitis and endocarditis is also recommended (23).

The treatment of gonorrhea involves a concern for NG resistance to multiple antibiotics including cephalosporins, sulfonamides, penicillins, tetracyclines, macrolides and fluoroquinolones. NG utilizes several mechanisms for resistance through both plasmid-mediated and chromosomal changes; these include enzymatic antimicrobial inactivation, reduced permeability and enhanced efflux of antimicrobials. Because dual therapy with ceftriaxone plus azithromycin is the only recommended treatment for gonorrhea, increases of the minimum inhibitory concentration in azithromycin and cephalosporin are cause for concern that resistance to these antimicrobial agents might be emerging (25).

In addition, oropharyngeal gonorrhea is thought to play a central role especially for asymptomatic and untreated infection. Pharyngeal infection is more difficult to eradicate compared to other sites (26). In 2007, fluoroquinolone-resistant NG emerged in the United States. Treatment failures with oral cephalosporin have been reported worldwide. There are also numerous reported cases of treatment failure to ceftriaxone worldwide, all with pharyngeal involvement. The role of pharyngeal infections is emphasized in the resistance of NG.

Table 2 summarizes current treatment recommendations for uncomplicated and DGIs. In patients with β-lactam allergy, gemifloxacin 320 mg orally or gentamicin 240 mg IM plus azithromycin 2g orally should be given. Recommendations for treatment of patients with a β-lactam allergy are similar treatment recommendations for HIV and pregnant patients. However, it is recommended that infectious disease and allergy immunonology specialists be both involved with pregnant women for penicillin desensitization consideration (11). For a patient with azithromycin allergy, a 7-day course of doxycycline can be used although this is not preferred given the high rates of tetracycline resistance. For patients with DGI, hospitalization and consultation with an infectious disease specialist should be considered.

Table 2. Recommended and alternative treatment regimens for gonococcal infections

Gonococcal infections	Treatment regimens
Uncomplicated cervicitis, urethritis, or proctitis	**Ceftriaxone** 250 mg IM in a single dose PLUS **Azithromycin** 1g orally in a single dose *Alternative:* If ceftriaxone is not available: **Cefixime** 400 mg orally in a single dose PLUS **Azithromycin** 1 g orally in a single dose
Uncomplicated pharyngitis	**Ceftriaxone** 250 mg IM in a single dose PLUS **Azithromycin** 1g orally in a single dose
Conjunctivitis	**Ceftriaxone** 1 g IM in a single dose PLUS **Azithromycin** 1g orally in a single dose
Disseminated	
-Arthritis and arthritis-dermatitis syndrome	**Ceftriaxone** 1 g IM or IV every 24 hours PLUS **Azithromycin** 1 g orally in a single dose ***Alternative:*** **Cefotaxime** 1 g IV every 8 hours, or **Ceftizoxime** 1 g IV every 8 hours PLUS **Azithromycin** 1 g orally in a single dose
-Meningitis and endocarditis	**Ceftriaxone** 1–2 g IV every 12–24 hour PLUS **Azithromycin** 1 g orally in a single dose

In order to maximize adherence with treatment, medications for gonococcal infection should be provided on site and directly observed. In order to minimize disease transmission, persons treated for gonorrhea should be instructed to abstain from sexual activity for seven days after treatment and until all sexual partners are adequately treated. Repeat testing is not needed for patients with uncomplicated urogenital or rectal gonorrhea, who are treated with recommended regimens; however, any patient with pharyngeal gonorrhea who is treated with an alternative regimen should return 14 days after treatment for culture or NAAT to confirm resolution of infection. All patients treated for gonorrhea should be retested at 3 months after therapy due to high rates of reinfection (11). Refractory symptoms are most often from reinfection not treatment failure. Suspected treatment failure should be reported to the CDC. All persons with gonorrhea should be tested for other STIs including chlamydia, syphilis, and HIV infection.

Management of sexual partners is recommended. They should be referred for evaluation and treatment. Sexual partners up to 60 days from the last sexual activity should be contacted. Partners also should abstain from unprotected sex until seven days post-treatment and until symptoms resolve (11). The US Preventive Services Task Force (USPSTF) recommends routine screening in adults and adolescents ages 15-65 years.

Populations that are considered at higher risk are those who have a new sex partner, more than one sex partner, a sex partner with concurrent partners, or a sex partner who has an STI (11). Additional risk factors for gonorrhea include inconsistent condom use among persons who are not in mutually monogamous relationships; previous or coexisting sexually transmitted infections; and exchanging sex for money or drugs. More frequent screening at 3–6 month intervals is indicated for MSM, including those with HIV infection with risky behaviors and multiple partners. Pregnant women who remain at high risk should be retested in the third trimester. Women and men in correctional facilities upon intake should get an initial test.

Other recommendations, among MSM, include at least annual pharyngeal screening for those who have receptive oral intercourse, urethral screening for those who have insertive intercourse, and rectal screening for those who have receptive anal intercourse. There are no routine screening recommendations for extragenital infections among other populations and risk groups (11, 29). Several studies showed that screening rates for gonorrhea at rectal and pharyngeal sites can be as high as 10%.

Syphilis

Syphilis is caused by the corkscrew-shaped bacterial spirochete, *Treponema pallidum* (TP) (see Figure 4) and this is a reportable disease in every state. First recognized as a sexually transmitted disease in the 1400s, syphilis can have serious, significant complications if left untreated (2, 30). In 2018, at least 35,000 primary and secondary syphilis cases were reported to the CDC with continued increasing rates in the United States; six in 10 cases were among MSM (2, 30). Syphilis is transmitted via direct contact with mucocutaneous lesions called chancre and condyloma lata. It can also be transmitted perinatally from mother to fetus (11). In 2016, 628 cases of congenital syphilis, including 41 syphilitic stillbirths, were reported to the CDC; this was a 28% increase from 2015 (31).

A 2017 CDC report showed 1 in 2 newborn syphilis cases in the United States occur due to gaps in testing and treatment during prenatal care (32). Cases occur when mothers are not tested early during prenatal care (10%), are diagnosed but not adequately treated for syphilis (31%), and acquired syphilis later in pregnancy after an initial negative test (11%) (32). The incubation period is 10-90 days with average incubation time of 3 weeks (11). Risk factors include MSM, HIV infection, having a partner with syphilis infection, previous syphilis infection, high risk sexual behavior and high prevalence of syphilis infection in the population (33, 34).

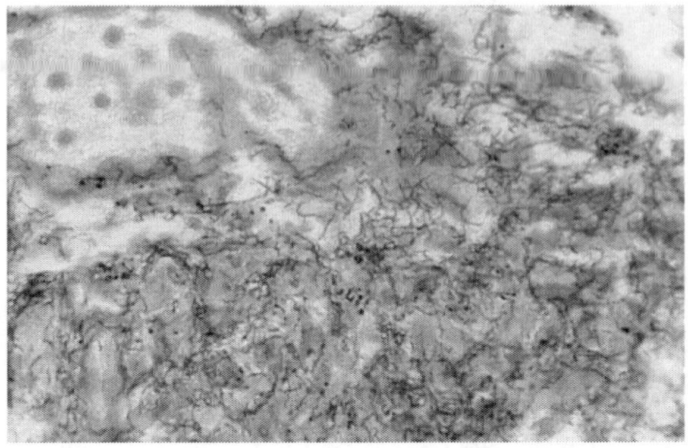

Figure 4. Numerous corkscrew-shaped *T pallidum* seen using Steiner silver stain method.

Primary syphilis

Primary syphilis typically presents with a painless ulcer or chancre at the site of infection appearing after the incubation period (see Figure 5). It can either be single or multiple. The chancre is very infectious, may last for weeks, and will heal spontaneously without treatment (33). The differential diagnosis for primary syphilis includes herpes simplex, chancroid, granuloma inguinale (Donovanosis), and lymphogranuloma venereum (LGV) (11).

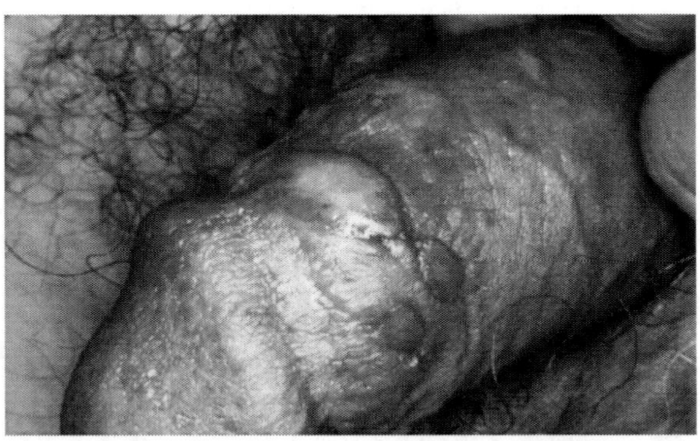

Figure 5. Penile painless ulcer seen in primary syphilis.

Secondary syphilis

Secondary syphilis typically presents several weeks after primary syphilis infection. It usually manifests as skin rash, mucocutaneous lesions with swollen lymph nodes and constitutional symptoms; the latter includes sore throat, fevers, anorexia, myalgia and hair loss. The infectious rash is notable in the trunk, palms (see Figure 6) and soles; also, it can be macular, papular or papulosquamous in appearance and can be diffuse, bilateral, symmetrical as well as following skin creases. The rash must be differentiated from pityriasis rosea, tinea versicolor, or scabies (11, 33).

Mucocutaneous lesions present as mucous patches or condyloma lata described as raised gray or white lesions on the affected sites; they may be seen in the mouth and genitals but may also appear on the underarm and perineal region (33). Condyloma lata is non-pruritic and classically involves the palms and soles. The lesions are often small, red-brown colored lesions that can be either macular or popular (11). However, the rash has a wide variety of presentations. Like primary syphilis, the symptoms will resolve spontaneously without treatment. Symptoms may recur over a year timeframe (11). Without treatment, secondary syphilis will progress to latent syphilis and possibly tertiary syphilis (11, 33).

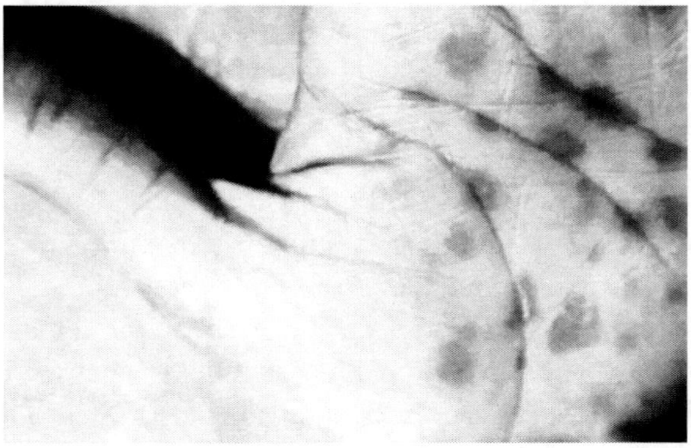

This image is in the public domain and thus free of any copyright restrictions. As a matter of courtesy we request that the content provider be credited and notified in any public or private usage of this image. URL: https://phil.cdc.gov/Details.aspx?pid=20177.

Figure 6. Characteristic palmar rash of secondary stage caused by *T. pallidum.*

Latent syphilis

Latent syphilis is defined by the absence of clinical manifestations in the setting of serologic detection of syphilis; this stage occurs when the manifestations of primary and secondary syphilis resolve (33). Latent syphilis can be either early or late; early latent syphilis is defined as infection acquired within the preceding year while late latent syphilis is infection acquired more than one year prior (11, 33). Latent syphilis is not sexually transmitted and can last for years to decades (11). Approximately 15% of untreated individuals will progress to the tertiary stage of syphilis (33).

Tertiary syphilis

The presentation of tertiary syphilis can be categorized into 1) cardiovascular syphilis, 2) gumma lesions, and 3) tertiary neurosyphilis. The devastating effects of tertiary syphilis are irreversible and can lead to aneurysms, heart disease, death, mental conditions, and neurologic problems such as dementia, blindness and deafness (11, 33). Neurosyphilis can occur at any stage of syphilis. It is the involvement of the central nervous system during syphilitic infection. Concomitant HIV infection and early syphilis are risk factors to developing this condition (11). Signs or symptoms suggesting neurologic or ophthalmic disease should prompt further evaluation. Routine analysis of the cerebrospinal fluid (CSF) in the absence of symptoms is not recommended, however, except in tertiary syphilis (11).

Clinical presentation of early neurosyphilis may include cranial nerve dysfunction, meningitis, stroke, acute onset of altered mental status, auditory deficits, and/or ophthalmic abnormalities (ocular syphilis) (11, 33). Early neurologic symptoms typically present within the first few months of infection; however, symptoms may occur after a few years (11, 33). Late neurologic symptoms may cause tabes dorsalis. This is secondary to gradual demyelination of spinal cord nerves that can lead to neuropathic pain, sensory deficits, balance problems, blindness and ataxia. This usually occurs in tertiary syphilis. These neurologic findings typically occur decades after initial infection (11). Patients will have higher nontreponemal serologic titers than those without neurosyphilis (35).

Diagnosis

Diagnosis is made by serologies or darkfield microscopy (11, 36). Darkfield examination of a lesion exudate or tissue in early syphilis may support a diagnosis of syphilis (11). However, due to the difficulty of darkfield examination, serology is now more typically utilized (33). The diagnosis is made with combination of a nontreponemal and a treponemal serologic test (11, 33, 36). There are high rates of both false positives and false negatives in either nontreponemal and treponemal test (11). Screening is done by doing a nontreponemal test first, and if positive, a treponemal test is performed (11, 36). Nontreponemal tests include Rapid Plasma Reagin (RPR) and Venereal Disease Research Laboratory (VDRL). Treponemal antibodies are detectable earlier than nontreponemal tests (33). Sensitivity of the nontreponemal tests is 78-86% for detecting primary syphilis and 100% for detecting secondary infection with specificity ranging from 85 to 99% for all stages (34).

Treponemal tests include fluorescent treponemal antibody absorbed (FTA-ABS), TP passive particle agglutination (TP-PA) assay, enzyme immunoassays (EIAs), chemiluminescence imunoassays (CIA), and rapid treponemal assays (33). The sensitivity of the FTA-ABS test is 84% for primary syphilis and 100% for syphilis in other stages with a specificity of 97% (34). The TP-PA assay has similar sensitivity and specificity to the FTA-ABS test (36). Treponemal studies are detectable for life even after successful treatment. Nontreponemal tests, on the other hand, become non-reactive after successful treatment (33, 36). In some cases, however, the nontreponemal studies can remain reactive for years known as the serofast reaction (11).

Interpretation of serologic testing is similar for those with HIV infection compared to those without HIV infection (31). Some clinical laboratories are now performing reverse sequence algorithms (RSA) where a treponemal test is performed first, and if positive, a nontreponemal study is performed. If the nontreponemal test is negative, a second treponemal study is performed (11, 33, 34, 36). If the second treponemal test is positive in a patient with a history of treatment for syphilis, no further management is necessary. However, those without a history of treatment for syphilis should be treated (11, 31, 32, 36). There is likelihood of high false positive results with this method (36). RSA may have role and have more benefit with early primary syphilis, previously treated syphilis, or longstanding untreated infection. Despite this, it is not currently recommended for the diagnosis of syphilis (11, 34). The CDC recommends traditional screening with a nontreponemal serologic study first followed by a confirmatory treponemal test. Rapid syphilis screening tests have been available in the United States since 2015. The rapid test allows for point-of-care testing in HIV and STI clinics (34,36).

For patients with signs and symptoms of neurosyphilis, further testing with a lumbar puncture and CSF analysis is indicated as follows: CSF cell count, protein, glucose, and CSF-VDRL. A reactive CSF-VDRL is considered diagnostic of neurosyphilis in a patient with neurologic sign (11). If the CSF-VDRL is non-reactive in a patient with neurologic signs and symptoms, the diagnosis of neurosyphilis should still be considered when serologic results are reactive. The CSF-VDRL has a low sensitivity, but high specificity. A CSF FTA-ABS test may be used in patients with a negative CSF-VDRL. This test is highly sensitive for neurosyphilis. If the CSF FTA-ABS is negative, then neurosyphilis is unlikely. For ocular syphilis, further evaluation with a slip lamp examination is warranted (11).

Management

The patient can be empirically treated for syphilis before laboratory results are available when history, local epidemiology and/or clinical exam are suggestive of the infection. Early treatment of syphilis helps to prevent further transmission (11). Parenteral penicillin G (benzathine penicillin) is the recommended treatment for all stages (30). After treatment, repeat testing should be performed. Nontreponemal tests generally are used to follow treatment response. A change in the ratio (1:16-1:4) that is four-fold is considered significant improvement (11). Table 3 summarizes the treatment recommendations for syphilitic infections. During latent stage of syphilis, it is important to treat early to prevent tertiary syphilis and vertical transmission during pregnancy.

Table 3. Recommended and alternative treatment regimens for syphilitic infections

Syphilitic infection	Treatment regimens
Primary, secondary (including among persons with HIV infection) and early latent	**Benzathine** penicillin G 2.4 million units IM in a single dose
Late latent or latent of unknown duration and tertiary with normal CSF exam	**Benzathine** penicillin G 7.2 million units total, administered as 3 doses of 2.4 million units IM each at 1-week intervals
Neurosyphilis and ocular infection	**Aqueous crystalline penicillin G** 18–24 million units per day, administered as 3–4 million units IV every 4 hours or continuous infusion, for 10–14 days ***Alternative:*** **Procaine penicillin G** 2.4 million units IM once daily PLUS **Probenecid** 500 mg orally four times a day, both for 10–14 days

Clinical and serologic follow-up is recommended at 6-month interval following treatment until 1 year after treatment (11, 35). A closer follow-up is recommended for HIV patients at 3-month interval until one year after treatment, then at two years after treatment (11, 34). Reinfection is considered for patients who do not clinically improve, have persistent symptoms, those with increased nontreponemal test titers, and those with failure of nontreponemal test titers to decline fourfold (11). It is challenging to determine treatment failure and reinfection based on repeat testing. Further evaluation with CSF analysis is often indicated in these cases (34). Jarisch–Herxheimer reaction is most seen in early syphilis where the spirochete burden is higher (11). It is an acute reaction including fever, myalgia, and headache within the first 24 hours of treatment (11, 31, 34). Treatment is supportive and symptomatic with antipyretics if needed (11).

Nontreponemal serologic follow-up is recommended at 6, 12, and 24 months following treatment in patients with a more frequent interval for those with HIV. CSF analysis should be done if there is a fourfold increase in titers, a lack of four-fold decline of high titers after 12 months, or if there are new symptoms. If CSF abnormalities are present, the patient should be treated for neurosyphilis. A second treatment for latent syphilis is recommended if CSF analysis is normal (11).

Neurosyphilis CSF abnormalities are common, especially in early syphilis and in those with HIV infection (11, 33-35). Treatment for neurosyphilis is not indicated in the absence of symptoms with the exception of tertiary syphilis (11, 33). In tertiary neurosyphilis, treatment is recommended if CSF analysis is consistent with neurosyphilis, even in the absence of symptoms (11). This is why all patients with tertiary syphilis should receive a CSF examination to evaluate for neurosyphilis (35). Ocular syphilis is treated even if CSF examination is normal (11, 34). It may occur in association with neurosyphilis. Follow-up lumbar puncture should be performed every 6 months until CSF cell count is normal. Also, CSF VDRL and CSF protein levels tend to normalize slower than cell count. Retreatment should be considered If CSF pleocytosis does not improve in 6 months (11).

All sexual partners in the 90 days prior to the time of diagnosis should be treated for early syphilis regardless of serologic results (11). Sexual partners that were over 90 days prior to the diagnosis also need serologic testing and treatment if results are positive based on the stage of syphilis. Latent syphilis is not transmitted sexually (35). However, long-term sexual partners of those with late latent and tertiary syphilis will need to be evaluated. Treatment is based on clinical and serologic findings (11). Presumptive treatment for early syphilis is recommended for the sexual partners of those with late latent syphilis and high titers in areas with increased prevalence (11).

Pregnancy and syphilis

All pregnant women are screened preferably on the initial visit for syphilis with a nontreponemal test at least once during their pregnancy (11, 33, 36, 37). The highest risk for fetal transmission is with primary and secondary syphilis, though risk still remains significant for pregnant women with late latent syphilis. The only recommended therapy for syphilis during pregnancy is parenteral penicillin G (11). No other treatments are known to be effective. Therefore, pregnant women with penicillin allergy should be desensitized (11). There is some evidence that additional therapy is beneficial in pregnant women in early syphilis. A second dose of benzathine penicillin G 2.4 M units IM may be administered one week after the initial dose. If a dose of penicillin is missed during late latent syphilis during pregnancy, the entire treatment course needs to be repeated (11, 35).

Fetal ultrasound is necessary if syphilis infection occurs and the pregnant woman acquires syphilis during the second half of pregnancy. This is necessary to look for congenital syphilis. Jarisch Herxheimer reaction can occur from treatment during the second half of pregnancy. However, these are not reasons to delay treatment. This reaction may lead to preterm labor or fetal distress. Follow-up should include repeated serologic titers at 28–32 week gestation and at the time of delivery (11).

HIV

Patients who have syphilis should always be tested for HIV. Abstinence from sexual contact or a monogamous relationship with a partner free of syphilis are the best ways to prevent infection (33). The use of latex condoms also reduces the risk of transmission. Screening for syphilis is recommended for MSM and those with HIV infection (34). The CDC recommends at least annual screening for high risk patients that include MSM and HIV-infected patients. Partner-based interventions during treatment can lead to reduced rates of re-infection (33). More frequent screening every 3 months in MSM and HIV-infected patients may improve early diagnosis and treatment of syphilis infection.

Lymphogranuloma venereum

Lymphogranuloma venereum (LGV) is an ulcerative disease of the genital area caused by the gram-negative bacteria *Chlamydia trachomatis*, especially serovars L1, L2, and L3. It is transmittable by vaginal, oral or anal sex and can be asymptomatic (38). There are increasing numbers of reports in MSM with likely presentation of proctocolitis and LGV can present similarly to inflammatory bowel disease. Clinical presentation includes rectal discharge that is mucoid or bloody, constipation, fever, anal pain and tenesmus (11). In MSM, it can present as systemic infection and may be invasive. LGV can lead to chronic rectal fissures and strictures if not treated immediately.

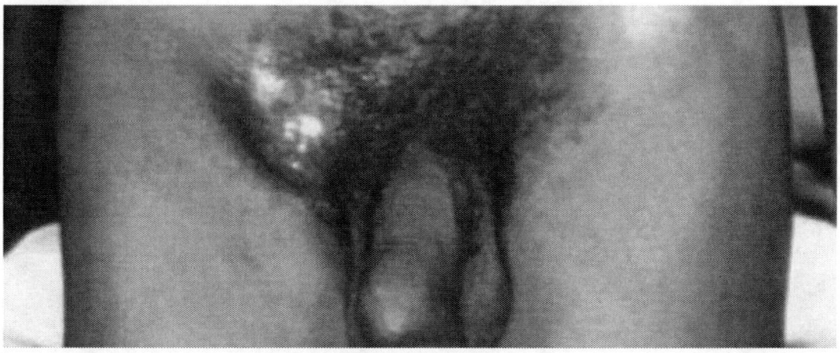

Figure 7. Right inguinal tender lymphadenopathy characteristic of LGV.

Characteristically, LGV has three stages of infection. The first stage is a self-limited genital ulcer or papule sometimes occurring at the site of inoculation. However, by the time patients seek care, the lesions have often disappeared. The second stage which is the most common clinical manifestation of LGV among heterosexuals is tender inguinal and/or femoral lymphadenopathy that is typically unilateral (see Figure 7). The third stage is the late stage and may have fistulas, strictures and fissures (24, 38). If left untreated, ulcerations can lead to necrosis and ruptured lymph nodes, anogenital fibrosis/strictures and anal fistulae. There have been rare reports of elephantiasis of the genitals, pneumonia and hepatitis (38).

Diagnosis

Diagnosis of LGV is based on clinical suspicion, epidemiologic information, and the exclusion of other etiologies for proctocolitis, inguinal lymphadenopathy and genital/rectal ulcers (38). Culture of genital lesions, rectal specimens, and lymph node swab as well as aspirate can be done. However, it is technically difficult and not readily available. Direct immunofluorescence or nucleic acid detection can also be utilized (11). NAATs for CT perform well on rectal specimens, but are not FDA cleared for this purpose. Many laboratories have performed validation studies needed to provide results from rectal specimens for clinical management.

MSM presenting with proctocolitis should be tested for chlamydia; NAAT performed on rectal specimens is the preferred approach to testing. Additional molecular procedures (e.g., Polymerase chain reaction (PCR) based genotyping) can be used to differentiate LGV from non-LGV CT in rectal specimens. However, these tests are not widely available, and a delay in results would not influence acute clinical management. Chlamydia serology may not be diagnostically helpful and are not recommended (24, 38).

Treatment

Table 4 summarizes treatment regimens for LGV. Persons with symptoms consistent with LGV, including proctocolitis or genital ulcer disease with lymphadenopathy, should be presumptively treated (24). Cases should be reported to the state health department and these persons should be tested for HIV, gonorrhea, and syphilis. Partners who had sexual contact with the patient within the 60 days before onset of the symptoms should be examined, tested and presumptively treated with azithromycin or doxycycline (24). Pregnant and lactating women should be treated with erythromycin and doxycycline should be avoided due to staining of teeth and bones. HIV-infected patients with LGV are treated with the same chlamydia regimen. However, prolonged therapy is most often required, and delay in resolution of symptoms is observed. Patients should be followed clinically until signs and symptoms have resolved (11, 38).

Chancroid

In the United States, chancroid is a rare cause of STI described as a genital ulcer disease caused by the fastidious gram-negative bacteria *Haemophilus ducreyi.* This bacterium has recently been associated with non-sexually transmitted, chronic skin ulcers in Africa and the Pacific; however, it has not been reported in the United States (39). It can cause significant morbidity and can increase transmission of HIV, especially in heterosexual populations (40).

Symptoms of chancroid start 4-7 days after exposure, primarily through sexual contact. It typically manifests as erythematous papules at the sites of microabrasions. Lesions are often very painful. The papular lesions progress to pustules and become ulcerated over several days. Ulcers typically occur in multiple numbers with a necrotic exudate covering the base; these lesions are tender, well circumscribed, non-indurated and have ragged borders (41, 42).

They are mostly found in the genital area, on the distal penis in males, and the vulva or cervix in females. They may present on the perianal region with patients engaged in anal intercourse. Through autoinoculation, ulcers may occur on non-genital region (42, 43). Patients may experience painful, unilateral inguinal adenopathy that can reach up to 50% of cases and will be associated with bubo formation; also, a portion of these will suppurate and can spontaneously rupture (44). See Figure 8. Patients with HIV tend to have slower healing, atypical appearing, and more numerous ulcers (41).

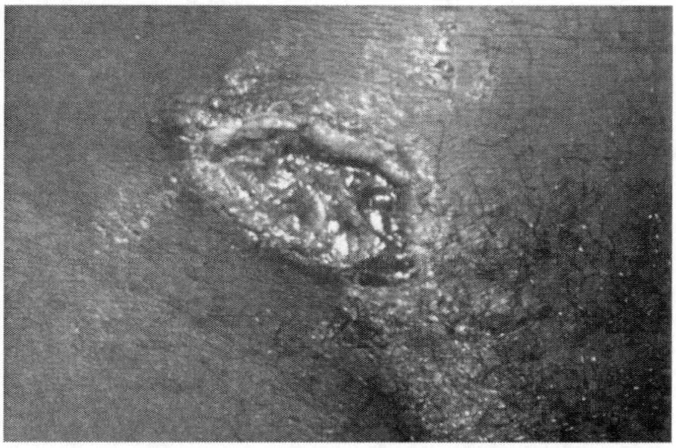

This image is in the public domain and thus free of any copyright restrictions. As a matter of courtesy we request that the content provider be credited and notified in any public or private usage of this image. URL: https://phil.cdc.gov/Details.aspx?pid=3701.

Figure 8. A necrotic swollen lymph node, called bubo, in the right inguinal region caused by *H ducreyi.*

Diagnosis

Diagnosis of chancroid is challenging and is mainly based on clinical findings. The combination of a painful genital ulcer and tender suppurative inguinal adenopathy suggests the diagnosis of chancroid. It is important to do microbiological diagnosis if possible in all cases of suspected chancroid. Polymerase chain reaction (PCR) is the most sensitive diagnostic method and some tests have the added advantage of testing simultaneously for other pathogens that cause genital ulcer disease such as donovanosis, syphilis and herpes simplex virus (HSV). Unfortunately, PCR is not readily available.

There are no FDA-approved assays commercially available (11, 42). Culture of *H. ducreyi* can be challenging and is difficult to perform. Gram stain is used but has poor sensitivity. It may show typical small gram-negative rods in a chain. Culture, if performed, requires more than one medium to increase chances of organism growth and recovery. Special culture medium is not widely available from commercial sources and even when these media are used, sensitivity is 80% (44).

Due to challenges of microbiologic studies, the CDC proposed case definition for chancroid. They define a probable case as having: (1) one or more painful genital ulcers; (2) presentation and physical appearance of ulcers and lymphadenopathy typical for chancroid; (3) no evidence of *T. pallidum* on darkfield examination of ulcer exudate and/or no serological evidence of syphilis at least 7 days after ulcer onset; and (4) negative HSV PCR or culture from the ulcer exudates (11). However, clinical diagnosis maybe unreliable and coinfections with other causes of genital ulcer disease do occur (43).

Treatment

Table 4 summarizes treatment regimens for chancroid. Resistance has emerged against antibiotics, specially ciprofloxacin and erythromycin as well as tolerability/compliance issues, making these antibiotics second-line options (11, 43, 44). Patients should be re-examined 3–7 days after initiation of therapy. If treatment is successful, ulcers improve symptomatically within three days and objectively within seven days after therapy. Further testing for other causes, medication compliance, co-infection, antibiotic resistance and incorrect diagnosis are the reasons for failure of treatment.

The time required for complete healing depends on the size of the ulcer. Large ulcers might require 42 weeks to heal. Healing is slower for some uncircumcised men who have ulcers under the foreskin. Treatment duration is longer in patients with buboes (43-45).

Patients should be tested for HIV infection at the time chancroid is diagnosed (11). Persons with HIV infection who have chancroid should be monitored closely because they are more likely to experience treatment failure and to have ulcers that heal slowly. Treatment failure in patients with HIV is usually not due to antimicrobial resistance (41, 42). The CDC recommends close monitoring with consideration of repeated or longer courses of therapy (11, 46).

Regardless of treatment response, patients should be retested for syphilis and HIV infection three months after diagnosis (11, 44). Clinical resolution of fluctuant lymphadenopathy is slower than that of ulcers and might require needle aspiration or incision and drainage, to prevent spontaneous rupture, despite otherwise successful therapy. Incision and drainage might be preferred because of reduced need for subsequent drainage procedures, which may predispose to sinus tract formation (11).

Patients with chancroid need to be counseled to avoid sexual contact until they have completed treatment. Partners should also abstain until completely treated. Partners from up to 10 days prior to ulcer formation need to be notified and treated regardless of symptomatology (11). Chancroid is a reportable disease to the local or state health department. Patients with chancroid should be offered testing for other STIs including HSV, syphilis, and HIV (11, 44). The World Health Organization (WHO) recommends syndromic management of genital ulcer disease which includes empiric therapy for chancroid where prevalence is high (45). Prevention consists primarily of STI education emphasizing appropriate and effective condom use (11, 44). There is also an increased risk for HIV transmission so patients should be counseled on this (40). There is currently no vaccine available for prevention.

Donovanosis (granuloma inguinale)

Donovanosis is caused by the intracellular gram-negative bacteria *Klebsiella granulomatis,* formerly known as *Calymmatobacterium granulomatis*. It is a genital ulcer disease that can cause severe scarring and destruction of involved areas; also, it can cause significant morbidity. Donovanosis can also increase transmission of HIV, especially in heterosexual populations

(40). In the United States, it is a rare cause of STI and is not a notifiable disease. Some cases are not sexually transmitted. The exact prevalence is unknown and epidemiological data for this disease is lacking in most of the world (47). Risk factors for an increased number of ulcerative lesions are uncircumcised men with poor hygiene and prior outbreaks (48, 49).

Donovanosis is estimated to present 1-360 days after exposure, with average incubation period of 50 days (2, 49). Lesions appear as papules or firm nodules that become ulcers. It is gradually progressive and can get worse quickly. Ulcers are beefy red, and non-tender with a fragile base (48, 49). Less commonly, it can present with irregular ulcers that are hard to distinguish from verrucous lesions of condyloma lata or condyloma accuminata, foul smelling, necrotic destructive ulcers, and sclerotic ulcers with scars (48-50). Ulcers can cause significant disfigurement. Ulcers tend to occur on the distal penis in men and the labia minora, fourchette and cervix in women; ulcers can occur in the anus in those who engage in anal intercourse. Pseudo-elephantiasis and dissemination to liver and bone are known complications (51). Dissemination usually occurs from cervical lesions in pregnant women (48-50). Patients who have concomitant HIV infection have lesions that heal slower and they tend to have more complications (52).

Diagnosis

Confirmation of donovanosis is primarily done via direct microscopy or histopathology with the visualization of Donovan bodies; see Figure 9 (49, 50, 52). Donovan bodies appear as bipolar rods within mononuclear cells with a classic "safety pin" appearance. Biopsy may be necessary in some cases, especially in chronic or atypical cases or to exclude other processes such as malignancy (49-52). Culture does not have any role as it is very difficult to perform. Also, there is no FDA-cleared molecular tests for the detection of *K. granulomatis* (2). Serology has no role in diagnosis (48).

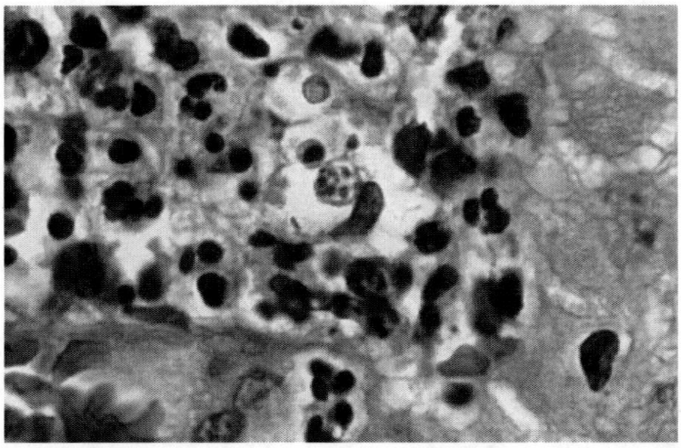

This image is in the public domain and thus free of any copyright restrictions. As a matter of courtesy we request that the content provider be credited and notified in any public or private usage of this image. URL: https://phil.cdc.gov/Details.aspx?pid=16205.

Figure 9. Intracellular Donovan bodies with mononuclear cells caused by *K granulomatis.*

Treatment

Patients should be screened for HIV and syphilis when diagnosed with donovanosis. Partners within 60 days before onset of the patient's symptoms should be examined and offered therapy. However, the value of empiric therapy in the absence of clinical signs and symptoms has not been established (2). Several antimicrobial regimens have been effective but only a limited number of controlled trials have been published. No microbiological susceptibility testing is available for *K. granulomatis*.

Table 4. Recommended and alternative treatment regimens for common ulcerative sexually transmitted infections/diseases

Ulcerative diseases	Treatment regimen
LGV	Doxycycline 100 mg orally twice a day for 21 days *Alternative:* Erythromycin base 500 mg orally four times a day for 21 days
Chancroid	Azithromycin 1 g orally in a single dose, OR Ceftriaxone 250 mg IM in a single dose, OR Ciprofloxacin 500 mg orally twice a day for 3 days, OR Erythromycin base 500 mg orally three times a day for 7 days
Granuloma inguinale	Azithromycin 1 g orally once per week or 500 mg daily for at least 3 weeks and until all lesions have completely healed *Alternative:* Doxycycline 100 mg orally twice a day for at least 3 weeks and until all lesions have completely healed, OR Ciprofloxacin 750 mg orally twice a day for at least 3 weeks and until all lesions have completely healed, OR Erythromycin base 500 mg orally four times a day for at least 3 weeks and until all lesions have completely healed, OR Trimethoprim-sulfamethoxazole one double-strength (160 mg/800 mg) tablet orally twice a day for at least 3 weeks and until all lesions have completely healed

Azithromycin has emerged from practical experience as the agent of choice for the major treatment guidelines. Other options include doxycycline, fluoroquinolones, erythromycin, and trimethoprim–sulfamethoxazole. Table 4 summarizes the treatment regimen for granuloma inguinale. Recommended treatment for patients with HIV will be the same. However, duration of treatment is longer. Surgical intervention may be needed in severe cases, such as pseudo-elephantiasis (53). The disfiguring nature of this illness may lead to psychosocial problems.

Several antimicrobial regimens have been effective, but only a limited number of controlled trials have been published (2). Treatment has been shown to halt progression of lesions and the patient should be followed closely until all lesions have healed. Relapse can occur 6-18 months after effective therapy and the patient should be counseled about this possibility (54). The relative infrequency of donovanosis with the difficulty in confirming the diagnosis necessitates a high index of suspicion in appropriate individuals. It can occur alone or with other STIs. Failed treatment should increase suspicion for other causes.

Bacterial vaginosis

Bacterial vaginosis (BV) is the most common cause of abnormal vaginal discharge; it is also called nonspecific vaginitis and *Gardnerella vaginalis* vaginitis (55, 56). The etiology of BV is unknown, but it is thought to be due to overgrowth of opportunistic bacteria (polymicrobes) and a decrease in the levels of *Lactobacilli* (56, 58, 59). The prevalence of BV can range from 20% to 60% by country and cultural factors may play a role in the prevalence of BV. It is highest in Sub-Saharan Africa; also, the prevalence of BV is higher in South East Africa when compared to West Africa (55). In US, the prevalence of BV was 29.2% as of 2004 (11, 60).

Symptomatic BV is characterized by increased vaginal pH, foul vaginal odor, and vaginal itching (57). Approximately 50% of cases of BV are asymptomatic and it is not known why the rate of asymptomatic status is so high (56, 61). The USPSTF does not currently recommend the screening of asymptomatic pregnant women for BV due to a lack of data supporting the benefits of screening (62).

Numerous risk factors are associated with BV, such as sexual history, intravaginal practices, contraceptive use, and antibiotic use. There's no sufficient data regarding risk factors for recurrent BV (63). Current literature suggests that there is an increase in the risk of BV with increased number of lifetime sex partners, women who have sex with women (WSW), use of a sex toy, early sexual activity, frequency of vaginal intercourse, recent partner change, oral sex, anal sex and history of bacterial STIs (55, 58, 63-65). There is a strong association between BV and penile-vaginal sex with multiple sex partners (63). Intravaginal practices such as douching have also been determined to increase the risk of BV infection (55, 58, 63-65). Studies have shown protective factors against BV include the use of combined oral contraceptives, progestin only contraceptives, and condom use (55, 58, 65).

Diagnosis

BV is diagnosed using either Amsel's criteria or Nugent score (see Table 5). Amsel's criteria is faster and more affordable making it the more commonly used method in clinical settings. The presence of 3 out of 4 positive criteria is required for diagnosis. It is considered particularly helpful during situations in which the provider's microscopic experience, availability of microscope tools, or time may be a limiting factor. There are four parameters used to determine the presence or absence of BV (11, 66-69). Figure 10 shows the clue cells with stippled appearance characteristic of BV in which bacteria adhere to the epithelial cells of the vagina.

Table 5. Amsel's criteria in BV diagnosis

1.	Vaginal secretion pH > 4.5
2.	Increased homogeneous thin vaginal discharge
3.	Positive whiff test - amine or fishy odor when potassium hydroxide 10% solution is added to a drop of vaginal secretions
4.	Presence of clue cells in wet mount

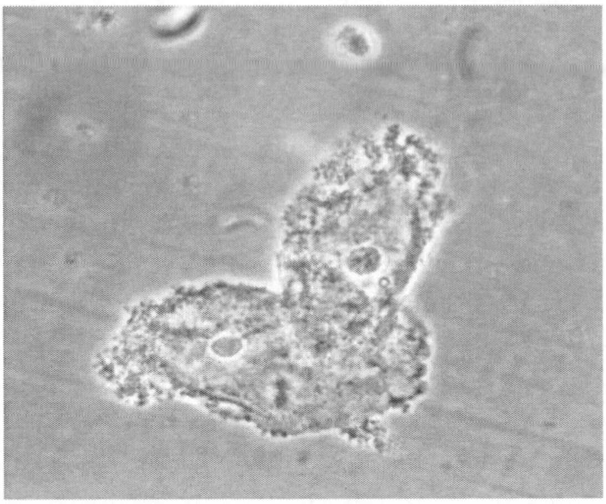

Figure 10. Clue cells are bacteria adhered to the vaginal epithelial cells seen in BV infection.

Treatment

Treatment is only recommended for symptomatic situations in both non-pregnant and pregnant women due to a lack of sufficient evidence to support treatment of asymptomatic women (11, 60). Table 6 summarizes current treatment recommendations for BV. Women with asymptomatic BV often experience high recurrence rates due to a lack of treatment. Though treatment for BV is only recommended for symptomatic cases of the disease, some studies report that treatment of asymptomatic BV may reduce the risk of adverse sequelae (71).

Recurrent BV occurs if infection recurs one or more times after the completion of an episodic regimen (11, 72). BV recurrence rates are high, despite effective treatment; indeed, recurrence occurs up to 80% three months after effective treatment (73). Nocturnal application of topical metronidazole twice a week for six months is the only approved treatment for recurrent BV (73). Currently, the treatment of the partners of women with recurrent BV is not recommended. Treatment of male sexual partners do not improve outcomes of initial BV. It also did not provide beneficial effect on BV recurrence in women (74).

Clinical guidelines do not recommend routine test of cure after treatment of an initial BV infection; also, follow-up visits are unnecessary if symptoms resolve (73). However, because persistent or recurrent BV is common, women should be advised to return for evaluation if symptoms recur (11). There is a lack of diagnostic tests which predict BV recurrence after treatment (75). There is an increased risk of getting other STIs with the presence of BV (76). BV increases the risk of HPV, HIV as well as HIV viral shedding. There is a twofold increased risk of herpes simplex virus type 2 (HSV-2) among women with BV (60). When pregnant women acquire BV, it may cause preterm delivery, intrauterine infection and pelvic inflammatory disease (11).

Table 6. Recommended and alternative treatment regimens for BV

Recommended	**Metronidazole** 500 mg orally twice a day for 7 day, OR **Metronidazole** gel 0.75%, one full applicator (5 g) intravaginally, once a day for 5 days, OR **Clindamycin** cream 2%, one full applicator (5 g) intravaginally at bedtime for 7 days
Alternative	**Tinidazole** 2 g orally once daily for 2 days, OR **Tinidazole** 1 g orally once daily for 5 days, OR **Clindamycin** 300 mg orally twice daily for 7 days, OR **Clindamycin** ovules 100 mg intravaginally once at bedtime for 3 days*

Mycoplasma genitalium

Mycoplasma genitalium (MG) belong to a species of bacteria well known for their small size. See Figure 11. MG in particular has a flask shape under electron microscopy and is becoming an increasingly common pathogen implicated in STIs. This bacterium was first discovered in the 1980s and is estimated to have an infection rate of up to 4% in men and 6.4% in women globally (77).

Its virulence factors include an organelle specific for adhesion, distinguishing it from other *Mycoplasma* species, and its gliding motility. MG adheres to genital epithelial cells as quickly as within two hours of infection (77). Invasion of the cells occurs shortly after adherence. Infection can be managed through phagocytosis by macrophages; however, invasion into epithelial cells allows evasion of this immune response, leading to chronic infection. General symptoms include fever with elevated inflammatory markers and leukocytosis. Interestingly, compared to other common causes of PID such as CT and GC, MG is less likely to have the very elevated ESR and CRP rates. Other symptoms include bilateral adnexal tenderness, vaginal bleeding outside of normal menstrual cycle, and abnormal vaginal discharge (78, 79).

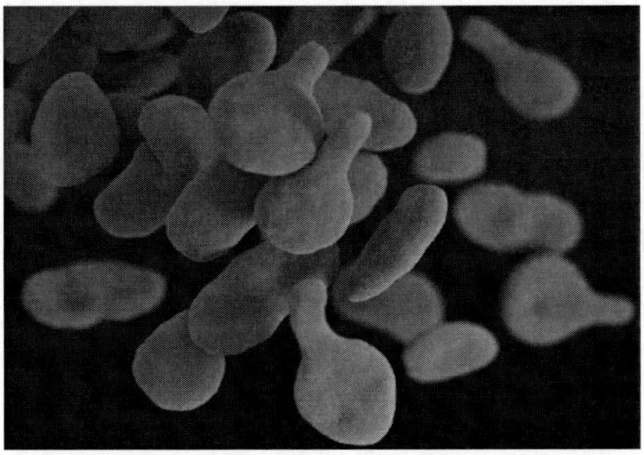

Figure 11. Medical illustration of *M genitalium* bacterium.

Diagnosis

PCR and NAAT are the primary diagnostics for MG. Culture of the bacterium is not performed due to poor yield from clinical samples. Endocervical sampling can be performed, but vaginal swabbing has been found to be as effective, and simpler, at collecting desquamated cervical cells for diagnosis of MG cervicitis. First-void urine samples have shown to be good for diagnosis of urethritis. Often, diagnosis of PID is missed due to lack of routine testing for MG. This often leads to inappropriate treatment (79).

Treatment

All *Mycoplasma* species are difficult to treat due to a lack of cell wall, eliminating effectivity of many antibiotics with mechanisms of actions against components of the cell wall. Antibiotics that are effective for MG infection include tetracyclines, macrolides, and fluoroquinolones. Tetracycline is often considered a first-line treatment, although it has therapeutic failure rates of up to 60% (77). Azithromycin is a preferred antibiotic for MG infection, however, recent studies are showing increased resistance. Azithromycin is still considered first line for upper and lower genital tract infection. Moxifloxacin can be used as first-line treatment for upper genital tract infection. Regardless of which treatment is implemented, PCR testing following treatment should be performed to confirm eradication (77).

Complications

Complications occur following treatment failure or lack of treatment. Chronic pelvic pain is a consequence in an estimated 42%. Further, this infection can cause inflammation and scarring of the fallopian tubes leading to possible infertility (22%). These complications can be easily avoided by proper diagnosis and treatment of this rising cause of PID (77, 78).

STI caused by protozoa

Trichomoniasis is the most prevalent non-viral STI in the United States, affecting an estimated 3.7 million persons (80). It is due to *Trichomonas vaginalis* (TV), a motile organism (protozoan) that lives in the lower genitourinary tract of females and males. TV is among the most common causes of protozoal infections and almost all cases are due to sexual transmission.

Risk factors for acquiring the infection include multiple sexual partners and the concomitant simultaneous presence of other STIs in the patient. In one study with 4,057 participants, trichomoniasis infection was found in 0.5% of males and 1.8% of females in the study population. They found prevalence among African American study participants to be higher, with 4.2% and 8.9% infection rates noted in African American males and females, respectively (81). According to another article, the estimated infection rate of is 3.2%. TV infection rates in the United States are higher than combining NG and CT infection rates.

Trichomoniasis is most prevalent among women ages 40 to 49, compared to the rate of chlamydia infections, which peaks in the 19 to 24-year-old age group (82).

The incubation period for trichomoniasis is 5-28 days. Most infected persons (70%–85%) have minimal or no symptoms, and untreated infections might last for months to years (83). Women with infection may present with vaginal discharge that might be diffuse, malodorous, or yellow-green with or without vulvar irritation. Figure 12 shows the white purulent exudate from the affected female's cervix. Dyspareunia, urinary frequency, dysuria, and/or vulvar pruritus or erythema can occur. In men, it often does not cause symptoms; however, if they become symptomatic, symptoms of urethritis which is the most common, epididymitis, or prostatitis can occur (80).

Other STIs should always be tested for when a patient presents with complaints concerning for trichomoniasis. PID should always be evaluated for in this situation because of the significant implications, including infertility, when not diagnosed and treated early. Significant morbidity can also occur during pregnancy if not treated such as preterm delivery, low birth weight infants, and premature rupture of membranes. Trichomonas, nevertheless, is not known to cause PID. If left untreated, trichomoniasis may remain subclinical or may resolve with host-immunity (82).

There are no recommended screening practices for trichomoniasis in the United States. Some suggest performing TV screening in specific populations, including populations at high risk for HIV infection, patients attending STI clinics, men with urethritis, sexual partners of an infected patient, women living in endemic areas, and women living in correctional facilities. Trichomonas infection has been shown to increase the risk of acquisition and transmission of HIV; it is, for example, associated with two- to threefold increased risk for HIV acquisition (82-84).

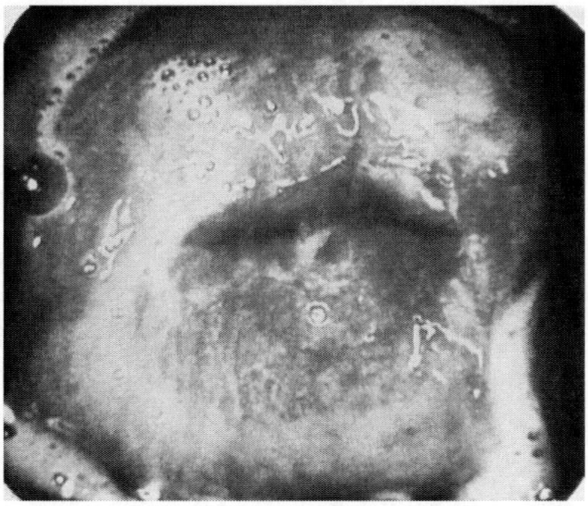

Figure 12. Cervicitis caused by *T vaginalis.*

Diagnosis

The most common diagnostic testing performed is wet prep microscopy because of its convenience and low cost. Trichomonads can be seen moving in the preparation when viewed under the microscope; see Figure 13. This test has been shown to be only 40- 60% sensitive (85). NAATs are gaining favor for TV testing as they have become the gold standard when testing for GC and CT. Many of the NAATs available have been shown to have greater than 90% sensitivity and specificity when testing for Trichomonas (83). NAAT is highly sensitive, often detecting three to five times more Trichomonas infections than wet-mount microscopy (86). Before NAATs and other point-of-care options were developed, the gold standard was a culture when testing for TV with a negative wet prep and a symptomatic patient.

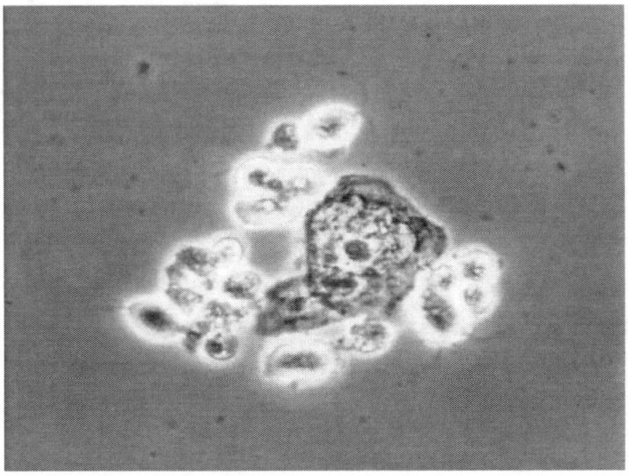

This image is in the public domain and thus free of any copyright restrictions. As a matter of courtesy we request that the content provider be credited and notified in any public or private usage of this image. URL: https://phil.cdc.gov/Details.aspx?pid=17912.

Figure 13. Group of trichomonads in a vaginal discharge wet mount.

Treatment

According to current treatment guidelines, there are three recommended strategies for treatment of trichomoniasis. These include a single 2-gram dose of metronidazole or a single 2-gram dose of tinidazole. An alternative regimen is a 7-day course of 500 mg metronidazole twice daily. When a patient has a known allergy to nitroimidazoles, there is a desensitization protocol that may be used, and a consultation with a specialist is recommended. Specialists should also be consulted when concerns exist for resistant TV.

In patients with known HIV infection, the recommended treatment regimen is a 7-day course of metronidazole 500 mg twice daily. Patients should be counseled on side effects of these medications. It is important to discuss alcohol abstinence when nitroimidazoles are used because they cause a disulfiram-like reaction when patients use alcohol simultaneously while on these antibiotics. The recommendation is 24-hours of alcohol abstinence following metronidazole and 72-hours of alcohol abstinence following tinidazole (11). According to a study, the percent of women positive for trichomoniasis on their test of cure was 19% when given a single dose of metronidazole vs. 11% when patients completed a 7-day course of metronidazole (87).

Patients infected with TV need to abstain from sex until they and their sex partners are treated – that is when therapy has been completed and any symptoms have resolved. The CDC recommends performing a test of cure for all women treated for trichomoniasis within 3 months of treatment due to high rates of reinfection. NAAT can be completed as soon as two weeks following treatment which is the recommended method for test of cure.

Many states allow expedited partner therapy. Providers may be able to prescribe treatment to their patients' partners without performing establishing a provider/patient relationship. Complete list of states that allow this can be found on the CDC website.

Because of high rates of reinfection, it is important to educate patients about safe sex practices. Patients diagnosed with trichomoniasis should be screened for other STIs, including HIV; however, the CDC does not recommend for or against treating for CT and NG while treating trichomoniasis. The decision depends on provider-patient relationship. A major factor that may dictate this is reliability of this patient for follow up as well as risks and benefits of treatment (11).

STIs caused by viruses

The human papillomavirus (HPV), a double stranded DNA virus, is the most common STI globally, affecting the oropharynx and anogenital regions transmitted via intimate contact. The pathogenesis of this virus is linked to the expression of viral oncogenes, which interact with host cell growth regulation, and leads to transformation of proteins such that affected individuals remain undetected for years from initial acquisition of the virus (11).

HPV causes mucocutaneous warts (oral, genital) and genitourinary cancers in both men and women (88). Despite the availability of HPV vaccination and that such vaccination is known to be effective, cervical cancer remains one of the leading causes of death in women (89). Increased risk of HPV infection in men includes having at least 3 lifetime partners who have sex with women and being an HIV-positive MSM particularly with involvement of the anal region (90).

The genomic makeup of the viral capsid protein characterizes the different HPV strains and are typically divided into "high-risk" or "low-risk" based on cancer predisposing ability. The high risk or oncogenic types 16 and 18 lead to cervical changes. These changes are usually asymptomatic and in immunocompetent individuals, the infection frequently resolves on its own within 1-2 years of infection (91). At least 60% of cervical cancers worldwide are caused by HPV-16 and around 10% from HPV-18 (90). Carcinomas of the anus, vagina, oropharynx, penis, and vulva are predominantly caused by HPV-16 (88).

Other relatively common high-risk strains include types 31, 33, 35, 45, 52 and 58. HPV-positive squamous cell carcinomas can be attributed to all the high-risk strains mentioned (90). Genital warts or condyloma acuminata are common manifestations of the low-risk strains, types 6 and 11, which account for up to 90% of warts in the anogenital region; see Figure 14 (90). Warts found in the respiratory tract can lead to recurrent respiratory papillomatosis (RRP) which can be devastating as it may require surgical intervention (90, 92).

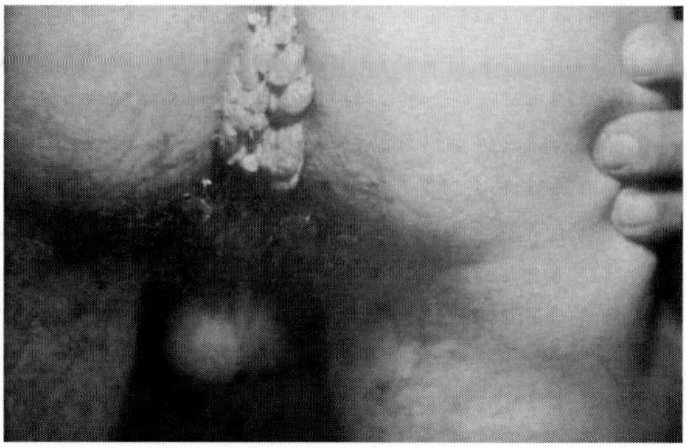

Figure 14. Anal warts caused by HPV.

Disease expression of HPV includes common warts (verruca vulgaris), genitourinary pre-cancerous lesions (such as low-grade squamous intraepithelial lesions) and high-grade intraepithelial lesions and cancers such as vulvar intraepithelial neoplasia, vaginal intraepithelial neoplasia, and cervical intraepithelial neoplasia (88). Other associated conditions include pre-cancerous lesions and cancers in the rectum and penis, certain oropharyngeal cancers and RRP (88, 93).

Diagnosis

HPV diagnosis is through testing of cervical specimens via the Papanicolaou (Pap) smears and initial screening is recommended at age 21 years regardless of sexual activity along with repeated Pap smears every three years in young adult women for early detection of atypical cervical changes. If there is persistence of such lesions, it is important for close follow-up given its potential progression through various stages from precancerous to cancerous lesions over time. Because of self-resolving infections in younger females, HPV testing is only recommended in females age 25 years or older. More frequent screening is recommended in immunocompromised women such as those who are HIV-positive or on immunosuppressant therapy. Currently, there are no FDA approved tests for detection of oropharyngeal, anal, or vaginal/vulvar HPV (11).

Treatment

In healthy immunocompetent individuals, there is spontaneous resolution of most HPV infections. For external anogenital warts most likely caused by HPV-6 and HPV-11, the CDC has listed certain topical treatments that includes imiquimod cream, podofilox solution or gel and sinecatechin ointment. Table 7 summarizes CDC recommendations for treating external warts in the anogenital regions, including the penis, groin, scrotum, vulva, perineum, and anus. Cryotherapy can be used as well.

These, however, do not treat the underlying virus and there is potential reoccurrence of warts (11). Internal warts may be present as well. For the oncogenic types that lead to persistent infections and life-threatening conditions, target treatment is warranted based on the stage of disease. Ablative methods such as thermal coagulation and freezing may be curative for pre-invasive cervical lesions (11, 94). For advanced lesions, cryotherapy and surgical techniques such as loop electrosurgical excision procedure or cone biopsy may be warranted (11, 94).

Table 7. CDC recommended treatment of external anogenital warts

Patient application	Imiquimod 3.75% or 5% cream, or Podofilox 0.5% solution/gel, or Sinecatechins 15% ointment
Health care provider application	Cryotherapy using liquid nitrogen/cryoprobe, or Surgical removal (tangential scissor/shave excision, curettage, laser or electrosurgery), or Tri/bichloroacetic acid 80-90% solution

With the HPV vaccination, prevention is still key. There are several HPV vaccines available – bivalent, quadrivalent, and 9-valent with the latter offering more protection than just the high-risk strains. The current recommendation is to vaccinate all males and females at age 11-12 years, and this can be given as early as age 9. Immunogenicity is best if the HPV vaccine is administered to younger adolescents. All previously unvaccinated males and females can be vaccinated up to age 45 years. With recent changes, the HPV vaccine can be administered as a 2-dose series if initiated before age 15, and 3-dose series if started at 15 years old (95).

Herpes simplex virus

Herpes simplex virus (HSV) is a double stranded DNA with type 1 (HSV-1) causing orolabial infections and type 2 (HSV-2) causing anogenital infections. It is prevalent causing genital herpes and is a life-long infection. Unlike GC and CT, HSV is not a reportable disease. Most cases are caused by HSV-2 although there is an increasing number of cases caused by HSV-1 due to oral-genital transmission. About 1 in 6 individuals from ages 14 to 49 years old have genital herpes (2, 11, 96).

The incubation period typically takes 2-12 days (average of 4 days) after initial exposure. Early coitarche and having multiple sexual partners increase one's risk of acquiring HSV. Primary infection refers to person without pre-existing antibodies to either HSV-1 or HSV-2 who develops an infection (96, 97). Non-primary infection of genital HSV-1 refers to a person with pre-existing antibodies to HSV-2 (or vice versa). Recurrent infection refers to the reactivation of genital HSV in which the HSV lesion type is the same type as the antibodies in the serum. Each of these types can be symptomatic or asymptomatic (subclinical) (97).

Clinically, manifestations of primary HSV infection are highly variable from asymptomatic to symptomatic and viral shedding occurs regardless of symptoms. The lesions start out as vesicles that develop into pustules and subsequently, the characteristic painful, eroding ulcerations emerge; these can affect various areas in men (i.e., the glans, coronal sulcus, penile shaft, urethra, or perianal area) and women (i.e., labia, vaginal introitus, perineal and perianal areas—see Figure 15). Such can extend into the inner thighs or buttocks.

Aside from ulcers, there can be constitutional symptoms such as fever and malaise, and other known presentations that can include urethral discharge, dysuria, vaginal discharge, and tender inguinal lymphadenopathy (97, 98). In others, the initial infection can even progress to lumbosacral radiculomyelitis, which presents as acute urinary retention with loss of sacral sensation. Non-primary infections are typically less severe, presumably due to antibodies of the other HSV type offering protection. Recurrent infections are less severe than both primary and non-primary infections, with a shorter mean duration of lesions (10 vs 19 days) (98).

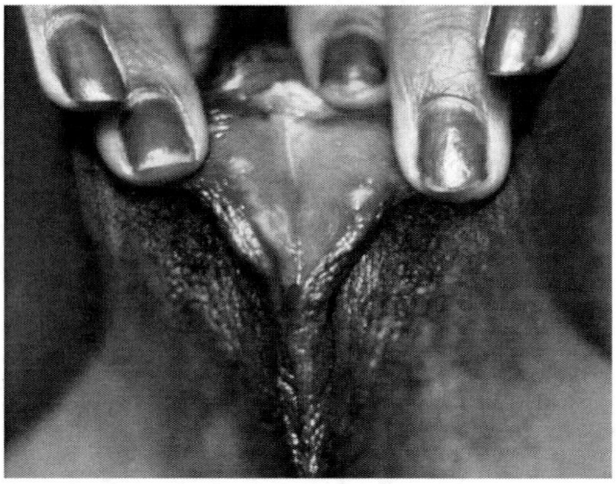

Figure 15. Herpetic outbreak on a female's perineum.

Differential diagnosis

It is important to differentiate between herpetic and non-herpetic ulcers. Other etiologies to consider include infectious causes discussed earlier such as syphilis, chancroid, LGV and granuloma inguinale. More systemic infections such as Epstein-Barr virus and adenovirus may present with genital ulcers. Also, traumatic causes should be ruled out.

Diagnosis

The clinical diagnosis based on history and physical examination of herpetic infections should be confirmed with laboratory testing. For patients with active lesions, PCR is the most sensitive test and effective with results coming back immediately, though this can be expensive compared to viral culture of the lesions. Currently, there are two FDA-cleared PCR tests available. For patients without active disease, type-specific serologic testing can be done (11, 98). For atypical ulcers, consider biopsy particularly if there is a lacking response to initial treatment. HIV must be done on everyone with anogenital or perianal ulcers if not yet checked (11).

Treatment

All patients with primary HSV infection should be treated with antiviral therapy due to the risk of prolonged clinical illness with severe genital lesions. Treatment should be started as soon as lesion appearance is seen and within 72 hours. Antivirals decrease the length and severity of disease by days to weeks, but does not eradicate latent virus. Treatments that can be used with duration from 7-10 days are acyclovir, famciclovir, and valacyclovir, Intravenous (IV) therapy is used for complicated infections such as involvement of the central nervous system, sacral nerve, and in disseminated cases. Persons with HSV encephalitis should be treated for 21 days of IV therapy and renal function must be monitored given the possibility of acyclovir nephrotoxicity (11).

Topical therapy has shown no proven benefit. In recurrent infections, antiviral therapy can reduce severity of symptoms as well as risk of transmission. It should be started at the first sign of prodromal symptoms (i.e., paresthesia, pruritus). Chronic suppressive therapy can be used for those with very frequent or severe recurrences (11). Table 8 summarizes recommendations for genital HSV treatment.

Recurrence of lesions is a common complication. For those not on suppressive therapy, the rate of recurrence is about 4 times per year for HSV-2 and 1 time per year for HSV-1 (98). Other more severe complications include aseptic meningitis, lumbosacral radiculomyelitis (as discussed above), and proctitis (97, 98). An important part of managing infected persons and their sexual partners is providing counseling particularly for those who find it difficult to cope with a lifelong infection. There should be emphasis that even if asymptomatic, there is potential risk of transmitting or acquiring the virus and thus, assertive protection during intercourse is recommended (11).

Table 8. Recommended and alternative treatment regimens for genital herpes

Genital herpes	Treatment regimens
First clinical episode	Acyclovir 400 mg orally three times a day for 7–10 days, or Acyclovir 200 mg orally five times a day for 7–10 days, or Valacyclovir 1 g orally twice a day for 7–10 days, or Famciclovir 250 mg orally three times a day for 7–10 days
Recurrent: suppressive therapy	Acyclovir 400 mg orally twice a day, or Valacyclovir 500 mg orally once a day, or Valacyclovir 1 g orally once a day, or Famiciclovir 250 mg orally twice a day
Recurrent: episodic therapy	Acyclovir 400 mg orally three times a day for 5 days, or Acyclovir 800 mg orally twice a day for 5 days, or Acyclovir 800 mg orally three times a day for 2 days, or Valacyclovir 500 mg orally twice a day for 3 days, or Valacyclovir 1 g orally once a day for 5 days, or Famciclovir 125 mg orally twice daily for 5 days, or Famciclovir 1 gram orally twice daily for 1 day, or Famciclovir 500 mg once, followed by 250 mg twice daily for 2 days
Severe disease	Acyclovir 5–10 mg/kg IV every 8 hours for 2–7 days or until clinical improvement is observed, followed by oral antiviral therapy to complete at least 10 days of total therapy

Human immunodeficiency virus

Human immunodeficiency virus (HIV) is a single stranded RNA retrovirus that can be acquired through sexual activity by anorectal methods in MSM and vaginal/penile methods in heterosexuals who comprise most HIV infections reported in the world. Non-sexual acquisition occurs via perinatal transmission, infected milk, infected blood (transfusion, injection in IV drug users), and organ transplantation (99). Recent CDC data revealed stabilization or decreased HIV incidence in the United States though there is continued increase in high risk groups (100). Individuals who were found to have an STI are at higher risk of acquiring HIV due to similar risky sexual behaviors such as promiscuity and lack of condom use for protection. Some STIs such as syphilis may potentially coexist in those with HIV, hence screening in high risk groups is highly recommended (11).

The pathogenesis of HIV is related to its target of CD4 T-cells resulting in immunodeficiency (11, 99). During the early infection stage around 6 months following HIV exposure, some people can be asymptomatic. However, others can develop acute retroviral syndrome which is a constellation of symptoms consisting of fever, lymphadenopathy, sore throat, rash, myalgias, diarrhea, weight loss, and headache (101). The time from exposure to the development of symptoms is about 2-4 weeks. The development of chronic HIV is typically asymptomatic, though some can have generalized symptoms. Other manifestations of chronic HIV include candidiasis, seborrheic dermatitis, bacterial folliculitis, and recurrence of HSV, varicella zoster virus, or HPV lesions (102).

Diagnosis

A variable period when there is no existing test to diagnose nor detect HIV after an exposure is called the eclipse period. Measuring the HIV RNA is important as it is the first dependable marker of infection with levels said to peak in 20-30 days. Two weeks after infection, the HIV-1 capsid protein p24 can be detectable followed by raising antibodies with eventual clearance of the antigen by week 6 (103).

The window period is referred to the time from infection to first detectable test result. In 1985, the first test to diagnose HIV was approved by the FDA and more tests have been developed over time (103). Initial testing for HIV should be conducted with an FDA approved antigen/antibody immunoassay that detects HIV antibodies and the HIV p24 antigen (11). If these are non-reactive, no further testing is needed. However, if there is a possibility of very early infection that may lead to an initial non-reactive immunoassay, then an HIV-NAAT should be performed (11).

The early diagnosis of HIV is crucial, as rapid initiation of anti-retroviral therapy reduces both transmission as well as viral load. Chronic HIV is diagnosed when there is a stable viral load level, with a progressive decline in CD4 cell count (102). There are available point-of-care tests approved by the FDA which allows for anonymous testing; however, the other tests discussed have greater sensitivity particularly in making the diagnosis early once infected (103).

Treatment

The CDC provides updated guidelines in prevention and treatment of HIV which entails use of antiretroviral therapy (ART) in reducing the amount of viral load. Though there is no formal cure, if taken correctly, ART can significantly slow the progression of HIV, as well as reduce the risk of transmission. ART is usually taken as a combination of 3 or more drugs typically comprised of two nucleoside or nucleotide reverse transcriptase inhibitors (NRTI) such as abacavir or tenofovir and a third drug like a protease inhibitor (such as indinavir or ritonavir), a non-NRTI (such as efavirenz or nevirapine), or an integrase inhibitor (such as raltegravir) (11, 104). There are ongoing investigational HIV treatment strategies and it is important for infected individuals to find providers who specializes in this area of medicine as counseling is equally important to avoid future complications.

Aside from the possible manifestations of chronic HIV that were mentioned above, the most feared complication of HIV is AIDS (acquired immunodeficiency syndrome). This is the outcome of chronic HIV, if not well controlled. It is defined as CD4 cells <200, or the presence of an AIDS defining condition. Some (but not all) AIDS defining conditions include candidiasis of the esophagus, cryptococcal infection, cytomegalovirus retinitis, Kaposi sarcoma, *Mycobacterium avium complex*, and *Pneumocystis carinii* pneumonia (102).

Hepatitis viruses

Hepatitis A virus (HAV) is a single stranded non-enveloped RNA virus that is spread by the fecal-oral route (105). The pathophysiology of the virus is biphasic. The first stage is the noncytopathic stage, in which viral replication occurs in the hepatocyte, resulting in the virus being released in the bile. It is in this phase where fecal shedding begins. The second stage is the cytopathic stage, in which there is portal zone infiltration and necrosis, as well as immune mediated hepatocellular destruction (105).

The clinical presentation of hepatitis A is similar in both males and females. Symptoms develop between 15-50 days from initial exposure. Initial symptoms are non-specific and include fever, malaise, anorexia, vomiting, diarrhea, and abdominal pain (106). During this time, both liver enzymes and bilirubin are elevated. About 1 week after symptom onset, jaundice, mild hepatomegaly, and choluria occurs (106). There can also be development of extrahepatic manifestations such as rash and arthralgias. In most patients, full recovery occurs in 2-3 months (107).

The gold standard for diagnosing acute hepatitis A is the detection of hepatitis A IgM antibodies; these antibodies are present at the onset of symptoms, and remains positive for 4-6 months (108). Another method of detection is hepatitis A RNA in the stool, though the detection of antibodies is easier and less expensive.

The most important prevention of hepatitis A is with routine vaccination. The vaccine is administered in a 2-dose schedule for children at 12 months of age. The vaccine is also recommended for high risk groups (MSM, international travel to endemic areas, IV drug abusers, homelessness, and others) (109). Treatment of acute hepatitis A infection, is mostly supportive, mainly hydration (11). For those who develop signs of acute liver failure, hospitalization is needed (11).

Though complications are rare (<1% of cases), the most feared complication is acute liver failure and this is more common in those with underlying liver disease. For adolescents and young adults, the case fatality rate is 0.1% (110). Acute hepatitis A does not become chronic, though relapse of the disease can occur. It can also trigger autoimmune hepatitis in some cases (111).

Hepatitis B virus (HBV)

HBV is a partially double stranded DNA virus that can be spread through sexual transmission and blood exposure. The liver injury sustained from this virus is largely due to immune mediated processes involving damage of hepatocytes by cytotoxic T cells (112).

The majority of individuals (~70%) have subclinical (anicteric) hepatitis, while 30% develop icteric hepatitis (113). The acute phase of hepatitis B occurs after an incubation period of ~1-4 months (114). In the acute phase, individuals can develop serum sickness like illness (fever, rash, arthralgias), followed by constitutional symptoms. This presentation can also be accompanied by anorexia, jaundice, and right upper abdominal pain. During this time, there are elevations in liver enzymes. The symptoms and lab abnormalities typically resolve in 1-3 months.

The persistent elevation of liver enzymes (especially ALT [alanine aminotransferase]) for >6 months indicates possible progression to chronic hepatitis. Chronic hepatitis is typically asymptomatic, while others can have nonspecific symptoms such as fatigue). Laboratory studies may be normal, but can also have mild to moderate elevations in liver enzymes. There can also be extrahepatic manifestations, the major ones being polyarteritis nodosa and glomerular disease (114).

Diagnosis

The diagnosis of acute hepatitis B infection involves the detection of HBsAg (hepatitis B surface antigen) as well as IgM antibodies to hepatitis B core antigen (anti-HBc). During the acute phase, markers of replication are also present – HBeAg and HBV DNA. The disappearance of HBV DNA, conversion of HBeAg to anti-HBe, and conversion of HBsAg to anti-HBs signal recovery. Past infection is diagnosed with anti-HBs and IgG anti-HBs. Chronic infection is diagnosed with the presence of HBsAg for >6 months (11).

Treatment

The treatment for acute hepatitis B infection is mainly supportive (11). It is important to manage any coagulopathy and/or encephalopathy that may result from acute liver failure. For chronic infections, there are several antiviral medications that may be used, and these patients should be referred to specialized providers that are experienced in the management of chronic hepatitis B infection (11). The complications of hepatitis B infection are fulminant hepatic failure, cirrhosis, hepatocellular carcinoma, and death (114). Table 9 summarizes the CDC recommendations for hepatitis B screening.

Table 9. Hepatitis B screening recommendations

• Screen all women and men who are at increased risk
• Pregnant women should get tested for HBsAg at first prenatal visit of each pregnancy regardless of past testing and should be retested at delivery if deemed high risk
• All MSM should get tested for HBsAg
• For persons with HIV, test for HBsAg and anti-HBc and/or anti-HBs

Hepatitis C virus (HCV)

HCV is an enveloped RNA virus that is commonly spread by parenteral exposures. This makes HCV common among drug users and in the medical community who may experience needle stick injuries. Additionally, there is recent research showing that HCV incidence is increasing among MSM. Interestingly, outside of the MSM population, sexual transmission of HCV is uncommon with prevalence of sexually transmitted HCV among monogamous heterosexual couples at 0.6% (115-117).

HCV invades hepatocytes that causes cell necrosis and liver disease. Patients who are infected with HCV can take 3 different paths: spontaneous complete viral clearance in 15% (median clearance time by 108 days following infection), chronic infection with fluctuating viremia in 37.5%, or chronic infection with plateau viremia in 47.5% (116, 118). HCV induced hepatic steatosis is common and can occur through three mechanisms: impaired hepatocyte lipid secretion, increased free fatty acid synthesis, or impaired fatty acid breakdown. HCV coinfection with HIV is an increasingly common cause of morbidity and mortality. It is estimated that coinfection rates of up to 30% exist for HCV and HIV in the United States (118).

The majority of people infected with HCV are asymptomatic. When symptoms present, anywhere from 2 weeks to 6 months following infection, they are often non-specific influenza-like symptoms such as fever, fatigue, vomiting, joint pain, nausea. Jaundice can be the key symptom differentiation of a viral upper respiratory tract infection ("cold") or influenza from HCV infection (119).

Diagnosis

Diagnosis of HCV is separated into identifying a chronic infection from an acute infection. Chronic HCV diagnosis is made by the presence of antibodies against HCV. However, the presence of antibodies does not differentiate between chronic and acute infection; therefore, HCV-RNA test must be performed to separate past from present infection. Core antigen has been commonly used for chronic HCV detection.

Acute infection is more difficult to diagnose due to the long seroconversion time, up to 90 days, until antibodies can be identified. In addition to antibodies not being present at time of testing for acute first-time infections, in cases of acute reinfection, the presence of antibodies may not be diagnostic since they may be present from a previous infection. In clinical settings, first line labs include liver function tests as a screening, with elevated levels warranting further work up (118, 119).

Treatment

Management of HCV Infection depends on a variety of factors such as the presence of liver cirrhosis, chronic infection, or firsttime infection. First line treatment is a combination of pegylated interferon and ribavirin, which act to activate gene transcription or act as a nucleoside inhibitor, respectively, to inhibit viral replication. There are a number of drugs that act directly on the virus such as sofosbuvir, simeprevir, and daclatasavir. There is increased efficacy when these drugs are combined with each other or in combination with the pegylated interferon and ribavirin therapy. Concerns with all these drugs include toxicity and frequently a lack of access due to cost (120).

Complications

Primary complications of HCV infection are related to the liver, causing damage, fibrosis, cirrhosis, and increased risk for hepatocellular carcinoma. Other organs and body systems that can be impacted by HCV infection include the kidneys, bone, skin, lymph nodes, and the immune system leading to autoimmune conditions (121). Table 10 summarizes the CDC recommendations for hepatitis B screening.

Table 10. Hepatitis C screening recommendations

• Screen all women (including those pregnant) and men (including MSM) born between the years 1945 to 1965 and if with identifiable risk factors
• Yearly HCV testing in MSM with HIV infection
• For persons with HIV, serologic testing must be done at initial evaluation

STIs caused by fungi and parasites

Candida is a single-celled fungus, otherwise known as a yeast. Vulvovaginal candidiasis is caused by a variety of *Candida* species, primarily *Candida albicans,* and is the second leading cause of vaginitis after bacterial causes. In males, *Candida* spp. can cause balanitis, infection of the glans penis. Candidiasis is transmitted sexually and is predominant in women during childbearing years with 75% being affected by vulvovaginal candidiasis (122). Many asymptomatic women, about 20%, are colonized by *Candida* in the perianal region, leading to easy access to the vagina and infection.

These yeast species infect the vaginal epithelial cells by sexual transmission, or by direct access from the perianal area in those who are colonized by *Candida*. Most women who are asymptomatically colonized typically have a risk factor. These factors include pregnancy, use of estrogen oral contraceptives, uncontrolled diabetes mellitus, HIV infection, or frequent coitus. Pregnancy and estrogen oral contraceptives increase ease of adherence to vaginal epithelial cells. Diabetes mellitus has been shown to be associated with increase colonization, but the mechanism is unclear. HIV infection causes an immunocompromised state, leading to reduced cell-mediated immunity and lack of response to a *Candida* infection. Frequent coitus increases the chances of transferring yeast in asymptomatic colonized women from the perianal area to the vagina, as well as the risk of male infection leading to balanitis (122).

Candidiasis more frequently affects females. Vulvovaginal candidiasis presents similarly to balanitis, with severe pruritis, erythema, and swelling of the labia. While "cottage cheese" discharge is often associated with vaginal candidiasis, most symptomatic women present with pruritis only – not discharge. Other symptoms patients may complain of include vulvar burning, pain with sexual intercourse, and pain with urination (dysuria). If infection occurs within a week of menstruation, symptoms may be worse, but are relieved with menstrual flow. Candidiasis is less common in males, but can cause balanitis. True infection presents with extreme pruritis, edema, and erythema of the glans. These symptoms can spread to the penile shaft and in some cases, to the scrotum. This occurs most frequently in uncircumcised diabetic males.

There is a milder form of infection that results from a hypersensitivity to *Candida* in vaginal secretions of asymptomatic colonized females. This form also presents with pruritis and erythema, but can be easily treated with proper washing of the penis, or with topical corticosteroids. In order to avoid recurrence, the female partner must be treated and *Candida* must be eradicated (122, 123).

Diagnosis

Microscopic examination of vaginal secretions and identification of germinated yeast is diagnostic of candidiasis. Due to BV and trichomoniasis being common causes of vaginitis, a simple way to differentiate them from candidiasis is to measure vaginal pH; a normal pH (4.0-4.5) is consistent with candidiasis, while a more basic pH is suggestive of other causes. Culture is the most sensitive method of identifying *Candida* spp. but many women who are colonized may have positive cultures, regardless of whether the infection is due to yeast (122, 123).

Treatment

Management of candidal infections is split up into treatment of acute isolated episodes and recurrent episodes. For an acute vaginitis, topical options are preferred. Nystatin creams, while effective, have a cure rate of 80%; topical azoles, a class of antifungals, are superior to nystatin with cure rates up to 90%. Acute infections can also be treated with oral medications, which most patients prefer over topical options. The primary concerns with oral therapies are toxicity and adverse effects, thus, for these reasons, they are not primary treatments for pregnant women. Recurrent episodes, more than four in a year, are treated with oral agents. First, the acute infection is treated with an azole, such as fluconazole. Relapse prevention is done with weekly oral fluconazole. Again, while topical treatment can be used as a preventative measure, most women prefer oral over topical agents (124).

While candidiasis does not typically cause complications, aside from the possibility of having recurrent infections, disseminated candidiasis may occur in rare cases. This presents with non-specific symptoms such as fevers and chills that do not improve with antibacterial treatments. In cases of symptoms refractory to antibiotics, fungal causes such as *Candida* species should be considered (125).

Pediculosis Pubis

Pediculosis pubis, commonly referred to as "pubic lice" and "crabs," is caused by the parasite *Pthirus pubis*. While it is not required to report a diagnosis of pediculosis pubis, it is estimated to affect up to 10% of the population worldwide. Evidence demonstrates that this parasite has been infecting humans for 10,000 years (126, 127). Outbreaks are related to a lack of sanitation, close quarters, and poor access to treatment options, such as seen in prisons and developing countries (128).

Pubic lice are transmitted sexually or by close genital contact. It has been reported to recur frequently in specific populations, such as MSM. Unlike many other STIs, condoms are not an effective form of protection against contracting pubic lice. The lice attach to the hair shaft and have the ability to travel across hairless body parts; see Figure 16. This unique ability leads to patients being affected in additional areas such as the axilla and abdominal hair, as well as the face, on beards and eyelashes. Lice lay nits that contain hundreds of eggs that hatch after a week. The newly hatched nymphs will become adults after 10 days survive by feeding on blood from the host and cannot survive after removal (129).

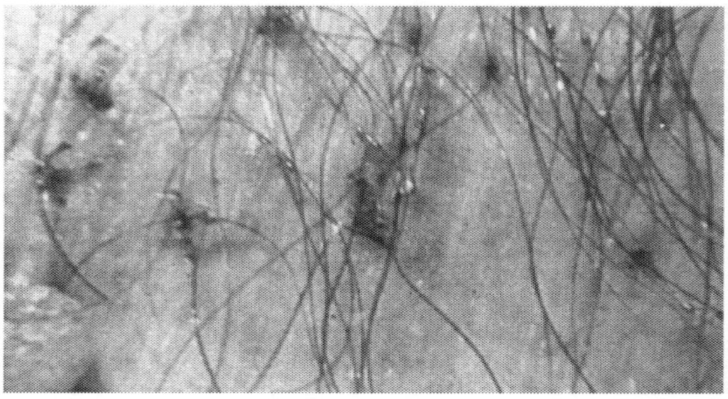

Figure 16. Crab lice seen in the pubic area.

The primary symptom, that people quickly notice, is itching in the pubic area. In some cases, the pruritus does not manifest until months after the infection. Lice and nits can be visualized with the naked eye with close inspection of the affected areas. It is important to examine the person thoroughly to ensure the lice have not traveled and infected other areas of the body (126). There is no lab test to diagnose pediculosis pubis. Diagnosis is made solely based on the visualization of nits and lice on inspection. A louse comb can be used to isolate live lice (127).

Treatment

The primary basis of treatment includes treating the patient in all areas of the body with hair, except eyelashes if they are unaffected, as well as their sexual partners. Commonly used insecticides for eradication of pubic lice include pyrethrins, permethrin, malathion, lindane, and DDT. Of these, permethrin is a synthetic version of pyrethrin and is more potent. Malathion inhibits cholinesterase and is broken down more quickly in humans than insects, making it a relatively safe treatment. Lindane and DDT are being phased out as common treatment forms due to increasing resistance to these agents. If eyelashes are affected, 1% permethrin cream of Vaseline can be applied to the area. Patients need to be informed of the importance of cleaning their clothing and bedding in hot water to decrease risk of reinfection (130).

Complications

While complications of pubic lice are not very common, long-term infection can have mild consequences. Some people may experience skin color changes at regions where lice were feeding long term. The pruritus can lead to intense scratching giving access to other pathogens and possible wound infections. In cases where eyelashes are affected, typically in children, conjunctivitis may develop. Conjunctivitis secondary to pubic lice has been treated with petroleum jelly and permethrin shampoo (131).

Scabies

Scabies is caused by a mite, *Sarcoptes scabiei var humanus*. This species can only use humans as a host, which it has done for more than 2,500 years. It is transmitted through skin to skin contact, making sexual transmission a common cause (127, 129). Annually this mite infects 300 million people worldwide and outbreaks are typical in long term care institutions such as nursing homes (132).

Scabies mites are known for their skin to skin contact transmission; however, they can also spread by fomites due to their ability to survive for up to 36 hours without a host. This makes eradication of scabies infestations particularly difficult. Chances of transmission is proportional to the number of parasites on the infected individual or fomite. Once the mites have found a host, they cause infection by burrowing into the skin, leaving feces as they go. Female mites additionally deposit eggs as they burrow, causing further irritation and inflammation. These eggs hatch within 4 days, but 90% do not survive to become mature mites (129, 132).

Scabies prefer warm moist areas such as the interdigital web spaces of the hands, axillae, genitalia (see Figure 17), breasts, and flexor surfaces of wrist and elbows. Symptoms do not present until after 4-6 weeks as our immune system does not mount a response for that long. Once lesions present, they are intensely pruritic and increase in severity at night. Typically, the pruritic lesions will affect entire families and that can be a primary indicator that scabies is the potential culprit. There are a variety of forms of scabies infections including crusted scabies (Norwegian scabies), bullous scabies, and nodular scabies.

Crusted scabies is dominant in the immunocompromised population and can lead to nail hyperkeratosis. Bullous scabies typically presents in patients over 65 years old. This form of scabies can present with lesions consistent with bullous pemphigoid, an autoimmune disorder of the subepidermal layer of the skin. The treatment of bullous scabies and bullous pemphigoid is drastically different and accurate diagnosis is crucial. Nodular scabies is particular in how it primarily affects areas of the body that are covered, such as the axillae and groin (132).

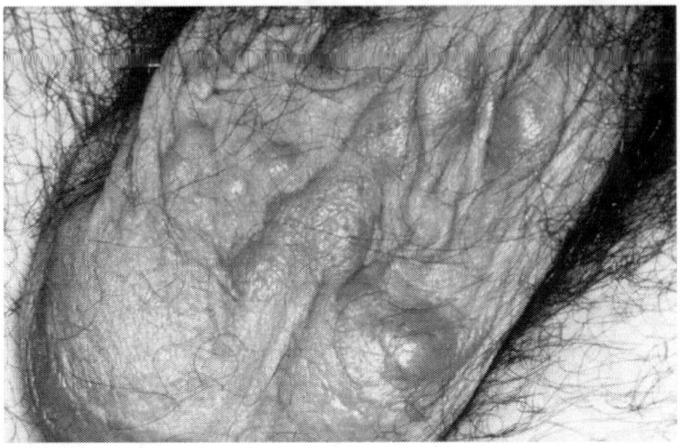

This image is in the public domain and thus free of any copyright restrictions. As a matter of courtesy we request that the content provider be credited and notified in any public or private usage of this image. URL: https://phil.cdc.gov/Details.aspx?pid=15347.

Figure 17. Scrotal papules infested with scabies.

Diagnosis

A scabies diagnosis relies on visualization of a mite, feces, or eggs. Typically, microscopic evaluation is done of a skin scraping from the lesion. Solvents used for visualization include mineral oil, saline, or potassium chloride. While some solvents are superior with regards to image quality, like potassium chloride, it has been found to dissolve mite feces; this could lead to a false negative result (132).

Treatment

The patient and any close contacts should be treated, regardless of having symptoms present, due to the high infectivity rate. Lindane lotion has been the first line treatment until recent research demonstrates central nervous system toxicity in animal studies. Permethrin cream is preferred over lindane due to its low toxicity due to low skin absorption; there is 40 times less risk of toxicity with 5% permethrin cream than 1% lindane lotion. Other treatments include sulfur (not commonly prescribed due to odor) and benzyl benzoate lotion, which has been used since 1937. In addition to the pharmacological treatment, patients should receive guidance and information on how to clean their home and clothing to ensure eradication of the mites (132).

Complications

There are few known complications that can result from a scabies infection. Aside from the mental toll it can take from impacting quality sleep, the excessive pruritus and itching can lead to breaks in the skin. Once the protective barrier of our skin is broken, infection can occur leading to further complications. (133)

Pelvic inflammatory disease

Pelvic inflammatory disease (PID) is an infection that affects the female upper genital tract, with frequent involvement of pelvic organs (134). It is classically initiated by an STI. Endocervical infection by these pathogens results in disruption of the endocervical canal barrier; this barrier normally protects the upper genital tract, which is sterile, from normal vaginal flora. Therefore, disruption of this barrier allows vaginal flora to make contact with upper genital organs, as well as the pelvic peritoneum (134). The most common organisms are *N gonorrhoeae, C trachomatis,* and *M genitalium*. However, in most cases, the exact organism is unknown, and is considered to be caused by a mixed or polymicrobial infection (134, 135).

Table 11. Clinical diagnosis of PID

Minimum criteria	One or more of the following: uterine tenderness, adnexal tenderness, or cervical motion tenderness
Additional criteria	Fever Mucopurulent discharge from the vagina or cervix Leukocytosis in vaginal discharge Elevated inflammatory markers (ESR, CRP) Laboratory presence of NG or CT
Most specific criteria	Biopsy of the endometrium with histopathologic evidence of endometrial infection/inflammation Imaging: transvaginal US or MRI showing evidence of pyo/hydrosalpinx, free-fluid or tubo-ovarian complex/abscess PID findings on laparoscopy

Table 11 summarizes the criteria in making the clinical diagnosis of PID (11). The main presenting symptom is bilateral lower abdominal pain. Patients can also present with abnormal uterine bleeding, dysuria, dyspareunia, abnormal vaginal discharge (134). On physical examination, patients can have lower abdominal tenderness to palpation. Rebound tenderness and fever are typically only seen in severe cases. The most defining characteristic on bimanual pelvic exam is acute cervical motion, uterine, and adnexal tenderness (134).

Diagnosis

When patients present with symptoms described above, the index of suspicion for PID should be high (134, 135). Evaluation should include urine pregnancy, microscopy of discharge, chlamydia/gonorrhea/mycoplasma testing, HIV and syphilis testing (135). Pelvic ultrasound can help to evaluate for alternate causes of pelvic pain, or to assess for complications of PID (i.e., pelvic abscess). A presumptive diagnosis of PID is made in at risk patients (sexually active women or women at risk for STI) with pelvic/lower abdominal pain, who also have evidence of cervical/adnexal/uterine tenderness on bimanual examination. Other findings that can support but are not necessary for the diagnosis of PID include: oral temperature >101 degree F, abnormal cervical/vaginal discharge, cervical friability, high amounts of white blood cells on microscopy of vaginal discharge, and/or documented infection with common organisms (11, 134, 135).

Treatment

There is a low threshold for treatment of PID, due to the risk of long-term sequelae if left untreated. Outpatient treatment includes a single intramuscular (IM) dose of long acting cephalosporin, plus doxycycline and metronidazole (for 14 days). Close follow-up is essential to ensure clinical improvement. The following are indications for hospitalization: severe clinical illness (high fever, severe pain, vomiting), complicated PID with pelvic abscess, need for surgical intervention (ruptured abscess), oral intolerance, lack of response to oral medications, pregnancy, and/or concern for noncompliance. Inpatient treatment involves IV antibiotic therapy with a second-generation cephalosporin or doxycycline. Clinicians can also use clindamycin in combination with gentamicin. If there is a pelvic abscess, metronidazole is added. Patients can be transitioned to oral therapy after 24 hours of sustained clinical improvement (11). Table 12 summarizes treatment recommendations.

Table 12. Treatment recommendations for PID

IM/Oral	**Ceftriaxone** 250 mg IM in a single dose PLUS **Doxycycline** 100 mg orally twice a day for 14 days WITH* or WITHOUT **Metronidazole** 500 mg orally twice a day for 14 days, or **Cefoxitin** 2 g IM in a single dose and **Probenecid**, 1 g orally administered concurrently in a single dose PLUS **Doxycycline** 100 mg orally twice a day for 14 days WITH or WITHOUT **Metronidazole** 500 mg orally twice a day for 14 days, or
	Other parenteral third-generation **cephalosporin** (e.g., ceftizoxime or cefotaxime) PLUS **Doxycycline** 100 mg orally twice a day for 14 days WITH* or WITHOUT **Metronidazole** 500 mg orally twice a day for 14 days
Parenteral	**Cefotetan** 2 g IV every 12 hours PLUS **Doxycycline** 100 mg orally or IV every 12 hours, or **Cefoxitin** 2 g IV every 6 hours PLUS **Doxycycline** 100 mg orally or IV every 12 hours, or **Clindamycin** 900 mg IV every 8 hours PLUS **Gentamicin** loading dose IV or IM (2 mg/kg), followed by a maintenance dose (1.5 mg/kg) every 8 hours. Single daily dosing (3–5 mg/kg) can be substituted
Alternative	**Ampicillin/Sulbactam** 3 g IV every 6 hours PLUS **Doxycycline** 100 mg orally or IV every 12 hours

Complications

Tubo-ovarian abscess is the most dangerous complication of acute PID and this can result in rupture, which is a surgical emergency. Fitz-Hugh – Curtis Syndrome is also a complication of acute PID; it involves inflammation and formation of adhesions in the liver capsule (i.e., violin string adhesions). Long term complications include: recurrent PID, hydrosalpinx, chronic pelvic pain, ectopic pregnancy, and infertility (due to injury to fallopian tube) (11, 134-136). Providers caring for affected patients must deliver non-judgmental care given the potential of severe health consequences and social stigma (137).

Epididymitis

Epididymitis is inflammation of the epididymis in males and in the outpatient setting, it is the most common cause of scrotal pain. The most common etiology is from sexually transmitted pathogens; however, it can also be from trauma or autoimmune conditions as well. The most common pathogens responsible for epididymitis are *C. trachomatis* and *N. gonorrhoeae* (138). These pathogens are believed to travel in a retrograde fashion via the ejaculatory ducts to the epididymis.

Patients with epididymitis present with unilateral, localized testicular pain and swelling, along with tenderness on palpation of the affected epididymis (which is located on the posterior testes). Some patients may have scrotal wall erythema and a reactive hydrocele. There may be a positive Prehn sign (i.e., relief of pain with manual elevation of affected testis). Severe illness (i.e., severe pain/swelling, fever, lower urinary tract symptoms) is rare (138).

Diagnosis

The presumptive diagnosis of epididymitis is made clinically by history and physical. It is important to first rule out urgent surgical causes of testicular pain first (i.e., testicular torsion). Urinalysis, urine culture, and NAAT for *N. gonorrhoeae* as well as *C trachomatis* should be performed. Identification of a pathogen supports the presumptive diagnosis. If there is uncertainty regarding the diagnosis, a Doppler ultrasound can be helpful. It will show increased blood flow to the affected epididymis; also, it will help with ruling out testicular torsion (138, 139).

Treatment

Most cases are treated outpatient with antibiotics, non-steroidal anti-inflammatory drugs, local ice application, and scrotal elevation to relieve pain. An empiric antibiotic regimen can be used to treat both chlamydia and gonorrhea (IM ceftriaxone plus doxycycline or azithromycin) (11, 138).

CDC recommendations for STI screening

Once a thorough, confidential sexual history has been obtained, it is important to discuss preventative care that particularly includes screening. Often, the adolescent or young adult may have no complaints yet be infected with an STI. Table 13 summarizes current recommendations according to the CDC for STI screening (11).

Table 13. CDC recommendations for screening chlamydia, gonorrhea, syphilis, trichomonas, herpes and HIV

		Chlamydia	**Gonorrhea**	**Syphilis**	**Trichomonas**	**Herpes**	**HIV**
Women	Sexually active women under 25 years of age	✓	✓				
	Sexually active women aged 25 years and older if at increased risk	✓	✓				
	All from ages 13 to 64 years old						✓
	All seeking evaluation and treatment for STIs						✓
	Retest 3 months after treatment	✓	✓				
	In high-prevalence settings (i.e., STI clinic, correctional facilities) and high risk sexual behaviors (i.e., multiple sexual partners, illicit drug use, past history of STI)				✓		
	Type-specific HSV serologic testing as indicated*					✓	
Pregnant women	All < 25 years old	✓	✓				
	All > 25 years old if at increased risk	✓	✓				
	All regardless of age at first prenatal visit			✓			✓
	Retest during the 3rd trimester • for women under 25 years of age • for women at high risk	 ✓ ✓					 ✓
	Test-of-cure 3-4 weeks after treatment	✓					
	Retest 3 months after treatment	✓	✓				
	Not routinely recommended but consider type-specific HSV serologic testing as indicated*					✓	
Men	Consider screening young men in high prevalence clinical settings or in populations with high burden of infection (e.g., MSM)	✓					
	All ages 13 to 64 years old						✓
	All seeking evaluation and treatment for STIs						✓
	Type-specific HSV serologic testing as indicated *					✓	
MSM	At least annually			✓			✓
	At least annually at sites of contact regardless of condom use • Urethra • Rectum • Pharynx	 ✓ ✓	 ✓ ✓ ✓				
	Every 3 to 6 months if at increased risk	✓	✓				
	Type-specific serologic tests as indicated					✓	
Persons with HIV	For sexually active individuals, screen at first HIV evaluation, and at least annually thereafter	✓	✓	✓			
	More frequent screening for might be appropriate depending on individual risk behaviors and the local epidemiology	✓	✓	✓			
	Recommended for sexually active women at entry to care and at least annually thereafter				✓		
	Type-specific HSV serologic testing as indicated*					✓	

*Indications: women and men presenting for an STI evaluation especially those with high risk sexual behaviors, persons with HIV infection, and MSM at increased risk for HIV acquisition. In pregnancy, can help guide counseling with emphasis on risk of acquiring genital herpes.

Behavioral considerations

After discussing the different STIs and related conditions/diseases, it is important to recognize again the variety of behavioral factors that can potentially impact an adolescent's likelihood of contracting an STI. The developmental changes that occur during adolescence as mentioned earlier, such as ongoing plasticity, synaptic pruning, and hormonal changes may play a role in risk-taking behavior and thus STI exposure (140). Adolescents have increased attraction to new and exciting experiences, and are prone to both risk-taking behaviors as well as greater emotional reactivity (141, 142). Hare et al. found that the prefrontal cortex of the adolescent was less active in an emotional context relative to adults, implying decreased regulation. They also demonstrated that adolescents had increased activity in the amygdala in response to emotionally evocative stimuli, compared to adults and younger children (143). The authors proposed a possible imbalance between emotional processing and impulse control during adolescence, suggesting that adolescent decision making may be more influenced by emotions compared to adults.

Another study found that given a hypothetical scenario, adolescents tend to use more intellectual, logical reasoning, but facing a quick decision that involved them personally, they were more likely to rely on emotions (142). Adolescents may be aware they are engaging in risky activities, but may choose to engage in them in the moment for a variety of reasons, including emotions and peer influence. Though the adolescent might have the knowledge and ability to reason and make good choices, they may be heavily influenced by feelings and context, and lack sufficient impulse control (142). For example, even when adolescents strongly intend to use condoms during sex, they may have challenges doing so in the moment (140). There is, of course, great individual variability in executive control, and other behavioral factors may be implicated as well.

A study used a nationally representative sample of students from eighty high schools and associated middle schools to examine risk patterns in adolescent sexual behavior (144). Overall most 16-18 year olds fell into either abstinent or low-risk classifications for sexual behavior. Certain demographic factors were associated with differing likelihood of belonging to a higher-risk group. Black adolescents were more likely to have multiple partners and have had early sexual activity, but overall were more likely to fall under low-risk classification. Adolescents who identified as gay or bisexual were less likely to be abstinent. Those in the lowest socioeconomic group were more likely to have multiple partners and engage in early sexual activity. As for substance use, experimental drinking or marijuana use was associated with higher likelihood of vaginal intercourse, but not risky sexual behavior. However, heavy drinking and marijuana use were related to increased odds of having multiple partners. Those with symptoms of depression were also more likely to have multiple partners. Interestingly, engaging in more risky behaviors was associated with higher STI risk in men, but rates of STIs were similar in sexually active women across risk classes (144).

A systematic review of 64 peer-reviewed studies looked at characteristics of adolescent's sexual partners and how they related to likelihood of STI diagnosis (145). Seven of the studies found that having an older partner was associated with increased prevalence of STIs for both males and females, but did not consistently find the same for incidence. Ten out of eleven studies that looked at Black partner race found significant association with likelihood of STI diagnosis, but only four of them performed adjusted statistical analysis. Of those four, only two found significant associations after adjustment. Seven out of ten cross-sectional studies looking at adolescents who had a partner with multiple partners found a significant positive association with STI diagnosis, which was more prominent in female subjects. Only two of four cross-sectional studies looking at partner substance use and STI diagnosis found significant results; one found that having a partner who was under the influence of drugs or alcohol during sex in the last sixty days was positively associated with odds of having an STI. The impact of a partner's history of past STI was inconsistent among studies, but several found an increased risk if the partner's sexual behaviors were unknown, highlighting the importance of communication. The partner's education was not consistently found to have an association with STI risk. As for sexual orientation, a study in the United States found that a greater proportion of males with HIV had had sex with another man. A study in Scotland found that both males and females who had a same-gender partner were more likely to have gonorrhea. Though the review provides valuable insight into partner characteristics, there was no standard definition of "partner" between papers (145).

Adolescents with positive social support at home and school may be at lower risk for STIs. A multivariable analysis using data from the National Longitudinal Study of Adolescent to Adult Health found that higher levels of school connectedness - such as feeling close to peers at school and feeling teachers care about you - were associated with lower odds of risk behaviors, having multiple sexual partners, and STI diagnosis (146). They found the same for higher levels of family connectedness, such as feeling close to parents and that they care about you. However, neither family nor school connectedness were protective for condom nonuse. Potential ideas to utilize these findings include programs that improve communication between parents and children, encouragement of parental monitoring, efforts by teachers and school staff to create a welcoming environment, and school staff aiding with access to safe sex resources (146).

Various other interventions have also been suggested to reduce STI risk in adolescents. A review looking at behavioral sexual risk reduction counseling found that high-intensity interventions, defined as including over 2 hours of material, showed a pooled effect of reducing odds of contracting an STI by 62% in adolescents (147). Most of the studies targeted adolescents determined beforehand to be at increased risk for STI. Consistent with this, recent USPSTF evidence-based recommendations suggested behavioral counseling for those at higher risk of acquiring STIs, including all sexually active adolescents, noting that evidence was stronger for a larger preventative effect in "high-contact" interventions lasting over two hours (148). The USPSTF notes that these interventions can come from the primary care physician, or they can refer the adolescent to counseling in other settings or to premade materials. This can take the form of in-person or telephone counseling, informational videos and websites, written resources, group sessions, or texting. The content should include background on STIs, assessment of the individual's risk, and "training in condom use, communication about safer sex, problem solving, and other pertinent skills", as well as aim to increase the individual's motivation to engage in safe sex practices (148).

To accurately identify those who would benefit from behavioral counseling, the USPSTF also recommends physicians regularly ask adolescents about their sexual history. Additionally, the USPSTF noted the need for further research in LGBTQ+ populations in regards to behavioral counseling for STI prevention in adolescents. Another strategy is examining and improving barriers to condom use (145). A global review looking at condom availability programs (CAP) in high schools found that CAP did not lead to users having more sexual partners, earlier onset of intercourse, or more sexual activity (149). In most of the studies, CAP did increase condom use and decrease STI rates, though the impact on HIV rates was unclear. Other potential suggestions include encouraging communication with one's partner about sexual behaviors, focusing more on males due to greater impact of risk behaviors, and encouraging more testing in adolescents who engage in risky sexual behaviors or those with partners possessing higher risk attributes (145).

Conclusion

Adolescent and young adults are at increased risk of acquiring STIs during their lifetime. Several behavioral/developmental, biological, and sociocultural factors have been identified and exert a significant role in transmission as well as treatment. Despite decline of incidences of most STIs, affected young individuals still suffer the medical and psychological complications of this disease. The different etiologies of STIs discussed could be bacterial, viral, protozoal, parasitic and fungal. Being adept with current guidelines, particularly the CDC recommendations, and ever-changing public health advisories is very important and must be routinely provided in any clinical visit. All STIs are preventable, most are treatable, but not all are curable. Hence, it is really important to involve the adolescent or young adult in the provision of their sexual reproductive health.

References

[1] Incidence, prevalence, and cost of sexually transmitted infections in the United States. CDC Fact Sheet. Atlanta, GA: National Center for HIV/AIDS, Viral Hepatitis, STD, and TB Prevention, 2013.

[2] Centers for Disease Control and Prevention. Sexually transmitted disease surveillance. Atlanta, GA: US Department Health Human Services, 2018.

[3] Steinberg L. Cognitive and affective development in adolescence. Trends Cogn Sci 2005; 9(2):69-74.

[4] Kann L, McManus T, Harris WA, Shanklin SL, Flint KH, Queen B. et al. Youth risk behavior surveillance—United States, 2017. MMWR Surveill Summ 2018;67(8):1-114.

[5] Cuffe KM, Newton-Levinson A, Gift TL, McFarlane M, Leichliter JS. Sexually transmitted infection testing among adolescents and young adults in the United States. J Adolesc Health 2016;58(5):512-9.

[6] Shannon CL, Klausner JD. The growing epidemic of sexually transmitted infections in adolescents: A neglected population. Curr Opin Pediatr 2018;30(1):137-43.

[7] Marcell AV, Burstein GR. Sexual and reproductive health care services in the pediatric setting. Pediatrics 2017;140(5):e20172858. doi: 10.1542/peds.2017-2858.

[8] Committee on Gynecologic Practice. Committee Opinion No 706: Sexual health. Obstet Gynecol 2017;130(1):e42-7.

[9] Adolescent health care, sexuality and contraception. American Academy of Family Physicians, 2017. URL: https://www.aafp.org/about/policies/all/adolescent-sexuality.html.

[10] Tulloch T, Kaufman M. Adolescent sexuality. Pediatr Rev 2013;34(1):29-38.

[11] Workowski KA, Bolan GA. Centers for Disease Control and Prevention. Sexually transmitted diseases treatment guidelines, 2015. MMWR Recomm Rep. 2015;64(RR-03):1–137

[12] Marrazzo JM, Martin DH. Management of women with cervicitis. Clin Infect Dis 2007; 44(suppl 3):S102–10.

[13] Centers for Disease Control and Prevention. Recommendations for the laboratory-based detection of Chlamydia trachomatis and Neisseria gonorrhoeae—2014.MMWR Recomm Rep. 2014;63(RR-02):1–19.

[14] Geisler WM. Diagnosis and management of uncomplicated Chlamydia trachomatis infections in adolescents and adults: summary of evidence reviewed for the 2015 Centers for Disease Control and Prevention Sexually Transmitted Diseases Treatment Guidelines. Clin Infect Dis 2015;61(suppl 8):S774–84.

[15] LeFevre ML, U.S. Preventive Services Task Force. Screening for chlamydia and gonorrhea: U.S. Preventive Services Task Force recommendation statement. Ann Intern Med 2014;161(12):902–10

[16] Steedman NM, McMillan A. Treatment of asymptomatic rectal Chlamydia trachomatis: is single-dose azithromycin effective? Int J STD AIDS 2009;20(1):16–8.

[17] Sherrard J, Barlow D. Gonorrhoea in men: clinical and diagnostic aspects. Genitourin Med 1996;72(6):422-6.

[18] Mayor M, Roett MA, Uduhiri KA. Diagnosis and management of gonococcal infections. Am Fam Physician 2012;86(10):931–8.

[19] Detels R, Green AM, Klausner JD, Katzenstein D, Gaydos C, Handsfield H, et al. The incidence and correlates of symptomatic and asymptomatic Chlamydia trachomatis and Neisseria gonorrhoeae infections in selected populations in five countries. Sex Transm Dis 2011;38(6):503–9.

[20] Wiesner PJ, Thompson SE III. Gonococcal diseases. Dis Mon 1980;26:1–44.

[21] Yi H, Shim CS, Kim GW, Kim JS, Choi IZ. Case of Fitz-Hugh-Curtis syndrome in male without presentation of sexually transmitted disease. World J Clin Cases 2015;3(11):965–69.

[22] de Vries HJ, Zingoni A, White JA, Ross JD, Kreuter A. European Guideline on the management of proctitis, proctocolitis and enteritis caused by sexually transmissible pathogens. Int J STD AIDS 2013;25(7):465-74.

[23] Rice PA. Gonococcal arthritis (disseminated gonococcal infection). Infect Dis Clin North Am 2005;19(4):853-61.

[24] Papp JR, Schachter J, Gaydos CA, Van Der Pol, Van Der Pol Barbara. Recommendations for the laboratory-based detection of Chlamydia trachomatis and Neisseria gonorrhoeae—2014 MMWR 2014;63(2):6–14.

[25] Kirkcaldy RD, Harvey A, Papp JR, Del Rio C, Soge OO, Holmes KK, et al. Neisseria gonorrhoeae Antimicrobial Susceptibility Surveillance — The Gonococcal Isolate Surveillance Project, 27 Sites, United States, 2014. MMWR Surveill Summ 2016;65(SS-7):1–19.

[26] Unemo M. Current and future antimicrobial treatment of gonorrhoea—the rapidly evolving Neisseria gonorrhoeae continues to challenge. BMC Infect Dis 2015;15:364.

[27] Lee H, Lee K, Chong Y. New treatment options for infections caused by increasingly antimicrobial-resistant Neisseria gonorrhoeae. Expert Rev Anti Infect Ther 2016;14(2): 243–56.

[28] Chisholm SA, Neal TJ, Alawattegama AB, Birley HD, Howe RA, Ison CA. Emergence of high level azithromycin resistance in Neisseria gonorrhoeae in England and Wales. J Antimicrob Chemother 2009;64:353–8.

[29] Kent CK, Chaw JK, Wong W, Liska S, Gibson S, Hubbard G, et al. Prevalence of rectal, urethral, and pharyngeal chlamydia and gonorrhea detected in 2 clinical settings among men who have sex with men: San Francisco, California, 2003.Clin Infect Dis 2005;41:67-74.

[30] Tampa M, Sarbu I, Matei C, Benea V, Georgescu SR. Brief history of syphilis. J MedLife 2014;7(1):4–10.

[31] Centers for Disease Control and Prevention. Congenital syphilis. CDC Fact Sheet. Atlanta, GA: National Center for HIV/AIDS, Viral Hepatitis, STD, and TB Prevention, 2017.

[32] Kimball A, Torrone E, Miele K, Bachmann L, Thorpe P, Weinstock H, et al. Missed opportunities for prevention of congenital syphilis — United States, 2018. MMWR 2020;69:661–5.

[33] Syphilis – CDC Fact Sheet (Detailed). Atlanta, GA: National Center for HIV/AIDS, Viral Hepatitis, STD, and TB Prevention, 2017.

[34] Cantor A, Nelson HD, Daeges M, Pappas M. Screening for syphilis in nonpregnant adolescents and adults: a systematic review to update the 2004 U.S. Preventive Services Task Force Recommendation. Evidence Synthesis No. 136. AHRQ Publication No. 14-05213-EF-1. Rockville, MD: Agency for Healthcare Research and Quality, 2015.

[35] Ghanem K. Management of adult syphilis: key questions to inform the 2015 Centers for Disease Control and Prevention sexually transmitted diseases treatment guidelines. Clin Infect Dis 2015;61(Suppl 8):s818–36.

[36] Centers for Disease Control and Prevention. Discordant results from reverse sequence syphilis screening—five laboratories, United States, 2006–2010. MMWR 2011;60(5):133–7.

[37] U.S. Preventive Services Task Force. Screening for syphilis infection in nonpregnant adults and adolescents. JAMA 2016;315(21):2321-7.
[38] Rawla P, Limaiem F. Lymphogranuloma Venereum. In: StatPearls. Treasure Island, FL: StatPearls Publishing, 2020.
[39] Lewis DA, Mitja O. Haemophilus ducreyi: from sexually transmitted infection to skin ulcer pathogen. Curr Opin Infect Dis 2016;29(1):52–7.
[40] Steen R, Dallabetta G. Genital ulcer disease control and HIV prevention. J Clin Virol 2004;29(3):143–51.
[41] Asin J. Chancroid; a report of 1402 cases. Am J Syph Gonorrhea Vener Dis 1952;36(5): 483–7.
[42] Lewis DA. Epidemiology, clinical features, diagnosis and treatment of Haemophilus ducreyi—a disappearing pathogen? Expert Rev Anti Infect Ther 2014;12(6):687–96.
[43] Trees DL, Morse SA. Chancroid and Haemophilus ducreyi: an update. Clin Microbiol Rev 1995;8(3):357–75.
[44] Kemp M, Christensen JJ, Lautenschlager S, Vall-Mayans M, Moi H. European guideline for the management of chancroid, 2011. Int J STD AIDS 2011;22(5):241–4.
[45] World Health Organization. Guidelines for the Management of Sexually Transmitted Infections. Geneva: World Health Organization; 2003.
[46] O'Farrell N, Lazaro NUK. National Guideline for the management of chancroid 2014. Int J STD AIDS 2014;25(14):975–83.
[47] Lewis DA, Muller E, Steele L, Sternberg M, Radebe F, Lyall M, et al. Prevalence and associations of genital ulcer and urethral pathogens in men presenting with genital ulcer syndrome to primary health care clinics in South Africa. Sex Transm Dis 2012;39(11): 880–5.
[48] O'Farrell N, Moi H. European guideline for the management of donovanosis, 2010. Int J STD AIDS 2010;21(9):609–10.
[49] Johnson LF, Coetzee DJ, Dorrington RE. Sentinel surveillance of sexually transmitted infections in South Africa: a review. Sex Transm Infect 2005;81(4):287–93.
[50] Velho PE, Souza EM, Belda Junior W. Donovanosis. Braz J Infect Dis 2008;12(6):521–5.
[51] Ballard RC.Klebsiella granulomatis (Donovanosis, Granuloma Inguinale). In: Bennett JE, Dolin R, Blaser MJ, eds. Mandell, Douglas, and Bennett's principles and practice of infectious diseases, vol 2, 8th edition. Philadelphia, PA: Elsevier Saunders, 2015:2664–6.
[52] Bowden FJ. Donovanosis in Australia: going, going. Sex Transm Infect 2005;81(5):365–6.
[53] Narang T, Kanwar AJ. Genital elephantiasis due to donovanosis: forgotten but not gone yet. Int J STD AIDS 2012;23(11):835–6.
[54] Richens J. United Kingdom national guideline for the management of donovanosis (granuloma inguinale) 2011.British Association of Sexual Health and HIV; 2011. URL: www.bashhguidelines.org/media/1061/3194.pdf.
[55] Bautista CT, Wurapa E, Sateren WB, Morris S, Hollingsworth B, Sanchez JL. Bacterial vaginosis: a synthesis of the literature on etiology, prevalence, risk factors, and relationship with chlamydia and gonorrhea infections. Mil Med Res 2016;3:4.
[56] Hay P. Bacterial vaginosis. Medicine 2014;42(7):359–63.
[57] Schwebke JR, Desmond R. Natural history of asymptomatic bacterial vaginosis in a high-risk group of women. Sex Transm Dis 2007;34(11):876–7.
[58] Ranjit E, Raghubanshi BR, Maskey S, Parajuli P. Prevalence of bacterial vaginosis and its association with risk factors among nonpregnant women: a hospital based study. Int J Microbiol 2018;2018:8349601.
[59] Holzman C, Leventhal JM, Qiu H, Jones NM, Wang J, Group BVS. Factors linked to bacterial vaginosis in nonpregnant women. Am J Public Health 2001;91(10):1664–70.
[60] Koumans EH, Sternberg M, Bruce C, McQuillan G, Kendrick J, Sutton M, et al. The prevalence of bacterial vaginosis in the United States, 2001-2004; associations with symptoms, sexual behaviors, and reproductive health. Sex Transm Dis 2007;34(11):864–9.
[61] Schwebke JR. Asymptomatic bacterial vaginosis: response to therapy. Am J Obstet Gynecol 2000;183(6):1434–9.

[62] Screening for bacterial vaginosis in pregnancy to prevent preterm delivery: U.S. Preventive Services Task Force recommendation statement. Ann Intern Med 2008; 148(3):214–9.
[63] Guédou FA, Van Damme L, Deese J, Crucitti T, Becker M, Mirembe F, et al. Behavioural and medical predictors of bacterial vaginosis recurrence among female sex workers: longitudinal analysis from a randomized controlled trial. BMC Infect Dis. 2013;13:208. Published 2013 May 8. doi:10.1186/1471-2334-13-208.
[64] Fethers KA, Fairley CK, Morton A, Hocking JS, Hopkins C, Kennedy LJ, et al. Early sexual experiences and risk factors for bacterial vaginosis. J Infect Dis 2009;200(11): 1662–70.
[65] Muzny CA, Sunesara IR, Austin EL, Mena LA, Schwebke JR. Bacterial vaginosis among African American women who have sex with women. Sex Transm Dis 2013;40(9):751–5.
[66] Mohammadzadeh F, Dolatian M, Jorjani M, Alavi Majd H. Diagnostic value of Amsel's clinical criteria for diagnosis of bacterial vaginosis. Glob J Health Sci 2014;7(3):8–14.
[67] Allsworth JE, Peipert JF. Severity of bacterial vaginosis and the risk of sexually transmitted infection. Am J Obstet Gynecol 2011;205(2):113.e1-113.e1136. doi:10.1016/j.ajog.2011.02.060.
[68] Martin DH, Marrazzo JM. The vaginal microbiome: current understanding and future directions. J Infect Dis 2016;214(Suppl 1):S36–41.
[69] Colonna C, Steelman M. Amsel criteria. In: StatPearls. Treasure Island, FL: StatPearls Publishing, 2020.
[70] Bradshaw CS, Sobel JD. Current treatment of bacterial vaginosis-limitations and need for innovation. J Infect Dis 2016;214(Suppl 1):S14–20.
[71] Gibbs RS. Asymptomatic bacterial vaginosis: is it time to treat? Am J Obstet Gynecol 2007;196(6):495–6.
[72] Klatt TE, Cole DC, Eastwood DC, Barnabei VM. Factors associated with recurrent bacterial vaginosis. J Reprod Med 2010;55(1-2):55–61.
[73] Marshall AO. Managing recurrent bacterial vaginosis: insights for busy providers. Sex Med Rev2015;3(2):88–9.
[74] Mehta SD. Systematic review of randomized trials of treatment of male sexual partners for improved bacteria vaginosis outcomes in women. Sex Transm Dis 2012;39(10):822–30.
[75] Sobel JD, Kaur N, Woznicki NA, Boikov D, Aguin T, Gill G, et al. Prognostic indicators of recurrence of bacterial vaginosis. J Clin Microbiol 2019;57(5):e00227-19.
[76] Bautista CT, Wurapa EK, Sateren WB, Morris SM, Hollingsworth BP, Sanchez JL. Association of bacterial vaginosis with chlamydia and gonorrhea among women in the U.S. army. Am J Prev Med 2017;52(5):632–9.
[77] McGowin CL, Totten PA. The unique microbiology and molecular pathogenesis of mycoplasma genitalium. J Infect Dis 2017;216(Suppl 2):S382-8.
[78] Cazanaev C, Manhart LE, Bebear C. Mycoplasma genitalium, an emerging sexually transmitted pathogen. Med Mal Infect 2012;42(9):381-92.
[79] Short VL, Totten PA, Ness RB, Astete SG, Kelsey SF, Murray P, et al. Clinical presentation of mycoplasma genitalium infections versus Neisseria gonorrhea infection among women with pelvic inflammatory disease. Clin Infect Dis 2009;48(1):41-7.
[80] Centers for Disease Control and Prevention. Trichomoniasis. CDC Fact Sheet. Atlanta, GA: National Center for HIV/AIDS, Viral Hepatitis, STD, and TB Prevention, 2020.
[81] Patel EU, Gaydos CA, Packman ZR, Quinn TC, Tobian AAR. Prevalence and correlates of Trichomonas vaginalis infection among men and women in the United States. Clin Infect Dis 2018;67(2):211-7.
[82] Van Der Pol B. Clinical and laboratory testing for Trichomonas vaginalis Infection. J Clin Microbiol 2016;54(1):7-12.
[83] Sutton M, Sternberg M, Koumans EH, McQuillan G, Berman S, Markowitz L. The prevalence of Trichomonas vaginalis infection among reproductive-age women in the United States, 2001-2004. Clin Infect Dis 2007;45(10):1319–26.
[84] Kissinger P, Adamski A. Trichomoniasis and HIV interactions: a review. Sex Transm Infect 2013;89:426–33.

[85] Kissinger P. Epidemiology and treatment of trichomoniasis. Curr Infect Dis Rep 2015; 17(6):484. doi: 10.1007/s11908-015-0484-7.
[86] Hollman D, Coupey SM, Fox AS, Herold BC. Screening for Trichomonas vaginalis in high-risk adolescent females with a new transcription-mediated nucleic acid amplification test (NAAT): associations with ethnicity, symptoms, and prior and current STIs. J Pediatr Adolesc Gynecol 2010;23:312–6.
[87] Kissinger P, Muzny CA, Mena LA, Lillis RA, Schwebke JR, Beauchamps L, et al. Single-dose versus 7-day-dose metronidazole for the treatment of trichomoniasis in women: an open-label, randomized controlled trial. Lancet Infect Dis 2018;18(11):1251-9.
[88] Holder N, Ahmed N, Cabral MD. Human papillomavirus infection in adolescents. Pediatr Med 2019;2:46.
[89] American cancer Society. Key statistics for cervical cancer. URL: https:// www.cancer.org/cancer/cervical-cancer/about/key-statistics.html.
[90] World Health Organization. Human papillomavirus vaccines: WHO position paper, May 2017-Recommendations. Vaccine 2017;35:5753-5.
[91] Kanodia S, Fahey LM, Kast WM. Mechanisms used by human papillomavirus to escape the host immune response. Curr Cancer Drug Targets 2007;7:79-89.
[92] Gissmann L, Wolnik L, Ikenberg H, Koldovsky **U**, Schnürch HG, zur Hausen **H**. Human papillomavirus types 6 and 11 DNA sequences in genital and laryngeal papillomas and in some cervical cancers. Proc Natl Acad Sci USA 1983;80:560-3.
[93] Human Papillomavirus (HPV). Genital HPV Infection Fact Sheet. Atlanta, GA: Centers for Disease Control and Surveillance, 2019.
[94] Castle PE, Murokora D, Perez C, Alvarez M, Quek SC, Campbell **C**. Treatment of cervical intraepithelial lesions. Int J Gynaecol Obstet 2017;138(Suppl 1):20-5.
[95] Meites E, Kempe A, Markowitz LE. Use of a 2-dose scheduled for human papilloma vaccination – Updated recommendations of the Advisory Committee on Immunization Practices. MMWR 2016;65:1405-8.
[96] Whitley RJ, Kimberlin DW, Roizman B. Herpes simplex viruses. Clin Infect Dis 1998; 26(3):541-55.
[97] Kimberlin DW, Rouse DJ. Clinical practice. Genital herpes. N Engl J Med 2004;350(19): 1970-7.
[98] Gupta R, Warren T, Wald A. Genital herpes. Lancet 2007;370(9605):2127-37.
[99] Lucas S, Nelson AM. HIV and the spectrum of human disease. J Pathol 2015;235:229–41.
[100] Hall HI, Song R, Tang T, An Q, Prejean J, Dietz P, et al. HIV trends in the United States: Diagnoses and estimated incidence. JMIR Public Health Surveill 2017;3(1):e8. doi:10.2196/publichealth.7051.
[101] Cohen M, Gay CL, Busch MP, Hecht M. The detection of acute HIV infection. J Inf Diseases 2010;202(S2):S270-7.
[102] Centers for Disease Control and Prevention. HIV: AIDS and Opportunistic Infections. Atlanta, GA: CDC, 2019. URL: https://www.cdc.gov/hiv/basics/livingwithhiv/opportunisticinfections.html.
[103] Hurt CB, Nelson JAE, Hightow-Weidman LB, Miller WC. Selecting an HIV test: A narrative review for clinicians and researchers. Sex Transm Dis 2017;44(12):739-46.
[104] Ghosn J, Taiwo B, Seedat S, Autran B, Katlama C. HIV. Lancet 2018;392(10148):685-97.
[105] Lemon SM. Type A viral hepatitis. New developments in an old disease. N Engl J Med 1985;313(17):1059-67.
[106] Kimberlin DW, Brady MT, Jackson MA, Long SS, eds. Hepatitis A. Red book: Report of the Committee on Infectious Diseases. Elk Grove Village, IL: AAP, 2018.
[107] Tong MJ, el-Farra NS, Grew MI. Clinical manifestations of hepatitis A: recent experience in a community teaching hospital. J Infect Dis 1995;171(Suppl 1):S15-8.
[108] Kao HW, Ashcavai M, Redeker AG. The persistence of hepatitis A IgM antibody after acute clinical hepatitis A. Hepatology 1984;4(5):933-6.
[109] Chapman LE, Sullivent EE, Grohnskopf LA, Beltrami EM, Perz JF, Kretsinger K, et al. Centers for Disease Control and Prevention. Prevention of hepatitis A through active or passive immunization: recommendations of the Advisory Committee on Immunization Practices (ACIP). MMWR Recomm Rep 2006;55(RR06):1-19.

[110] Centers for Diseaae Conrol and Prevention. Hepatitis surveillance report. Atlanta, GA: United States Department of Health and Human Services, Centers for Disease Control and Prevention, 2011.
[111] Skoog SM, Rivard RE, Batts KP, Smith CI. Autoimmune hepatitis preceded by acute hepatitis A infection. Am J Gastroenterol 2002;97(6):1568-9.
[112] Wright TL, Mamish D, Combs C, Kim M, Donegan E, Ferrell L, et al. Hepatitis B virus and apparent fulminant non-A, non-B hepatitis. Lancet 1992;339(8799):52-5.
[113] Liaw YF, Tsai SL, Sheen IS, Chao M, Yeh CT, Hsieh SY, et al. Clinical and virological course of chronic hepatitis B virus infection with hepatitis C and D virus markers. Am J Gastroenterol 1998;93(3):354-9.
[114] Centers for Disease Control and Prevention. Viral Hepatitis; Hepatitis B Questions and Answers for Health Professionals. Atlanta, GA: CDC. URL: https://www.cdc.gov/hepatitis/hbv/hbvfaq.htm#treatment.
[115] Nijmeijer BM, Koopsen J, Schinkel J, Prins M, Geijtenbeek TB, Nijmeijer BM, et al. Sexually transmitted hepatitis C virus infections: current trends, and recent advances in understanding the spread in men who have sex with men. J Int AIDS Soc 2019;22(Suppl 6):e25348.
[116] Chan DP, Sun HY, Wong HT, Lee SS, Hung CC. Sexually acquired hepatitis C virus infection: a review. Int J Infect Dis 2016;49:47-58.
[117] Terrault NA, Dodge JL, Murphy EL, Tavis JE, Kiss A, Levin TR, et al. Sexual transmission of hepatitis C virus among monogamous heterosexual couples: the HCV partners study. Hepatology 2013;57:881–9.
[118] Irshad M, Singh Makotia D, Irshad K. An insight into the diagnosis and pathogenesis of hepatitis C virus infection. World J Gastroenterol 2013;19(44):7896-909.
[119] CDC. Viral hepatitis: hepatitis C. Atlanta, GA: CDC, 2020. URL: www.cdc.gov/hepatitis
[120] Gonzalez-Grande R, Jimenez-Perez M, Gonzalez Arjona C, Mostazo Torres J. New approaches in the treatment of hepatitis C. World J Gastroenterol 2016;22(4):1421-32.
[121] Lo Re V. Extrahepatic complications of hepatitis C virus infection in HIV and the impact of successful antiviral treatment. Clin Infect Dis 2017;64(4):498-500.
[122] Sobel JD. Genital candidiasis. Medicine 2005;33(10);62-5.
[123] Sobel JD. Recurrent vulvovaginal candidiasis. Am J Obstet Gynecol 2016;214(1):15-21.
[124] Pappas PG, Kauffman CA, Andes DR, Clancy CJ, Marr KA, Ostrosky-Zeichner L, et al. Clinical practice guideline for the management of candidiasis: 2016 Update by the Infectious Diseases Society of America. Clin Infect Dis 2016;62(4):e1-50.
[125] CDC. Fungal diseases: invasive candidiasis. Atlanta, GA: CDC, 2019. URL: https://www.cdc.gov/fungal/diseases/candidiasis/invasive/index.html.
[126] Anderson AL, Chaney E. Pubic lice (Pthirus pubis): history, biology and treatment vs. knowledge and beliefs of US college students. Int J Environ Res Public Health 2009; 6(2):592-600.
[127] Orion E, Matz H, Wolf R. Ectoparisitic sexually transmitted diseases: Scabies and pediculosis. Clin Dermatol 2004;22(6):513-9.
[128] Bick JA. Infection control in jails and prisons. Clin Infect Dis 2007;45(8):1047-55.
[129] Chosidow O. Scabies and pediculosis: Neglected diseases to highlight. Clin Microbiol Infect 2012;18(4):311-2.
[130] Mayo clinic. Pubic lice (crabs). URL: https://www.mayoclinic.org/diseases-conditions/pubic-lice-crabs/symptoms-causes/syc-20350300.
[131] Karabela Y, Yardimci G, Yildirim I, Atalay E, Karabela SN. Treatment of phthiriasis palpebrarum and crab louse: Petrolatum jelly and 1% permethrin shampoo. Case Rep Med 2015;2015:287906. doi:10.1155/2015/287906.
[132] Orkin M. Scabies: what's new? Curr Probl Dermatol 1995;22:105-11.
[133] CDC. Parasites: scabies. 2010. URL: https://www.cdc.gov/parasites/scabies/index.html.
[134] Ford GW, Decker CF. Pelvic inflammatory disease. Dis Mon 2016:62(8):301-5.
[135] Soper DE. Pelvic inflammatory disease. Obstet Gynecol 2010;116(2 Pt 1):419-28.
[136] Curry A, Williams T, Penny ML. Pelvic inflammatory disease: Diagnosis, management, and prevention. Am Fam Physician 2019;100(6):357-364.

[137] Greydanus DE, Merrick J, Cabral MD. Pelvic inflammatory disease: Management requires a patient, prudent, prejudice-free provider. Int J Adolesc Med Health 2018; 32(1):/j/ijamh.2020.32.issue-1/ijamh-2018-0216/ijamh-2018-0216.xml. doi:10.1515/ijamh-2018-0216.
[138] Trojian TH, Lishnak TS, Heiman D. Epididymitis and orchitis: An overview. Am Fam Physician 2009;79(7):583-7.
[139] Wampler SM, Llanes M. Common scrotal and testicular problems. Prim Care 2010;37(3): 613-26.
[140] Feldstein Ewing SW, Ryman SG, Gillman AS, Weiland BJ, Thayer RE, Bryan AD. Developmental cognitive neuroscience of adolescent sexual risk and alcohol use. AIDS Behav 2016;20 Suppl 1(Suppl 1):S97-108.
[141] Romer D, Reyna VF, Satterthwaite TD. Beyond stereotypes of adolescent risk taking: Placing the adolescent brain in developmental context. Dev Cogn Neurosci 2017;27:19-34.
[142] Casey BJ, Jones RM, Hare TA. The adolescent brain. Ann N Y Acad Sci 2008;1124:111-26.
[143] Hare TA, Tottenham N, Galvan A, Voss HU, Glover GH, Casey BJ. Biological substrates of emotional reactivity and regulation in adolescence during an emotional go-nogo task. Biol Psychiatry 2008;63(10):927-34.
[144] Vasilenko SA, Kugler KC, Butera NM, Lanza ST. Patterns of adolescent sexual behavior predicting young adult sexually transmitted infections: a latent class analysis approach. Arch Sex Behav 2015;44(3):705-15.
[145] Swartzendruber A, Zenilman JM, Niccolai LM, Kershaw TS, Brown JL, Diclemente RJ, Sales JM. It takes 2: partner attributes associated with sexually transmitted infections among adolescents. Sex Transm Dis 2013;40(5):372-8.
[146] Steiner RJ, Sheremenko G, Lesesne C, Dittus PJ, Sieving RE, Ethier KA. Adolescent Connectedness and Adult Health Outcomes. Pediatrics 2019;144(1):e20183766.
[147] O'Connor EA, Lin JS, Burda BU, Henderson JT, Walsh ES, Whitlock EP. Behavioral sexual risk-reduction counseling in primary care to prevent sexually transmitted infections: a systematic review for the U.S. Preventive Services Task Force. Ann Intern Med 2014;161(12):874-83.
[148] US Preventive Services Task Force, Krist AH, Davidson KW, Mangione CM, Barry MJ, Cabana M, et al. Behavioral counseling interventions to prevent sexually transmitted infections: US Preventive Services Task Force Recommendation Statement. JAMA 2020;324(7):674-681.
[149] Algur E, Wang E, Friedman HS, Deperthes B. A Systematic Global Review of Condom Availability Programs in High Schools. J Adolesc Health 2019;64(3):292-304.

Section three: Eating disorders (editor: Donald E. Greydanus)

Chapter 9

Psychiatric perspectives in pediatric obesity

Stephen McLearie, MBBS, Sultan Albrahim, MBBS, Salma Malik, MD, Nehdia Hashemi, MD, Goran Petrovski, MD, PhD and Ahsan Nazeer*, MD

Department of Psychiatry, Division of Child and Adolescent Psychiatry, Sidra Medicine, Doha, Qatar, Institute of Living, Hartford, USA and WMU Homer Stryker MD School of Medicine, Kalamazoo, Michigan, United States of America

Abstract

Pediatric obesity is an international epidemic with exponential rises in prevalence over recent decades. There are serious consequences for physical health, including risk of metabolic syndrome and cardiovascular sequelae; also, there are complex neurobiological and psychiatric associations. Psychiatric associations include biological, psychological and social factors that include predisposing, precipitating, and perpetuating factors. Treatment approaches can be considered physical, pharmacological, psychological and social. An understanding of psychiatric factors can help in understanding etiological associations, and in developing holistic treatment approaches. This discussion elucidates these issues and considers complex interrelationships and homeostatic feedback loops.

Introduction

Obesity is defined as a BMI (body mass index) at or above the 95th percentile for children and adolescents of the same age and gender. Overweight is a BMI at or above the 85th percentile (and below the 95th percentile) for children and teens of the same age and gender (1).

The prevalence of obesity is already well above the critical threshold of 15%, which is recognized as an epidemic requiring intervention (2). Prevalence rates have increased dramatically worldwide during the last few decades, and global obesity rates have nearly tripled

* *Correspondence:* Ahsan Nazeer MD, Department of Psychiatry, Division of Child and Adolescent Psychiatry, Sidra Medicine, Doha, Qatar. Email: anazeer@sidra.org.

In: Behavioral Pediatrics II
Editors: Donald E. Greydanus, Dilip R. Patel, Ahsan Nazeer et al.
ISBN: 979-8-88697-019-7

since 1975, with more than 300 million children and adolescents aged 5-19 years considered overweight or obese by 2016.

Obesity is a major risk factor for multiple medical complications, including cardiovascular disease, insulin resistance, and type 2 diabetes, gastrointestinal (fatty liver) and pulmonary (sleep apnea) comorbidities, musculoskeletal complications, and some forms of cancer (3, 4).

Precision medicine approaches require an understanding of genetics, biomarkers, phenotypes, and psychosocial factors to inform and optimize care (5). This discussion elucidates some of these factors relating to obesity and how our increasing understanding of these can inform treatment.

Children and adolescents presenting with obesity are at particular risk of future medical and psychological complications (6, 7). Various factors can play an essential role in how susceptible an individual child or adolescent may be to develop obesity and will respond to interventions. These factors include depression, body image, anxiety, dieting history, parental attitudes to shape, weight, and culture. Although medical care is of paramount importance in obesity management, understanding the psychological factors associated with pediatric obesity and synergies in neurobiological factors can help design and deliver complex holistic treatment strategies.

Developmental factors

Given the rapid increase in obesity in a relatively short period, the rise in obesity is unlikely to be explained by limiting etiologic explanations to underlying genetically determined differences, increased availability of energy-rich foods, and increasingly sedentary lifestyles. Epigenetic processes can be affected by intrauterine and developmental factors, early life adversity, and exposure to chemicals as well as toxins, potentially impacting DNA methylation and gene transcription.

There may be critical periods *in utero* when the impact of various toxins may most significantly impact development. Obesity and type 2 diabetes mellitus in adults have been found to be associated with undernutrition during pregnancy and rebound early weight gain. There is an interest in the possibility that some environmental factors (including plastics and pesticides) may be considered endocrine-disrupting chemicals (EDCs) and impact obesity.

Furthermore, the imbalances in the hypothalamic–pituitary–adrenal (HPA) axis significantly impact metabolism; indeed, studies are increasingly looking at the influence of the diathesis-stress model on the developing brain and neuroendocrine systems. These important concepts are considered under the developmental origins of health and disease (DOHaD) approach (8).

Psycho-social factors

During young adulthood, psychosocial risk factors for obesity include fewer years of education, lower family income, higher poverty rates, and disruptive relationships. Overweight children, as young as age five, can develop low self-esteem and negative body image. It has also been demonstrated that "the greater the frequency of being teased about weight and shape while growing up, the more negative one's appearance is regarded, and the greater the degree of body dissatisfaction in adulthood (9-11)." Comments are now provided on self-esteem, quality of life, family, bullying, and abuse-neglect.

Self-esteem

Self-esteem is typically lower in all domains for overweight children and further varies by age and gender. Females are at greater risk for lower self-esteem, which is a particular challenge during the transitions from puberty into early and middle adolescence years. Some studies report that severely obese females express lower self-esteem than moderately obese females, suggesting that self-esteem relates to the obesity severity (12-15).

Quality of life

Children's quality of life with obesity is often significantly impacted and may be equivalent to that of children with cancer or diabetes mellitus (16).

Family

Parental attitudes and behaviors are critical in developing self-esteem and personality. Overly harsh parenting and negative comments can significantly impact self-esteem, which can lead to food restriction or binge eating (17-19).

Bullying

Teasing about body weight and shape has been reported by more than 50% of children with obesity (20). Moreover, those bullied reported high rates of abnormal eating behaviors, including skipping meals, binge eating, and "emotional eating" (20).

Abuse and neglect

Social factors associated with obesity may include neglect, abuse, and non-supportive home environments. Neglected children are significantly more likely than others to become obese. For adults seeking treatment for obesity, an increase in the prevalence of childhood sexual abuse and an increase in nonsexual abuse has been found, compared with a control population (21, 22). However, for adolescent obesity, a recently published birth cohort study has not found a correlation between child abuse and adolescent obesity (23). Thus, these associations require further longitudinal studies.

Psychiatric comorbidity

Many studies have found high psychological disorders and psychiatric illnesses in obese children and adolescents, particularly in females. Those seeking clinical treatment have been found to have increased levels of depression, anxiety, somatoform, and eating problems. According to one estimate, more than 40% met the criteria for a diagnosis of the DSM-IV (American Psychiatric Association's 1994 Diagnostic and statistical manual of mental disorders, 4th edition) among a group of obese adolescents seeking treatment for weight management.

However, it is also important to note that those who do not present medically may have a lower incidence of psychological problem; such a concept is fundamental in designing population-based interventions (24-26). Comments are now provided for obesity comorbidities of depression, eating disorders, ADHD, and complications of antipsychotic medications.

Depression

There is a complex interrelationship between childhood depression and obesity. Predisposing precipitating and perpetuating factors can have modulating and mediating effects. A meta-analysis by Sutaria et al. (27) found a 10% prevalence rate of depression among obese children in community samples. The odds of depression were 1.32 higher in obese children; the odds of depression were significantly higher for obese female children than normal-weight female children, a risk that persists into adulthood (27). However, an association was not found between male subgroups and depression (27).

The National Health and Nutrition Examination Survey (NHANES)-III data showed that for the most obese adolescents, the prevalence of major depression increased to highly significant levels – 20% for boys and 30% for girls (28). In clinical settings, atypical depressive symptoms may be a more common presentation. Hence it is recommended that physicians consider this psychopathology in obese children and make an appropriate referral for formal psychological assessment if there are on-going concerns in this regard. Timely evaluation and treatment are important as both obesity and depression have been independently associated with cardiovascular risk.

Eating disorders

The prevalence of eating disorders and of eating problems (i.e., weight preoccupation, binge eating, dieting, and purging) has been found to be significantly increased in obese patient groups. For example, an increased risk for a bulimic disorder has been found (OR=7.86) for obese adolescent males and obese adolescent females (OR=3.27) relative to normal weight subjects (29-31). Interestingly, although binge eating disorder has been associated with obesity in adults, this association has not been found in children (29-31). Also, clinicians should also beware that children who have treatment for obesity do not develop a rebound type of anorexia nervosa.

ADHD

Attention-deficit/hyperactivity disorder (ADHD) is one of the most frequent childhood-onset neurodevelopmental disorders and is a major public health concern. A limited body of research focuses on the relationship between ADHD and obesity; however, studies in both community and clinical samples suggest that children with ADHD have a higher prevalence of obesity than the non-ADHD cohort (32-34). This association remains when adjusted for confounding psychosocial factors including lower socioeconomic status, gender, country, and study quality.

However, it is important to note that a sizeable number of studies have not controlled for the confounding effects of other psychiatric comorbidities, hence the results are inconsistent among studies (32-34). Moreover, this limitation makes it difficult to understand the extent to which ADHD is accounted for and the impact of psychostimulants used for the treatment of ADHD. Studies have shown that the individuals who are treated with psychostimulants were not at higher risk of obesity, hence suggesting a protective effect of these medications.

So far, the underlying mechanisms in the relationship of ADHD and obesity are not clear. Some studies have identified abnormal eating patterns as a possible link; however, others have hypothesized a common biological dysfunction linking the emergence of obesity with sleep disorders, decreased physical activity and the direct contribution of ADHD.

There is also some evidence that treatment of ADHD by psychostimulants in individuals with refractory obesity may lead to weight loss. However, in the authors' clinical experiences, anorexigenic effects are most evident during the first two months of treatment and usually diminish in most individuals. It is quite possible that treatment of ADHD reduces novelty seeking, which helps ongoing adherence to a regular diet and resultant weight loss.

Antipsychotic Medications

Most physicians are well aware of the impact that antipsychotic medications often have on weight and appetite, as well as associations with later medical complications such as obesity, insulin resistance or type 2 diabetes mellitus. While these medications are often imperative for the treatment of schizophrenia or major mood disorders, the impact of obesity and associated medical comorbidities is a significant concern for prescribing clinicians.

It is well recognized that individuals with schizophrenia are considerably more likely to be obese than their non-schizophrenic peers. Factors contributing to weight gain include physical inactivity, depressed mood, unhealthy diet and impaired motivation. After starting antipsychotics, clinical experience is that patients gain the greatest amount of weight during the initial six months. Antipsychotics differ in their propensity to cause obesity but there is no clear relationship between the dose of the medication and weight gain.

The propensity for antipsychotic-induced weight gain is far greater in pediatric patients than in adults. Weight gain in drug naïve patients is significantly greater than in patients with prior antipsychotic medication exposure. The overall mean weight gain in medication naïve patients may be >10 pounds after three months of treatment irrespective of race, gender, pubertal status or age range.

Current research is evaluating whether antipsychotic medications can induce weight gain by increased appetite, decreased metabolism, or both acting synergistically. Issues that regulate appetite and energy homeostasis include neurotransmitters, neuropeptides, the neuroendocrine system, and inflammatory markers (such as cytokines); these are all considered part of the homeostatic systems (35). Such effects may be predisposed to by epigenetic, developmental and environmental vulnerabilities along with individual variants in psychokinetic and psychodynamic profiles. Furthermore, periods of protracted serious mental illness may further compound obesity risk by perpetuating effects such as predisposition to less active lifestyles.

These factors may be an excellent microcosm of the biological and psychosocial mechanisms associated with obesity. Research has increased our understanding of the mechanisms of therapeutic action of psychotropic medications, and the mechanisms of side effect action on appetite and weight gain; these are an excellent models of synergies in understanding the etiologies and treatment approaches between psychiatry and endocrinology.

Genetics

Genetics of obesity are complex and at present, approximately 7% of patients with severe obesity are thought to have genetic conditions or mutations driving their obesity (36). This number is likely to increase as our understanding of the molecular genetics develops. Genetic conditions can usefully be classified as:

- With developmental delay-autosomal dominant and recessive;
- Without developmental delay-autosomal dominant and recessive

Autosomal dominant conditions associated with developmental delay include Albright's inherited osteopathy and the Prader-Willi syndrome; Prader-Willi syndrome, in particular, is associated with marked hyperphagia (36). Autosomal recessive conditions with developmental delay include the Bardet Biedl syndrome. Melanocortin 4 receptor deficiency is an autosomal dominant condition without developmental delay and is associated with hyperphagia. Autosomal recessive disorders without developmental delay include syndromes affecting leptin (36). A discussion of neurobiological factors involved in obesity is now presented.

Neurobiological factors

The neurobiology of obesity is complex and there are many associations with psychiatric neurobiological pathways. Appetite is regulated by neuronal circuits and endocrine homeostatic feedback loops. Neuronal circuits between various central nervous system structures (i.e., hypothalamus, mesolimbic system and brainstem-dorsal vagal complex [DVC]) interact with endogenous hormones to regulate appetite. For example, centrally, there may be direct signaling to the arcuate nucleus in the hypothalamus or signaling to the DVC in the brainstem via the vagus nerve, which then communicates with the hypothalamus (37).

In the gastrointestinal system (GI), endogenous hormones and peptides can be orexigenic or anorexigenic. GI hormones act peripherally to modulate digestion and absorption of nutrients. However, they also act as neurotransmitters within the central nervous system to modulate food intake; in addition, the arcuate nucleus at the base of the hypothalamus is permeable to circulating hormones (38). Neuronal signals informed by complex neuroendocrine homeostatic feedback loops are central to energy balance. Factors usefully considered are central neuronal circuitry, neurotransmitters, neuropeptides, neuroendocrine system, and other mechanisms and are further described below (39). These factors are now considered.

Central neuronal circuitry

Hypothalamus

Neuronal projections from the arcuate nucleus communicate with the other hypothalamic areas involved in appetite regulation. Hypothalamic nuclei (i.e., the dorsomedial nucleus [DMN], the paraventricular nucleus [PVN] and the ventromedial nucleus [VMN]) have been implicated as control centers for appetite. Also having important roles are the neuropeptide Y and Agouti related peptide (NPY/AgRP) along with pro-opiomelanocortin as well as cocaine and amphetamine-regulated transcript (POMC/CART) expressing neurons.

Mesolimbic

Mesolimbic reward systems can also regulate appetite by neuronal signaling and projections to the hypothalamus. Dopamine systems also have a role in reward pathways.

Brainstem

In the brainstem, the DVC receives signals from peripheral satiety hormones and vagal afferents from the GI tract, relaying information with reciprocal circuitry with the hypothalamus. Vagal efferents with the sympathetic nervous system and hormonal mechanisms modulate nutritional homeostasis. Interestingly, vagal nerve stimulation in depression and in epilepsy has been found to suppress appetite (40).

Central neuropeptide signaling

Two specific arcuate nucleus neuronal subtypes are important for appetite regulation and metabolism: NPY/AgRP and POMC/CART (41).

NPY/AgRP

There are neurons that co-express neuropeptide Y (NPY) and Agouti related peptide (AgRP) that stimulate feeding. NPY effects are mediated by stimulation of hypothalamic Y1R and Y5R receptors, and by local inhibition of POMC neurons in the ARC (hypothalamic arcuate nucleus). AgRP acts as a selective antagonist at MC3R and MC4R (Melanocortin 3 and Melanocortin 4 receptors) in the hypothalamic paraventricular nucleus (PVN).

POMC/CART

There are also neurons that co-expressing pro-opiomelanocortin (POMC) and cocaine-and amphetamine-regulated transcript (CART) which suppress feeding._Within POMC neurons, α-melanocyte-stimulating hormone (α-MSH) is produced; α-MSH binds to Melanocortin-4 (MC4R) receptors in the PVN and suppresses appetite.

CART is a neurotransmitter and hormone which is involved in diverse areas including regulation of appetite, reward and addiction systems, as well as psychostimulant effects. Neuronal expression of CART in the hypothalamic arcuate nucleus co-localizes with POMC.

Neurotransmitters

Neurotransmitters play an important role in appetite regulation. Orexigenic neurotransmitters include $5HT_{2C}$ receptor antagonists/inverse agonists (such as mirtazapine), histamine receptor antagonists/inverse agonists (such as olanzapine and quetiapine), and dopamine antagonists (such as risperidone and haloperidol). Lorcaserin is a selective $5\text{-}HT_{2C}$ receptor agonist with proven weight loss efficacy and cardiovascular safety for adults (42, 43).

Other psychotropic medications that can be orexigenic include lithium, carbamazepine, and gabapentin. Gamma-aminobutyric acid (GABA) may have some anti-obesity effects via leptin modulated hypothalamic pre-synaptic GABA release. Central opioid and cannabinoid systems may also stimulate appetite.

Neuropeptides

Naturally occurring neuropeptide hormones that enhance hunger include ghrelin, orexin, and neuropeptide Y. In contrast, leptin is a hormone predominantly made by adipose cells that helps to inhibit hunger. Leptin opposes the actions of ghrelin, the so-called "hunger hormone." Leptin and ghrelin act on receptors in the arcuate nucleus of the hypothalamus. In obesity, a decreased sensitivity to leptin may occur, resulting in an inability to detect satiety despite high energy stores.

AMPK (adenosine monophosphate protein kinase) activation centrally leads to increased food intake; one of the effects of insulin is inhibition of AMPK. Also, cholecystokinin (CCK) is a peptide hormone secreted by the duodenum that both releases digestive enzymes and mediates satiety. CCK mediates satiety, opposing the actions of ghrelin by acting on widely distributed central nervous system CCK receptors (44-46).

Neuroendocrine

The neuroendocrine system includes insulin, glucagon, prolactin and tumor necrosis factor (TNF). Insulin is a pancreatic hormone (from beta cells) and is the main anabolic hormone of the body. Glucagon is a peptide hormone from the pancreas (alpha cells) that opposes the actions of insulin and is considered the main catabolic hormone.

Prolactin is increasingly understood to have a range of roles beyond lactation, including reproduction, pancreatic function, adipocyte control and immune modulation. Excess body fat can result in the metabolic syndrome with insulin resistance and is associated with reduced serum prolactin (47). TNF-alpha is a pro-inflammatory cytokine (i.e., a cell signaling protein) that is secreted by adipose tissue; its levels correlate with the degree of adiposity and the associated insulin resistance. Thus, TNF or its receptors are a potential treatment target in research efforts to deal with obesity (48).

Other factors

Resting metabolism may also account for some individual neurobiological differences in obesity profiles. Also, there is a growing interest in the brain-gut axis as a treatment target including for depression management (49). The concept of developing "psychobiotic" medications is informed by the high levels of tryptophan produced by the gastrointestinal tract (GIT), the importance of monoamines centrally in mood regulation, concern about potential neurotoxic cytokine release from permeable GIT tissues, and some treatment effect for patients presenting to liaison psychiatry services with conditions such as irritable bowel syndrome (50-52).

Obesity is a leading risk factor for impaired glucose tolerance and type 2 diabetes (T2D). Although the cause of the obesity epidemic is multi-factorial and not entirely clear, the recent acceleration in incidence is too rapid to be accounted for only by genetics, the wide availability of calorie-rich foods, and increasingly sedentary lifestyles. Accumulating data suggest that the important causes of the obesity epidemic may be related to developmental and early life environmental conditions. The concept of the developmental origins of health and disease (DOHaD) suggests that adverse influences early in development, particularly during intrauterine life, may result in permanent changes in the physiology and metabolism of the infant, which in turn result in an increased risk of non-communicable diseases in adulthood. For example, undernutrition during pregnancy and rapid postnatal weight gain are associated with obesity and T2D in the adult offspring. Moreover, increasing evidence suggests that early-life exposure to a wide range of chemicals has a significant impact on the causes of metabolic disorders. Although the underlying molecular mechanisms remain to be determined, these factors can affect epigenetic processes, such as DNA methylation, allowing the developmental environment to modulate gene transcription. The objective of this review article was to summarize recent progress in the biomedical implications of the DOHaD concept, focusing on the pathogenesis of obesity and T2D, and to discuss a future direction for preventive strategies from a public health perspective.

Interventions

The main principles of treatment are modifying energy intake coupled with increased energy expenditure. There are excellent guidelines from the European Society of Endocrinology and the Paediatric Endocrine Society (36). Interventions considered now include population-based options, lifestyle changes, multidisciplinary efforts, medications for obesity and bariatric surgery.

Population-based

International approaches that have shown some benefit include positive *behavioral* strategies such as "walk a mile" programs in schools, *legislative* approaches such as nutrient labeling, and effective *media communication* of risks as well as strategies; also useful in some jurisdictions are specific measures such as a "sugar tax." Interestingly breast feeding has not been demonstrated to have a robust effect on obesity, but it is, of course, recommended as it has many other benefits.

Lifestyle

Lifestyle approaches often prescribed by a clinician include increased exercise (at least 20 and up to 60 minutes daily), less video screen time, reduced junk food, increased intake of whole fruit rather than fruit juice, and reducing intake of high fructose corn syrup as well as saturated fats. Also, helpful measures are improved sleep hygiene and better family-based communication strategies to help self-esteem. A family component of modeling and supporting lifestyle change is intuitively important, while school-based programs for obesity reduction are also encouraged.

Multidisciplinary (MDT) approaches

Multidisciplinary holistic approaches have been developed in pediatric centers with teams that include primary care clinicians, nurse specialists, physiotherapists, occupational therapists, and psychologists/psychiatrists. Such programs typically include:

- Family based interventions;
- Nutritional and exercise advice;
- Behavioral, cognitive, motivational and interpersonal therapy type components;
- Decreasing sedentary activity;
- Social supports

Various MDT programs have demonstrated efficacy. For example, Braet in the United States developed a cognitive and behavioral treatment model for children, showing promising results (53). Family-based behavioral therapy programs have been developed as seen with Epstein and colleagues who elegantly describe a detailed approach with good and consistent efficacy (54). In Europe, family-based MDT outpatient treatment programs have also been shown to have good efficacy (55).

Medications

It is recommended that medication treatments are only considered for children who are obese rather than overweight typically following a trial of lifestyle and behavioral treatment approaches. Anti-obesity medications are then used in conjunction with ongoing behavioral and lifestyle treatment approaches. Medications to consider include orlistat, lisdexamfetamine, sibutramine, bupropion with naltrexone, and lorcaserin.

Orlistat is a lipase inhibitor that reduces fat absorption, is FDA-approved, and has some benefits; however, this drug can have unpleasant GI side effects. Lisdexamfetamine is a CNS stimulant and is approved for treatment of binge eating disorder in adults--though not in children; however, it is often used for ADHD in children.

Sibutramine is a monoamine reuptake inhibitor which was used as an adjunct treatment for obesity but has been withdrawn due to side effects including cardiovascular concerns. For bupropion with naltrexone, it is recommended to monitor for suicidality, paralleling concerns about use of selective serotonin reuptake inhibitors (SSRI's) in children It is recommended that use of such medication be reassessed if there has not been a significant improvement by 12 weeks (i.e., more than 4% of BMI).

Bariatric surgery

Surgical approaches should be used with caution for carefully selected patients with high BMI, medical complications, and who have not responded to other treatments. Untreated psychiatric illness is a relative contraindication to such surgery from a psychiatric perspective.

Efficacy of this procedure is encouraging for this subgroup of patients in the short to medium term; weight loss can range from 52 to 70 percent of excess body weight (56-58). Clinical benefits can include lower adiposity and insulin resistance, and improvements in quality of life as well as depression. However, longer term studies would be helpful including studies on the psychological impact including sense of self and identity.

Most pediatric teams have an awareness of the importance of holistic approaches and refer to psychiatry when there are concerns about well-being or a psychiatric illness. In view of the complex holistic considerations, it should be helpful to have psychology and psychiatry involved early in the design and implementation of multidisciplinary (MDT) stepped care treatment programs. For major centers where bariatric surgery is undertaken, it would be prudent to consider an assessment by the psychiatric team for all children pre and post-bariatric surgery (56-58).

Conclusion

The etiological associations of obesity are a complex interaction of genetic, neurochemical, endocrine, cognitive, behavioral, and environmental factors. It is useful to review how core factors (i.e., neurotransmitters, neuropeptides, the neuroendocrine system, and inflammatory markers) are involved in complex neurobiological feedback loops regulating appetite and energy homeostasis. Such issues are compounded by epigenetic vulnerabilities and individual variants including resting metabolism.

There are many parallels and synergies between the central nervous system factors affecting both child obesity and psychiatric conditions in children. There are striking similarities in factors associated with mood, reward, and addiction. Research is increasing our current understanding of epigenetic, neurobiological, psychosocial and environmental factors.

Furthermore, an integrated medical and psycho-social approach is helpful in addressing the medical and neuro-endocrine implications of childhood obesity. Also under research are population-based approaches and public education methods.

Stepped care interventions are helpful in treating the subgroup of those with obesity who present to medical services. Dealing with beneficial approaches to the global epidemic of child and adult obesity presents wonderful opportunities for psychiatry to contribute to multi-dimensional holistic approaches that include etiological understanding and treatment of associated psychiatric conditions. This will allow those in psychiatry and psychology to work closely with pediatric multidisciplinary teams in order to help design as well as deliver complex evidence-based treatment programs.

References

[1] Barlow SE. Expert Committee recommendations regarding the prevention, assessment, and treatment of child and adolescent overweight and obesity: Summary report. Pediatrics 2007; 120(Suppl):S164–92.

[2] WHO. Diet, nutrition and the prevention of chronic diseases. World Health Organ Tech Rep Ser 2003;916:i–viii,1-149.

[3] Hamann A. Obesity update 2017. Diabetologe 2017;13(5):331–41.

[4] World Health Organization. Obesity and overweight. 2018. URL: http://www.who.int/en/news-room/fact-sheets/detail/obesity-and-overweight.

[5] Frühbeck G, Kiortsis DN, Catalán V. Precision medicine: Diagnosis and management of obesity. Lancet Diabetes Endocrinol 2018;6(3):164–6.

[6] Davison KK, Birch LL. Weight status, parent reaction, and self-concept in five-year-old girls. Pediatrics 2001;107(1):46–53.

[7] Strauss RS. Childhood obesity and self-esteem. Pediatrics 2000;105(1):e15.

[8] Inadera H. Developmental origins of obesity and type 2 diabetes: molecular aspects and role of chemicals. Environ Health Prev Med 2013;18(3):185–97.

[9] Maffeis C, Tatò L. Long-term effects of childhood obesity on morbidity and mortality. Horm Res 2001;55(Suppl 1):42–5.

[10] Ebbeling CB, Pawlak DB, Ludwig DS. Childhood obesity: public-health crisis, common sense cure. Lancet 2002;360(9331):473–82.

[11] Grilo CM, Wilfley DE, Brownell KD, Rodin J. Teasing, body image, and self-esteem in a clinical sample of obese women. Addict Behav 1994;19(4):443–50.

[12] Manus HE, Killeen MR. Maintenance of self-esteem by obese children. J Child Adolesc Psychiatr Nurs 1995;8(1):17–27.

[13] Pesa JA, Syre TR, Jones E. Psychosocial differences associated with body weight among female adolescents: the importance of body image. J Adolesc Health 2000;26(5):330–7.

[14] Danielsen YS, Stormark KM, Nordhus IH, Mæhle M, Sand L, Ekornås B, et al. Factors associated with low self-esteem in children with overweight. Obes Facts 2012;5(5):722–33.

[15] Hill AJ. Obesity in children and the "myth of psychological maladjustment": Self-esteem in the spotlight. Curr Obes Rep 2017;6(1):63–70.

[16] Gray WN, Janicke DM, Ingerski LM, Silverstein JH. The impact of peer victimization, parent distress and child depression on barrier formation and physical activity in overweight youth. J Dev Behav Pediatr 2008;29(1):26–33.

[17] Taylor CB, Bryson S, Celio Doyle AA, Luce KH, Cunning D, Abascal LB, et al. The adverse effect of negative comments about weight and shape from family and siblings on women at high risk for eating disorders. Pediatrics 2006;118(2):731–8.

[18] Birch LL, Fisher JO, Davison KK. Learning to overeat: maternal use of restrictive feeding practices promotes girls' eating in the absence of hunger. Am J Clin Nutr 2003;78(2):215–20.

[19] Rollins BY, Loken E, Savage JS, Birch LL. Effects of restriction on children's intake differ by child temperament, food reinforcement, and parent's chronic use of restriction. Appetite 2014;73:31–9.

[20] Fairburn CG, Harrison PJ. Eating disorders. Lancet 2003;361(9355):407–16.

[21] Lissau I, Sørensen TI. Parental neglect during childhood and increased risk of obesity in young adulthood. Lancet 1994;343(8893):324–7.

[22] Felitti VJ. Childhood sexual abuse, depression, and family dysfunction in adult obese patients: a case control study. South Med J 1993;86(7):732–6.

[23] Hawton K, Norris T, Crawley E, Shield JPH. Is child abuse associated with adolescent obesity? A population cohort study. Child Obes 2018;14(2):106–13.

[24] Britz B, Siegfried W, Ziegler A, Lamertz C, Herpertz-Dahlmann BM, Remschmidt H, et al. Rates of psychiatric disorders in a clinical study group of adolescents with extreme obesity and in obese adolescents ascertained via a population based study. Int J Obes Relat Metab Disord 2000;24(12):1707–14.

[25] Vila G, Zipper E, Dabbas M, Bertrand C, Robert JJ, Ricour C, et al. Mental disorders in obese children and adolescents. Psychosom Med 2004;66(3):387–94.
[26] Erermis S, Cetin N, Tamar M, Bukusoglu N, Akdeniz F, Goksen D. Is obesity a risk factor for psychopathology among adolescents? Pediatr Int 2004;46(3):296–301.
[27] Sutaria S, Devakumar D, Yasuda SS, Das S, Saxena S. Is obesity associated with depression in children? Systematic review and meta-analysis. Arch Dis Child 2018 Jun 29. pii: archdischild-2017-314608. doi: 10.1136/archdischild-2017-314608.
[28] Stunkard AJ, Faith MS, Allison KC. Depression and obesity. Biol Psychiatry 2003;54(3): 330–7.
[29] Neumark-Sztainer DR, Wall MM, Haines JI, Story MT, Sherwood NE, van den Berg PA. Shared risk and protective factors for overweight and disordered eating in adolescents. Am J Prev Med 2007;33(5):359–69.
[30] Flament MF, Henderson K, Buchholz A, Obeid N, Nguyen HNT, Birmingham M, et al. Weight status and DSM-5 diagnoses of eating disorders in adolescents from the community. J Am Acad Child Adolesc Psychiatry 2015;54(5):403–11.
[31] Hudson JI, Hiripi E, Pope HG, Kessler RC. The prevalence and correlates of eating disorders in the National Comorbidity Survey Replication. Biol Psychiatry 2007;61(3): 348–58.
[32] Cortese S, Moreira-Maia CR, St. Fleur D, Morcillo-Peñalver C, Rohde LA, Faraone SV. Association Between ADHD and obesity: A systematic review and meta-analysis. Am J Psychiatry 2016;173(1):34–43.
[33] Cortese S, Tessari L. Attention-deficit/hyperactivity disorder (ADHD) and obesity: Update 2016. Curr Psychiatry Rep 2017;19(1):4. doi: 10.1007/s11920-017-0754-1.
[34] Rankin J, Matthews L, Cobley S, Han A, Sanders R, Wiltshire HD, et al. Psychological consequences of childhood obesity: psychiatric comorbidity and prevention. Adolesc Health Med Ther 2016;7:125–46.
[35] Wysokinski A, Kloszewska I. Mechanisms of increased appetite and weight gain induced by psychotropic medications. J Adv Clin Pharmacol 2014;1(1):12–33.
[36] Styne DM, Arslanian SA, Connor EL, Farooqi IS, Murad MH, Silverstein JH, et al. Pediatric obesity-assessment, treatment, and prevention: An endocrine society clinical practice guideline. J Clin Endocrinol Metab 2017;102(3):709–57.
[37] Browning KN, Verheijden S, Boeckxstaens GE. The vagus nerve in appetite regulation, mood, and intestinal inflammation. Gastroenterology 2017;152:730–44.
[38] Perry B, Wang Y. Appetite regulation and weight control: the role of gut hormones. Nutr Diabetes 2012;2(1):e26.
[39] Kim GW, Lin JE, Valentino MA, Colon-Gonzalez F, Waldman SA. Regulation of appetite to treat obesity. Expert Rev Clin Pharmacol 2011;4(2):243–59.
[40] de Lartigue G. Role of the vagus nerve in the development and treatment of diet-induced obesity. J Physiol 2016;594(20):5791–815.
[41] Suzuki K, Simpson KA, Minnion JS, Shillito JC, Bloom SR. The role of gut hormones and the hypothalamus in appetite regulation. Endocr J 2010;57(5):359–72.
[42] Food and Drug Administration. BELVIQ (lorcaserin hydrochloride) highlights of prescribing information, 2012.
[43] Bohula EA, Wiviott SD, McGuire DK, Inzucchi SE, Kuder J, Im K, et al. Cardiovascular safety of lorcaserin in overweight or obese patients. N Engl J Med 2018;379(12):1107-17.
[44] Brennan AM, Mantzoros CS. Drug Insight: the role of leptin in human physiology and pathophysiology--emerging clinical applications. Nat Clin Pract Endocrinol Metab 2006; 2(6):318–27.
[45] Pan H, Guo J, Su Z. Advances in understanding the interrelations between leptin resistance and obesity. Physiol Behav 2014;130:157–69.
[46] Kobelt P, Tebbe JJ, Tjandra I, Stengel A, Bae H-G, Andresen V, et al. CCK inhibits the orexigenic effect of peripheral ghrelin. Am J Physiol Regul Integr Comp Physiol 2005; 288(3):R751-8.
[47] Ruiz-Herrera X, de Los Ríos EA, Díaz JM, Lerma-Alvarado RM, Martínez de la Escalera L, López-Barrera F, et al. Prolactin promotes adipose tissue fitness and insulin sensitivity in obese males. Endocrinology 2017;158(1):56–68.

[48] Tzanavari T, Giannogonas P, Karalis KP. TNF-α and obesity. In: Kolloas G, Sfikakis PP, eds. TNF Pathophysiology. Molecular and cellular mechanisms. Basel, Switzerland: Karger, 2010:145–56.
[49] Liang S, Wu X, Hu X, Wang T, Jin F. Recognizing depression from the microbiota–gut–brain axis. Int J Mol Sci 2018;19:1592.
[50] Riehl ME. The emerging role of brain-gut therapies for irritable bowel syndrome. Gastroenterol Hepatol (NY) 2018;14(7):436–8.
[51] Dinan TG, Stanton C, Cryan JF. Psychobiotics: A novel class of psychotropic. Biol Psychiatry 2013;74(10):720–6.
[52] Carabotti M, Scirocco A, Maselli MA, Severi C. The gut-brain axis: interactions between enteric microbiota, central and enteric nervous systems. Ann Gastroenterol 2015;28(2): 203–9.
[53] Braet C, Van Winckel M. Long-term follow-up of a cognitive behavioral treatment program for obese children. Behav Ther 2000;31(1):55–74.
[54] Epstein LH, Paluch RA, Roemmich JN, Beecher MD. Family-based obesity treatment, then and now: twenty-five years of pediatric obesity treatment. Health Psychol 2007; 26(4):381–91.
[55] O'Malley G, Clarke M, Burls A, Murphy S, Murphy N, Perry IJ. A smartphone intervention for adolescent obesity: study protocol for a randomised controlled non-inferiority trial. Trials 2014;15(1):43.
[56] Inge TH, Courcoulas AP, Jenkins TM, Michalsky MP, Helmrath MA, Brandt ML, et al. Weight loss and health status 3 years after bariatric surgery in adolescents. N Engl J Med 2016;374(2):113–23.
[57] Zeller MH, Reiter-Purtill J, Ratcliff MB, Inge TH, Noll JG. Two-year trends in psychosocial functioning after adolescent Roux-en-Y gastric bypass. Surg Obes Relat Dis 2011;7(6): 727–32.
[58] Järvholm K, Olbers T, Marcus C, Mrild S, Gronowitz E, Friberg P, et al. Short-term psychological outcomes in severely obese adolescents after bariatric surgery. Obesity 2012; 20(2):318-23.

Chapter 10

Motivational interviewing and childhood obesity

Kalani A. Gates[1,2,*], MA, Kanhai Amin[3] and Sheryl Lozowski-Sullivan[2,4], MPH, PhD

[1]Department of Psychology, College of Arts and Sciences, Western Michigan University, Kalamazoo, Michigan, [2]Department of Pediatric and Adolescent Medicine, Division of Pediatric Psychology, Western Michigan University, Homer Stryker, MD School of Medicine, Kalamazoo, Michigan, United States of America , [3]Yale University, New Haven, Connecticut and [4]Integrated Behavioral Health Psychological Services, Kalamazoo, Michigan, United States of America

Abstract

The technique of motivational interviewing (MI) is considered in this discussion and is considered as a patient-centered, empathetic style of counseling originating from William R Miller's clinical model. The central pillar of this technique is the patient's self-introspection and articulation of reasons for change; individuals produce their own reasons for changing behavior to an empathetic, non-confrontational clinician, instead of the clinician providing reasons for altering behavior. Three clinical cases are presented to illustrate the utilization of MI in helping children and adolescents as well as their families deal with childhood and adolescent obesity.

Introduction

Childhood obesity endures as a major public health concern at the national and international levels. According to the World Health Organization (WHO), for children and adolescents aged 5-19 globally between 1975 and 2016, the prevalence of overweight or obese children and adolescents increased more than four-fold from 4% to 18% (**1**). Once considered a high-income country problem, it is now a low- and middle-income country issue, particularly in urban areas (1). In the United States, the Centers for Disease Control (CDC) shows a significant increasing

* ***Correspondence:*** Email: kalani.a.gates@wmich.edu.

In: Behavioral Pediatrics II
Editors: Donald E. Greydanus, Dilip R. Patel, Ahsan Nazeer et al.
ISBN: 979-8-88697-019-7

linear trend in prevalence rates from 13.5% to 18.5% for youth aged 2-19 years between 1999-2000 and 2015-2016 (2).

Childhood obesity, as defined by the *International classification of disease-10,* is characterized as a body mass index (BMI) score that either meets or exceeds the 95th percentile BMI score for same-aged children (3). BMI is age and sex-specific in children as well as adolescents and is referred to as "BMI-for-age." A BMI score that is 120% greater than scores of same-aged peers, in the 95th percentile, is indicative of a diagnosis of morbid (severe) obesity (3). In the United States, prevalence rates of childhood obesity are exceptionally high and continue to rise. Rates of childhood obesity have more than doubled within the last three decades (2). According to data collected from the National Health and Nutrition Examination Survey, 18.5% of the pediatric population suffers from obesity (3). When examining these data by age, adolescents and school age children (6-19 years of age) have higher rates of obesity than preschool age children (2-5 years of age) (3). In terms of gender differences, male children and adolescents have a higher likelihood of being obese than female children and adolescents (3).

Obesity's fundamental cause is an imbalance between calories consumed and calories expended. According to the WHO, global obesity exists due to the increased intake of calorie-dense foods and reduced activity due to increasingly sedentary jobs, changing forms of transportation, and urbanization (1). Several factors contribute to weight gain in children and adolescents. Lifestyle factors increase the likelihood of weight gain; these include an unbalanced diet (i.e., high-calorie, low-nutrient food, and sugary beverages) and lack of sufficient activity.

Socioeconomic factors also influence a child's weight. Children in families with limited financial resources or those unable to travel to a grocery store regularly are more likely to eat packaged and preserved foods; these foods are often more calorie-dense than freshly prepared foods. These socioeconomic factors may account for the higher rates of obesity among Hispanic (25.8%) and Black (22.0%) children and lower rates of obesity among White children (14.1%) (4, 5). This means one in four Hispanic children are obese compared to one in seven White children.

Psychological factors may lead to an excess in calorie intake and deficits in physical activity; these include elevated levels of stress or the presence of common mental health conditions (i.e., attention-deficit/hyperactivity disorder, anxiety, and depressive disorders) during this time of development.

Prescription medications are associated with weight gain among youth; these include steroids and some psychiatric medications, such as antidepressants and antipsychotics. Research also suggests that genetics increase the risk of obesity (6-11). It is estimated that roughly 2-5% of the variation in BMI comes from genetic variations according to genome-wide association studies (8). Twin studies, on the other hand, have found high heritability rates upward of 50-70%, indicating a stronger relationship between genetics and obesity at the individual level (9, 10).

Obesity and excess weight are linked to more deaths worldwide than malnutrition (1). There are not only physiologically deleterious risks but also psychosocial risks for obese youth. Children and adolescents who suffer from obesity have an increased risk of disease and dysfunction within various bodily systems such as the cardiovascular (e.g., hypertension, chronic inflammation), pulmonary (e.g., sleep apnea, asthma), endocrine (e.g., type 2 diabetes, precocious puberty), and musculoskeletal (e.g., Blout's disease, forearm fracture) (1, 3, 11). In addition, these youth are at an increased risk of unwanted psychosocial consequences (e.g., lowered self-esteem, mental health issues) (1, 11). These increased health risks may lead to unwanted consequences into adulthood not only due to their own delirious effects, but also due to the tendency of childhood obesity to carry on into adulthood (1).

Motivational interviewing

Motivational interviewing (MI) is a patient-centered, empathetic style of counseling originating from William R Miller's clinical model (12). The central pillar of this technique is the patient's self-introspection and articulation of reasons for change; individuals produce their own reasons for changing behavior to an empathetic, non-confrontational clinician, instead of the clinician providing reasons for altering behavior (12).

The clinical implementation of MI has evolved over time as more research has been conducted. However, the central spirit of MI has remained constant and is thoroughly noted in *behavioural and cognitive psychotherapy.* The summary of the key points are as follows. The clinician or counselor acts in an empathetic manner forming a non-hierarchical relationship with the individual. In turn, this creates an environment where the person can manifest their own reasons for change. The person must resolve their own ambivalence without direct persuasion from the clinician. The clinician's role is to guide the client's thoughts without imposing anything upon them; self-motivational ideas are reinforced while remaining cognizant of a client's willingness to change (13). Originally, it was thought that the clinician should provide "resistance" or counter arguments; however, this was determined to be counterproductive (12). Thus, MI is a technique of "dancing rather than wrestling" with the individual (14).

MI consists of four central processes: Engaging, Focusing, Evoking, and Planning. An extensive analysis of these four pillars is given in Miller's *motivational interviewing: Helping people change,* but this discussion provides a summary (14).

Engaging

The natural tendency and training of clinicians is to fix problems. However, the engaging process is dependent on reflective listening where the clinician abstains from providing or eliciting solutions. This stage aims to create trust and comfort while using open-ended questions to allow the client to reveal their thoughts and problems. The clinician strives to provide a comfortable environment where the patient does not feel judged. Ultimately, the goal is to establish a relationship where the client feels included in the therapy. Clients who feel involved are not only more likely to come back, but they are also less resistant. Whenever engagement is lost, it is crucial to re-engage before advancing forward.

Focusing

This stage is commonly known as the "What?" The purpose of this stage is to focus on a goal after uncovering the broad importance (e.g., health, ease of movement). This stage depends on the client as some may arrive with a goal in mind while others may require a couple of sessions before arriving at a goal. However, it is important for the clinician not to focus on behavior change too quickly. The point is to uncover what is important to the patient and the reasons motivating them to change. Ultimately, the clinician and client will arrive at the target behavior which requires changing. The clinician must ensure they are working with the client towards a common purpose instead of imposing one on the client. However, the goal may arise from directing, following, or guiding by the clinician.

Directing refers to the clinician directing the client to a particular motivating reason for behavior change. The clinician must make sure the client feels in charge; as a result, this mode is quite difficult. Following entails allowing the client to produce their own ideas. Meanwhile, guiding encompasses guiding the client to a particular goal; however, the patient still uncovers the direction by themselves. Focusing can be time-consuming; however, simply telling a person what they need to do does not result in behavior change.

Evoking

Evoking is also referred to as the "Why?" The purpose of this stage is to elicit and emphasize reasons for change. Clinicians want to ensure "change talk," or reasons for change, while directing away from sustain talk. In this stage, the clients are hopefully producing their own reasons for change, and it is the duty of the clinician to support the patients while recognizing which ideas the client seems the most motivated by. The client will likely have negative thoughts during this stage. However, the clinician must make sure they do not impose a tone of authority and try to fix their problems. Rather, the clinician must use what the patient has revealed about their motivations to guide them towards more positive thoughts. If the client requires help and the clinician feels they must provide ideas or solutions, they must ask the patient for permission before revealing their ideas for reasons to change. By doing this, the patient still feels a sense of control.

Planning

Planning is also referred to as the "How?" This process can only occur after significant engagement levels, a defined, measurable goal, and ample motivation for change. In this stage, the clinician facilitates the client into creating a specific plan of action. The clinician should ensure that there is a solid plan around the patient's own motivations.

Brief MI history

MI was originally conceived by Miller and Norwegian colleagues as a therapeutic method for individuals suffering from alcohol related problems. It was first published by Miller in a 1983 article in *Behavioral Psychotherapy.* Later, in 1991, Miller and Steve Rollnick proceeded to write a textbook on MI and two additional editions have been released. Since then, MI has been studied for a plethora of behaviors including obesity, drug use, gambling, smoking, abuse, rehabilitation, infection, and others (12, 13, 15-17).

MI was recently studied in various pediatric challenges, including but not limited to obesity, dental care, diabetes, reproductive health, smoking, and behavior. Suarez et al. analyzed many of these studies. Among the nine randomized control trials (RCT) considered, seven demonstrated positive findings while one showed mixed findings, and another demonstrated no statistical significance (18). Overall, more research needs to be conducted. However, there is promising evidence for the implementation of MI in a pediatric setting.

Research evidence on effectiveness of MI and childhood obesity

In the last two decades, a body of empirical literature has emerged examining the effectiveness of MI, either as a stand-alone treatment or as a supplement to other weight reduction interventions. In this section, this research is delineated by the age of the study's participants (i.e., children versus adolescents). The primary outcome measures for these studies are (i) a reduction in participants' BMI scores; or (ii) reductions of the participants' waist and limb circumference. Secondary measures including changes in lifestyle habits such as food selection and frequency of physical activity were examined as well.

Several studies have examined the effects of MI as a stand-alone treatment on obesity for children under the age of thirteen. A meta-analysis of original, peer-reviewed articles on MI and childhood obesity, published between 2007 and 2014, identified six studies on this topic. Three of these studies found significant positive effects of MI on children's BMI and lifestyle changes (19). The other three studies found no significant differences between the BMI scores and other related outcome measures at pre-post treatment or across treatment groups. However, as Borello and colleagues point out, these studies have important limitations including methodological issues such as small sample sizes, lack of randomization for clinicians and participants, unequal participant characteristics in comparison groups, low patient treatment adherence, and the lack of metrics on MI training as well as supervision for clinicians. In summary, the researchers argue that there is not enough data to support the effectiveness of MI on reducing obesity in younger children due to these methodological limitations and general scarcity of research.

In a second meta-analytic study, which examined RCTs on stand-alone MI interventions for youth 10 years and younger, researchers found positive changes in anthropometric measures (20). Of the seven identified studies, four studies reported significantly lower BMIs, waist circumferences, or waist-to-hip ratios of participants (or combinations of those outcomes) from pre-post when compared to controls. While there was overlap in the articles found in both reviews, the authors of the more recent review conclude that MI engenders positive behavior change among parents of younger children (20). Ultimately, these parental behaviors were found to lead to weight reduction among their children.

Other researchers hope to fill the gaps in the literature by continuing this line of research while utilizing more valid methodologies. In collaboration with the American Pediatric Association and the Children's Hospital of Philadelphia, Wright and colleagues are conducting an RCT in which pediatricians and nurse practitioners from multiple pediatric primary care sites are trained to implement a MI-focused weight reduction intervention when working with youths ages 3-11 (with a BMI $\geq 85^{th}$ percentile of their same-aged peers) (21). In this study, children will receive an enhanced motivational interview intervention, which consists of 12 didactic counseling sessions with expertly trained clinicians.

In terms of the research examining the effects of MI as a stand-alone treatment on adolescent obesity, the research appears to be unclear as well. A meta-analytic study examining the literature on MI interventions in adolescent obesity, between 1997 to 2018, found that MI alone did not appear to be effective in reducing the studies participants' BMI and other weight-related measures (22). Although, much like the studies on MI and weight reduction in younger age groups, the studies included in this review also had similar methodological limitations (e.g., insufficient sample sizes, "therapeutic dose", and training of clinicians). As a result, studies with stronger methodologies are needed to determine the effectiveness of MI on adolescent weight gain at this time.

Researchers have also examined whether MI is effective as an adjunctive treatment rather than a stand-alone treatment. In one randomized controlled trial, Black female adolescents between the ages of 11 to 18 were enrolled in TEENS, a 6-month evidence-based weight loss intervention (23). Participants in the intervention group also received MI Values, an adjunctive MI intervention, from trained and supervised clinicians. The BMI z-scores and food consumption intake significantly decreased at pre-post. Additionally, the time in which participants engaged in intensive exercise also increased across both groups. For participants in the intervention group, these changes remained at 6-months follow-up. At 3-months, the intervention group also reported consuming significantly less calories than the control group participants. In another RCT study, a single call of MI conducted by trained clinical psychologists increased parent attendance to the baseline session of an adjunctive adolescent obesity treatment when compared to parents in the control group (24).

Collectively, these findings suggest that more research is needed to determine the effectiveness of MI as a stand-alone treatment for children and adolescents. Research examining the effectiveness of MI as an intervention used in conjunction with other obesity treatments appears to be promising in encouraging positive behaviors that lead to patient weight loss.

Special challenges and considerations

There are several important considerations for health professionals who work with youth and their families from this population. Aside from the typical challenges that are seen when providing services to children and adolescents, providers may face additional obstacles when working with the parents or caregivers of youth who are obese. For example, children who suffer from obesity are more likely to have parents who are also obese when compared to children in a healthy BMI range (25). Although this association may arise from familial genetics or environmental factors (e.g., eating and lifestyle habits) or a combination of the two, health providers may find it to be difficult to facilitate positive behavior changes from the youth if the family's lifestyle habits are in opposition to the patient's treatment plan. Moreover, obese youth typically have very little autonomy when it comes to the prerequisites necessitated to engage in behaviors that mitigate weight gain. For example, as the authority of the household, parents and caretakers often purchase groceries and determine meal portions as well as mealtimes for their children. Even if parents and caregivers are amenable to the health provider's treatment recommendations for their children, they may be resistant to changing the family's lifestyle habits.

These changes may be more difficult for families due to the global food industry and prevailing calorie-dense, easily accessible food culture. The convenience and affordability of many fast-food options make it particularly challenging for youth and families to avoid consuming high-calorie and-low nutrient foods. With these considerations in mind, health providers could utilize MI techniques not only to address their patients' resistance, but also to address the patients' parents' and/or caregivers' resistance.

Providers' biases (i.e., implicit and explicit) is another important factor to consider when working with youths and families who are obese. Weight bias refers to negative attitudes or beliefs about an individual due to their body weight. Whether intentional or not, such bias manifests through stereotypes and/or discrimination toward these patients which, in turn, may negatively influence critical provider behaviors such as treatment decisions (26). Internalized weight stigmatization and anticipated provider discrimination are considerable concerns as well (27). Such perceptions may lead to reticent help-seeking behaviors from patients and their families, further limiting opportunities for intervention and treatment for health professionals (28, 29). Obese patients are keenly aware of weight-bias since they often experience this in their daily lives.

Therefore, it is important that providers receive the appropriate training and education about the etiological complexities (biopsychosocial factors) of obesity and take a holistic approach when determining the patients' likely causes of weight gain. By increasing education on the genetic, metabolic, and socioeconomic factors associated with weight gain, health providers may be less likely to attribute their patients' weight issues as an exclusive result of their own personal choices (30). Eliminating this component of blame may help to reduce implicit biases and patients' worries related to weight stigmatization and prejudice. Additionally, educational programming to teach providers to use respectful terminology and communicative styles when discussing their patients' body weight is warranted given these concerns (31, 32). Simply knowing the detrimental effects of weight biases on patients' health outcomes have been shown to decrease weight bias as well. Finally, structured evidence-based implicit bias training with components to address weight bias may also reduce providers' weight biases.

Motivational interviewing through case examples

In short, MI techniques often feel circular or repetitive to the clinician but unmistakably are not lecturing or wrestling with the individual; rather, the use of MI techniques should feel like a dance in which the clinician is the lead (14). In this section, we explore the "dance" through case examples. The two components of MI are relational and technical. Relational involves the interpersonal and empathic components highlighted in the Engage stage. Technical involves drawing out and reinforcing change talk **(12).** Importantly, when change talk does not exist, the clinician retreats; they do not double down on efforts falling into the familiar education or lecture style as this has been found to be counter-productive to behavior change.

Case example 1

Samantha "Sam" is an 8-year-old biracial female (Guatemalan and Euro-American) who lives with her mother, two younger sisters, and an older brother. The four children see their father on weekends where the father's live-in girlfriend has two male children close to Sam's and her older brother's ages. Occasionally these two sons visit their father or abuelos (grandparents) on the weekends, but the children are often together on the weekends. The boys tease Sam frequently because she is morbidly obese. Sam's pediatrician expresses concern with Sam's weight in part because the family members tend toward obesity. Sam has mild asthma and seasonal allergies.

The clinical psychologist met the patient and her mother in an integrated behavioral health (IBH) pediatric practice affiliated with a university hospital and medical school. The pediatric fellow provided a warm hand-off to the psychologist (i.e., the physician introduced the IBH model, the psychologist, and the topic of weight maintenance). The first 30-minute visit was used to establish engagement by playing a game with Sam while discussing their routines, eating habits, and determining whether the family wanted a referral for an intensive program for weight management or wanted to address her weight on their own. On the second brief intervention appointment with the psychologist, she introduces MI techniques:

Psych: The first time we met, mom, you indicated that you would like to lose weight and you would like to see Sam "grow into her current" weight which is what the pediatric fellow suggested as well. Mom, why is this important to you?

Mom: I would like to be healthy, look better, and for Sam to thin out so she isn't teased so much. I was teased as a child for being overweight and it was horrible. I don't want her to go through that.

Psych: Why is being healthy and looking better important to you?

Mom: Well, I was teased so much I think it affected, you know, my confidence. I don't want that for my Sammy.

Psych: Anything else?

Mom: Confidence affects everything in life, you know; I remember crying so much as a child. My mother would say, it's okay, they are just mean kids. And give me a treat. I really try not to do that with Sam, give her a cookie or ice cream to feel better. I talk to her and sit with her when she is upset and tell her how it will get better for her.

Sam breaks in: Yeah, when the boys were "oinking" at me, I hit them. I try to tell mommy, but they keep on doing it. It makes me sad.

Psych: Sam, I'm so sorry that the boys do that. You are lucky to have your mom. Sam, what is important to you?

Sam: I don't like to be teased.

Psych: I can understand Sam, no one likes to be teased. Do you think you might like some help not gaining more weight?

Sam: Yes.

Psych: Mom, is there anything else behind why you feel it is important?

Mom: Because being overweight as a child makes a life-long struggle with weight. I've tried so many diets and gained weight back because I didn't stick to the diet or felt deprived. I don't want that for Sam.

Psych: So, what I hear is you think it is important for Sam to reduce her weight gain because it affects her health, the way she looks, her confidence, and so she does not have a lifetime of dieting, losing, and gaining weight. Did I miss anything?

Mom: Yes, she has such a pretty face. I want people to see her pretty face, not an overweight girl.

Psych: Ah, she does have a beautiful smile and sparkling eyes. And Sam doesn't want to be teased, that doesn't feel good, does it Sam? Another reason underlying the why of addressing weight and food is how other people view the overweight person and how people judge Sam based on her weight not what her face looks like. These are all wonderful reasons to make some small changes. Recall that we talked about small changes that can make a big difference? Now let's talk about one small change we can try this week based on what Sam typically eats each day. Sam, we need you to be a part of this. We are not going to tell you what to do. Let's start with breakfast.

The psychologist, Sam, and mother identify a small, well-defined, and achievable goal for the week. Sam and mom will try a fruit (e.g., apples, strawberries, blueberries) rather than having bacon in the morning with her waffles and replace her full sugar syrup with a lite version or honey-sweetened version or use half the amount of syrup. Sam suggested she could try a different breakfast so they will consider yogurt or eggs with a little pinch of shredded "yellow" cheese but no coffee because that is "gross," according to Sam. They agreed to try these small changes in breakfast for 5 out of the next 7 mornings. Sam's mother stated the list of items to shop for and committed to a time to buy these items.

Case 1 illustrates that when working with children, working with parents is essential. Encouraging Sam to join the conversation is important but not as important as Focusing and Evoking with the mother of an 8- year-old. Planning a specific, well-defined behavior change and the timeframe is important. Replacement foods or limiting portions rather than deprivation or "never" eating certain foods is key. Sometimes non-food rewards (e.g., extra story, game with mom) that are *reinforcing to the child* are needed to encourage compliance with the goal behavior.

Case example 2

Jerome is a 15-year-old African American male who lives with his parents and brother. His parents and brother fall within the expected body mass index (BMI) based on height; Jerome's weight has been creeping upwards since middle school began. The maternal and paternal histories are positive for type I diabetes mellitus and stroke. Jerome likes sweets (cakes, cookies, donuts, sweet cereals, soda-pop, ice cream) and what his father calls "junk food" (fast food fries & burgers, potato chips, and pizza). Meals are often eaten as a family with meat, starches, and vegetables; however, meals often end with arguments regarding Jerome's eating habits. Arguments begin between Jerome and his father, then lead to conflict between the father and mother because the mother defends their son's eating habits, saying he will grow into his weight.

Jerome runs track in the spring and plays football in the fall. He shoots hoops with friends and skateboarded frequently in elementary and middle school. Recently, he expressed the desire to quit his high school sports. Jerome gained 20 pounds on his 5'11" frame in the past three months now weighing 164 lbs. (90th percentile). Jerome's paternal grandfather was "heavy" according to his father, expressing worry that Jerome is "following" his grandfather who struggled with weight and type I diabetes until his death at 65 years of age. Jerome has no medical conditions and does not take any medications.

Physician: Jerome, is it important to you to reduce the weight gain you had in the past three months?

Jerome: I guess, I mean...

Dad breaks in: You really need to get control of this eating, or you are going to be fat and sick like your grandad. Doc, you should see this kid eat all kinds of sweet stuff – donuts, candy, ice cream, and junk food – he eats fast food almost every day.

Physician: (noticing Jerome hang his head, the tension in the room escalates thinking dad does have a point and this kid could stand to lose weight), raises his hand to dad as if to say, "hold on" and interjects: It sounds like this is a hot button for dad.

Mom: It is and then I get to protecting Jerome and his dad and I start arguing.

Physician: Let's agree that Dad can't make Jerome change and that dad is worried, right?

Dad: Uh, huh. My father died at 65 from a stroke. He had high blood pressure, type I diabetes, and he would sneak sweets. That man did not take care of himself.

Physician: (Thinking Jerome is heading down that path & he is looking heavy). Well, Dad, I can see how you don't want those health problems for Jerome. And that you are worried about Jerome given that you don't think your father took care of his health. Is that correct? (Dad nods.) Jerome, what is important to you?

Jerome: Being healthy, losing weight.

Physician: OK, why are those important to you?

Jerome: I would feel better, probably play football better, feel better about myself.

Physician: Jerome, does it help you to hear how scared dad is for you? Do his comments help you?

Jerome: No.

Physician: Instead of telling you all the bad things that can happen to you when you are overweight, how about we work on this over the next couple of months? What do you say?

Jerome: Yeah. OK.

Physician: Dad, how about you talk to me about your worries privately? Jerome and I will work together. Now, Jerome, I hear you telling me that being healthy, losing some weight or not gaining more would feel better, help you play football better, what else?

Jerome: More confidence in the weight room, swimming in the summer, I don't want to take my t-shirt off, I don't even know about track this year...

Physician: Why are all these things important?

Jerome: Because I like doing these things, because I am good at these things, and I'd like to run track. Track is where I get to see most of my friends and hang out. You know, there is a lot of time between events. It's fun.

Physician: So, track is important because you like it and it is a fun time with friends, it's important for you to lose weight or not gain because you could be better at football, feel better in the weight room lifting, swim with your shirt off, and it sounds like you would feel less self-conscious. Is that right?

Jerome: Yep, I think that's it.

Physician: Is there one behavior you think you might want to change?

Jerome: I was thinking about instead of, you know, burger & fries for lunch, maybe try a sub sandwich. Maybe have less sweets.

Physician: Yes, that is a good start. Let's try one or two changes at a time. That is how we build new habits, in small changes, not big changes because big changes are hard to maintain. What one sweet thing have you thought about cutting back?

Jerome: Soda. I really like water; I don't know why I don't just have water.

Physician: Excellent. We have a sub sandwich once or twice a week and reduce soda intake by half? (Jerome nods.) For the next seven out of ten days? (Jerome nods.) I see Jerome can meet again in ten days. In the meantime, mom and dad, can we stay away from arguing over Jerome's eating?

Everyone nods in agreement.

Case 2 illustrates that MI techniques do not assume anything but ask "why?" "Why is that important?" And again, after the person responds, "And why is that important?" It can seem like asking the same question again, but it is about drilling down into deeper meaning. It also illustrates the inherent thoughts about weight bias that may pop into the provider's head. He resists allowing these thoughts to block his ability to effectively work with Jerome. Case 2 illustrates that there are often challenges within a family that thwart moving forward; these need to be addressed also. Often naming and acknowledging the emotions involved help diminish the tension surrounding the issue as the physician does with the father's worries about his son following his father down a similar path of weight gain and medical sequelae.

Case 2 shows how the physician typically needs to pivot away from describing all the negative health outcomes from obesity to what motivates the individual to want to change. Describing all the bad outcomes is not promoting change, it makes the patient feel badly and often berated. The physician checked in with himself during this dialogue and could have discouraged the patient if he had shown the weight-bias inner thoughts. He checked in with himself, engaged Jerome, focused on the "what?", evoked the "why?" And provided the mental space for Jerome to plan the "how?"

Case example 3

Zoe is a 17-year-old female of Euro-American and Chinese American descent. She lives with her mother, stepfather, maternal grandmother, older sister, and her sister's infant son. Zoe spends much of her time in her room, but she enjoys marching band (trumpet), jazz band, drama, and choir. Zoe is a strong student in all subjects except when a teacher is harsh or tries to be friendly by teasing. She instantly dislikes the subject when she dislikes the teacher. She is shy and withdrawn in school except when someone is teased or bullied and when people "say stupid things." Zoe lives with her biological mother and stepfather. She does not see her biological father. Zoe's parents and Zoe are overweight. Zoe's weight has increased slowly in the past two-three years to the 105th percentile BMI-for-age. Zoe was diagnosed with attention-deficit/ hyperactivity disorder, inattentive type (ADHD) when she was 10 years old. She takes methylphenidate, 5 mg twice daily. Her mother indicates that when her medication wears off, she starts to eat about 5 pm most days.

Her mother frequently finds wrappers (cheese sticks, chips), crumbs (sandwich) or other items on the counter in the morning, signs that Zoe ate late into the night. The resident physician established that Zoe does not eat breakfast and at most, eats chips or a granola bar for lunch. She doesn't usually have money on her school lunch account not because they do not have the money but because she doesn't eat. Zoe indicated there are days she might have eaten something if there was money on her school lunch account. The physician attempted to establish how much Zoe eats at night.

Physician: Zoe, Mom, do you have concerns about Zoe eating most of her calories in the evening?

Zoe: I never thought about it. Could that be why I have gained more weight? I don't understand because I don't eat most of the daytime.

Mom: No, Zoe, that isn't it. You are just big boned, you're fine.

Physician: Well, I think we might look at changing her ADHD medication if she is taking in most of her calories after 5pm. Zoe, what is important to you in terms of your weight?

Zoe: I don't know, I guess I'd like to lose weight. My clothes don't fit well.

Mom: I don't think she needs to lose weight; she is just fine. Her grandmother thinks so, too.

Physician: Well, I understand you think she is fine, but her weight is at the 105th percentile, and it sounds like Zoe might want to make some changes. Zoe, what is important to you?

Zoe: Being healthy.

Physician: That is a good start. Why is healthy important to you?

Zoe: I don't know, isn't that important to everyone?

Physician: Well, no, people do a lot of things that are not healthy for them, Zoe, like smoking, driving without a seat belt, eating lots of high fat foods, using drugs, lots of things. Why is being healthy important to you?

Zoe: So, I can do the things I like, band was rough this year, it is hard to march in a uniform that is too tight, I like to wear clothes I have, I like to feel like people aren't looking at me in the cafeteria, I don't like feeling like people are watching to see what I eat at lunch or trying to catch me eat a bunch of junk foods.

Physician: So, if I have this right, you are self-conscious about eating in front of people (Zoe shakes her head in agreement)? Do you think they are judging you based on what you eat (Zoe nods again)? And your clothes are tight, and you would like to be healthier? What do you think about just writing down what you eat?

Zoe: You mean everything? I guess I could do that.

Physician: Zoe, think about what we talked about today. Let's talk about it again next time. (Physician schedules a 1-2-month follow-up rather than 6 or 12 months to revisit Zoe's resistance versus change talk).

Case 3 illustrates that people often are not clear on what is important to them. Notice there is not change talk in this case but resistance talk. Case 3 shows that it is important to retreat when the patient is not producing change talk and resist the impulse to push the patient into the reasons for change. Giving the patient the reasons to change rather than help them produce these reasons is not effective **(15)**. Parental resistance to change can be challenging for physicians who want to launch into all the health implications of being obese.

Conclusion

In conclusion, with its roots in counseling psychology, motivational interviewing (MI) is an empathetic and non-confrontational technique used among clinicians to address resistance to behavior change by patients with a variety of different health issues. More recently, MI has been used in healthcare settings to address childhood obesity. Childhood obesity continues to be a major public health concern, particularly in the United States, as made evident by the steadily increasing rate of children and adolescents who struggle with their weight each year.

The current literature on the effectiveness of MI is mixed, in part, due to methodological concerns and subsequent limitations of previous studies. MI techniques utilized by health care providers, as a stand-alone treatment, appear to be effective in changing parental behaviors of young children thereby, reducing their children's weight. With respect to adolescents, the research on MI as a stand-alone treatment is less clear, highlighting a need for more research in this area. In spite of this, studies examining the effects of MI as an adjunctive treatment to other weight loss interventions have shown to be effective.

Clinical considerations when working with youth and families from this population are warranted. For example, providers should be aware of the causal factors of childhood obesity, familial and societal structures that encourage weight gain, and ways in which weight bias can affect patient outcomes. Additional education and training in these areas may lead to better patient outcomes. Overall, MI is a promising technique that can be used by health providers to facilitate positive weight-related changes among childhood patients who struggle with obesity.

References

[1] World Health Organization. Obesity and overweight. Geneva: WHO. URL: https://www.who.int/news-room/fact-sheets/detail/obesity-and-overweight.

[2] Hales C, Carroll M, Fryar C, Ogden C. Prevalence of obesity among adults and youth: United States, 2015–2016. Hyattsville, MD: National Center for Health Statistics, NCHS Data Brief Report No 288, 2017.

[3] World Health Organization. ICD-10: International statistical classification of diseases and related health problems: Tenth revision, 2nd edition. Geneva: World Health Organization, 2004.

[4] de Onis M, Blossner M, Borghi E. Global prevalence and trends of overweight and obesity among preschool children. Am J Clin Nutr 2010;92:1257–64.

[5] Ogden CL, Fryar CD, Hales CM, Carroll MD, Aoki Y, Freedman DS. Differences in obesity prevalence by demographics and urbanization in US children and adolescents, 2013-2016. JAMA 2018;319(23):2410–8.

[6] Brandkvist M, Bjørngaard JH, Ødegård RA, Åsvold BO, Sund ER, Vie GÅ. Quantifying the impact of genes on body mass index during the obesity epidemic: longitudinal findings from the UNT Study. BMJ 2019;366:l4067.

[7] Locke AE, The LifeLines Cohort Study, Kahali B, Berndt SI, Justice AE, Pers TH, et al. Genetic studies of body mass index yield new insights for obesity biology. Nature 2015; 518(7538):197–206.

[8] Yengo L, Sidorenko J, Kemper KE, Zheng Z, Wood AR, Weedon MN, et al. Meta-analysis of genome-wide association studies for height and body mass index in ~700000 individuals of European ancestry. Hum Mol Genet 2018;27(20):3641–9.

[9] Rokholm B, Silventoinen K, Tynelius P, Gamborg M, Sørensen TIA, Rasmussen F. Increasing genetic variance of body mass index during the Swedish obesity epidemic. PLoS One 2011;6(11):e27135.

[10] Silventoinen K, Jelenkovic A, Sund R, Yokoyama Y, Hur Y-M, Cozen W, et al. Differences in genetic and environmental variation in adult BMI by sex, age, time period, and region: an individual-based pooled analysis of 40 twin cohorts. Am J Clin Nutr 2017; 106(2):457–66.
[11] Lyon HN, Hirschhorn, JN. Genetics of common forms of obesity: A brief overview. Am J Clin Nutr 2005;82(1):215-7.
[12] Miller WR, Rose GS. Toward a theory of motivational interviewing. Am Psychol 2009; 64(6):527-37.
[13] Rollnick S, Miller, WR. What is motivational interviewing? Behav Cogn Psychother 1995;23(4):325-34.
[14] Rollnick S, Miller WR, Butler,CC. Motivational interviewing in health care: Helping patients change behavior. New York: Guilford, 2008.
[15] Miller WR, Rollnick S. Motivational interviewing helping people change. New York: Gulliford, 2013.
[16] Sanci L, Chondros P, Sawyer S, Pirkis J, Ozer E, Hegarty K, et al. Responding to young people's health risks in primary care: A cluster randomised trial of training clinicians in screening and motivational interviewing. PLoS One 2015;10(9):e0137581.
[17] Pirlott AG, Kisbu-Sakarya Y, Defrancesco, CA, Elliot, DL, Makinnon, DP. Mechanisms of motivational interviewing in health promotion: A Bayesian mediation analysis. Int J Behav Nutr Phy Act 2012;9(1):69.
[18] Suarez M, Mullins S. Motivational interviewing and pediatric health behavior interventions. J Dev Behav Pediatr 2008;29(5):417-28.
[19] Borrello M, Pietrabissa G, Ceccarini M, Manzoni GM, Castelnuovo G. Motivational interviewing in childhood obesity treatment. Front Psychol 2015;6:1732.
[20] Suire KB, Kavookjian J, Wadsworth DD. Motivational interviewing for overweight children: A systematic review. Pediatrics 2020;146(5):e20200193.
[21] Wright ME, Delacroix E, Sonneville KR, Considine S, Proctor T, Steffes J, et al. Reducing paediatric overweight and obesity through motivational interviewing: study protocol for a randomised controlled trial in the AAP PROS research network. BMJ Open 2020;10(7):e035720.
[22] Vallabhan MK, Jimenez EY, Nash JL, Gonzales-Pacheco D, Coakley KE, Noe SR, et al. Motivational interviewing to treat adolescents with obesity: A meta-analysis. Pediatrics 2018;142(5):e20180733.
[23] Bean MK, Ingersoll KS, Powell P, Stern M, Evans RK, Wickham EP, et al. Impact of motivational interviewing on outcomes of an adolescent obesity treatment: results from the MI Values randomized controlled pilot trial. Clin Obes 2018;8(5):323–6.
[24] Bean MK, Thornton LM, Jeffers AJ, Gow RW, Mazzeo SE. Impact of motivational interviewing on engagement in a parent-exclusive paediatric obesity intervention: randomized controlled trial of NOURISH+MI. Pediatr Obes 2019;14(4):e12484.
[25] Reilly JJ, Armstrong J, Dorosty AR, Emmett PM, Ness A, Rogers I, et al. Early life risk factors for obesity in childhood: cohort study. BMJ 2005;330(7504):1357.
[26] Phelan SM, Burgess DJ, Yeazel MW, Hellerstedt WL, Griffin JM, van Ryn M. Impact of weight bias and stigma on quality of care and outcomes for patients with obesity: Obesity stigma and patient care. Obes Rev 2015;16(4):319–26.
[27] Lee MS, Gonzalez BD, Small BJ, Thompson JK. Internalized weight bias and psychological wellbeing: An exploratory investigation of a preliminary model. PLoS One 2019;14(5):e0216324.
[28] Sutin AR, Terracciano A. Perceived weight discrimination and obesity. PLoS One 2013; 8(7):e70048.
[29] Drury CA, Louis M. Exploring the association between body weight, stigma of obesity, and health care avoidance. J Am Acad Nurs Pract 2002;14(12):554-561.
[30] Hilbert A. Weight stigma reduction and genetic determinism. PLoS One 2016;11(9): e0162993.
[31] Persky S, Eccleston CP. Medical student bias and care recommendations for an obese versus non-obese virtual patient. Int J Obes (Lond) 2011;35(5):728–35.
[32] Wear D, Aultman JM, Varley JD, Zarconi J. Making fun of patients: medical students' perceptions and use of derogatory and cynical humor in clinical settings. Acad Med 2006; 81(5):454–62.

Chapter 11

Pediatric obesity psychopharmacology: Quo vadis?

Flora Bacopoulou[1], MD, PhD
and Donald E. Greydanus[2,*], MD, DrHC(Athens)

[1]Center for Adolescent Medicine and UNESCO Chair on Adolescent Health Care, First Department of Pediatrics, School of Medicine, National and Kapodistrian University of Athens, Aghia Sophia Children's Hospital, Athens, Greece

[2]Department of Pediatric and Adolescent Medicine, Western Michigan University Homer Stryker M.D. School of Medicine, Kalamazoo, Michigan, United States of America

Abstract

Obesity is a major risk factor for child, adolescent and adult health. Though diet and exercise are the cornerstone of obesity prevention and treatment, many pediatric persons do not adhere to a nutrition-exercise approach. This review reflects on concepts of pharmacology for the management of obesity in children and adolescents in the early 21st century. Medications considered in the management of obesity include sympathomimetics (with or without topiramate), serotonin agonists, fat blockers (gastrointestinal lipase inhibitors), glucagon-like peptide 1 (GLP-1) agonists, antidepressant/opioid antagonist combination and others. Medications that were used for obesity management and later pulled from the market are also discussed. There are two drugs, orlistat and liraglutide, approved by the United States Food and Drug Administration (US-FDA) for adolescents ≥ 12 years of age with obesity. In the pediatric population there remains limited evidence on the safety and efficacy of anti-obesity medications used in adults and close monitoring for adverse effects is needed. The use of medications to assist in the management of overweight and obesity in pediatric and adult persons will increase as the 21st century continues. Clinicians should be vigilant about the current state of the art with regard to pharmacology of obesity and to its future.

* ***Correspondence:*** Professor Donald E Greydanus, MD, DrHC(Athens), Department of Pediatric and Adolescent Medicine, Western Michigan University Homer Stryker MD School of Medicine, 1000 Oakland Drive, Kalamazoo, MI 49008, United States. Email: donald.greydanus@med.wmich.edu.

In: Behavioral Pediatrics II
Editors: Donald E. Greydanus, Dilip R. Patel, Ahsan Nazeer et al.
ISBN: 979-8-88697-019-7

Introduction

Obesity is a major risk factor for child, adolescent and adult health. Though diet and exercise are core components to management of obesity in children and adolescents, the role of pharmacology in obesity treatment is a growing phenomenon in the 21st century (1-3). This review refers to medications that are being used and may be used in the near or far future to help with a growing worldwide problem with obesity in persons of all ages in all countries that affects 2.8 to 3.5 billion humans of all ages (1, 4). Though most of these drugs do not have approval of the United States Food and Drug Administration (US-FDA), they may be approved by agencies of countries (i.e., European Medicines Agency, EMA) or simply used by various clinicians even without any official approval (4-6).

Caution is always urged for clinicians utilizing various medications in this regard. Drugs have side effects that can be very detrimental to overweight and obese persons. In this regard, this treatise begins with former medications utilized for obesity control but withdrawn from the market because of adverse effects. This discussion does not consider medication for conditions co-morbid with obesity, such as polycystic ovary syndrome, diabetes mellitus and other endocrine disorders (1). Also, clinicians should be aware of use of some drugs for medical conditions that have side effects of weight gain such as use of some medications for diabetes mellitus (i.e., insulin, thiazolidinediones, sulfonylureas) or psychosis (i.e., some antipsychotic medications) (7-10).

Guidance suggests use of medications for obesity in adults with obesity i.e., a body mass index (BMI) ≥ 30 kg/m^2 or with overweight BMI ≥ 27 kg/m^2 if comorbid conditions are found (1, 11). Medications that are U.S. FDA-approved for obesity in those over 16 years of age are listed in Table 1 (11-13). These medications are not approved for management of obesity in pregnant or lactating persons. Weight loss that does occur is usually limited to 3-10% of the initial weight—such as 2 to 10 kilograms, noted during the first 6 months or less of starting the drug, and reversal of the weight loss may occur after stopping the drug (2, 14, 15).

Table 1. Classification of anti-obesity medications

Antidepressant/opioid antagonist combination
Gastrointestinal lipase inhibitors (fat blockers)
Glucagon-like peptide 1 (GLP-1) agonists
Serotonin agonists
Sympathomimetics (with or without topiramate)
Others: See text

Clinicians should be aware of the age limitations in children, the potential expense of such drugs, and their various adverse effects (1). Side effects may be known for adults but are usually unknown or limited in knowledge when applied to children and adolescents; such poor knowledge is worsened by limited research trials for pediatric persons (16, 17). Adverse effects of anorexigenic agents are key contributors to discontinuation by persons such as adolescents taking them (18).

Current status

From the viewpoint of the US-FDA, there are two drugs, orlistat and liraglutide, FDA-approved for pediatric persons ≥ 12 years of age with obesity (19). Liraglutide has recently been approved for chronic weight management of adolescents with obesity, as defined by specific BMI cut-offs for age and sex that correspond to a BMI 30 kg/m^2 or higher for adults, and with a body weight of at least 60 kg. There are a number of medications approved for adults with obesity, as listed in Table 2. Phentermine and other sympathomimietics, as listed in Table 2 are FDA-approved for short-term consumption (i.e., ≤ 12 weeks) while the others in Table 2 are acceptable for long-term usage (14, 20, 21).

Table 2. Medications with US-FDA approval for adult obesity

A.	Gastrointestinal lipase inhibitor: *orlistat* (starting at age 12 years)
B.	Glucagon-like peptide 1 (GLP-1) analog: *liraglutide* - diabetes mellitus drug (starting at age 12 years)
C.	Monoamine modulators
	1. *phentermine/topiramate ER*
	2. *naltrexone/bupropion ER*
D.	Sympathomimetics
	1. *phentermine,*
	2. *benzphetamine,*
	3. *diethylproprion*
	4. *phendimetrazine*

An interesting movement for anti-obesity drugs in the 21st century is the development of combination drug management that may contain medications initially utilized for indications apart from obesity per se (11, 14, 22-24). Also taken by obese persons are various over-the-counter herbal products (1-3). Research is occurring on the potential anorexigenic actions of plant diterpenes (diterpenoids) (25).

Many of these anti-obesity agents are considered in this discussion. However, first agents to be considered are medications that were once used/approved for obesity management, but approval was withdrawn because of serious adverse effects that were eventually identified. Such medications serve as a reminder of limits and risks associated with use of anti-obesity drugs (1, 26).

Previous anti-obesity drugs

Table 3 lists several drugs that were considered as anti-obesity medications but became withdrawn or not approved by the US-FDA usually due to concerns over adverse effects (1-3). The lessons of these chemicals are important for researchers and clinicians to keep in mind when considering pharmacology for obesity management in children and adolescents. For example, aminorex, an amphetamine-like chemical, was an anti-obesity drug withdrawn in 1968 due to its side-effect profile including increased pulmonary hypertension risk (1, 27).

Table 3. Withdrawn of proposed and/or formerly approved anti-obesity agents

1.	Aminorex
2.	Beloranib
3.	Dexfenfluramine
4.	Fenfluramine
5.	Lorcaserin
6.	Phenylpropanolamine (PPA)
7.	Rimonabant
8.	Sibutramine

Beloranib

The selective methionine aminopeptidase 2 inhibitor, beloranib, was under research as an anti-obesity agent until two individuals with Prader-Willi syndrome on this drug died and the studies were stopped in 2015 (1, 28). Such stories remind all physicians of their prime Hippocratic rule—primum, non nocere (29, 30).

Fenfluramine

The serotonergic chemical, fenfluramine, was combined with the amphetamine-like agent, phentermine, in a popular anti-obesity dual program or Phen-Fen diet (31). The use of fenfluramine and also dexfenfluramine, was found to have an increased risk for primary hypertension and valvulopathy—leading to the withdrawal of both as anti-obesity drugs in 1997 (32, 33). As noted below, phentermine has remained on the U.S. market since 1959 for short-term obesity management.

Lorcaserin

Lorcaserin is a selective serotonin 2C receptor agonist that received FDA approval for long-term obesity management in 2012 (1, 20). Research noted it is an appetite suppressant that decreased food intake with a mean weight loss of 5% after one year (1). However, the FDA withdrew its approval of lorcaserin for weight loss in February of 2020 because of concerns over an increase in cancer in adults taking this drug (34-38).

Phenylpropanolamine (PPA)

PPA is part of the phenethylamine drug family that became well-known for its decongestant and appetite suppressant effects. However, it was withdrawn by the FDA in 2000 because of research identifying increased risk of hemorrhagic cardiovascular accidents in 18- to 49-year-old females as well as the concern over birth defects if taken by pregnant females (39-41).

Rimonabant

Rimonabant is a CB1-selective cannabinoid receptor antagonist/inverse agonist) that was utilized in Europe for adult obesity treatment as well as management of nicotine use disorder (42, 43). Continued research on rimonabant revealed increased risk for adverse neuropsychiatric effects (i.e., depression, suicide) and the US-FDA did not approve of this chemical for obesity management and it was withdrawn from the European market in 2006 (44, 45).

Sibutramine

Sibutramine, a norepinephrine-5-hydroxytryptamine reuptake inhibitor, had been FDA-approved as an anti-obesity drug for persons ≥ 16 years of age (46). However, various adverse effects were identified that were cardiovascular, neuropsychiatric and carcinogenic along with a number of contraindications (1). This increasing adverse profile lead to the US-FDA withdrawal of sibutramine in 2010 for obesity management (1, 44).

Orlistat

Orlistat is a lipase (gastric and pancreatic) inhibitor that is derived from endogenous lipstatin that is isolated from *Streptomyces toxytricini* (47). Orlistat was approved by the US-FDA in 1998 for obesity in adults and it is also approved for persons with obesity ≥12 years of age; it is the only weight-reduction medication approved for obese adolescents (1, 48). The typical adult oral dose is 120 mg three times a day and there is a reduced fat absorption of 30% and mild to moderate weight reduction (49, 50). An over-the-counter dose was also FDA approved for weight loss at 60 mg three times a day with a resultant 25% decrease in fat absorption (50). Persons on orlistat have a decrease in fat-soluble vitamins; thus, they should take a daily multivitamin with fat soluble vitamins at least two hours before swallowing this medication.

Weight loss less than five kilograms has been noted for up to four years using the 120 mg dose; in one adult study a loss of 1.15 kilograms was seen in adults on a low fat and decreased calorie diet (1, 16, 51). Some research on adolescents taking orlistat revealed no significant benefit in terms of weight loss (52). However, other research in youth have noted a decrease in body mass index up to 4.09 kg/m^2 (53).

Some persons on this medication also have lower blood pressure, serum glucose and lipid levels; also, insulin sensitivity can improve (49, 54). Also, of importance is that adults diagnosed with nonalcoholic fatty liver disease (NAFLD) who are prescribed orlistat can have a demonstrated decrease in hepatic infiltration along with a rise in serum adiponectin and a reduction in serum periostin (55).

Side effect profile

Orlistat is an approved anti-obesity medication in the United States and Europe; also, a drug with similar action, cetilistat, has been approved in Japan since 2013 (1, 56). Orlistat, however, has a markedly high rate of discontinuation because of its side effect profile; particularly bothersome is its gastrointestinal adverse effects (see Table 4) (57, 58). Studies reveal that the discontinuation rate among obese youth is high (2, 15).

In persons on this medication, liver function testing should be done knowing that serious hepatic complications have been reported that include cholelithiasis, cholostatic hepatitis and the rare subacute liver failure in adults (58-61). Renal function should be monitored as well since there are uncommon reports in adults on orlistat who developed acute renal injury and even renal failure from orlistat-induced calcium oxalate nephropathy and renal stone disease; it should be avoided in those with renal insufficiency (61-64). Thus, persons taking orlistat as a medication for weight loss should be carefully monitored by their clinicians (1, 47, 65-68).

Table 4. Orlistat potential adverse effect profile (partial list) (1, 2, 15, 16, 47-64)

Gastrointestinal
Abdominal pain
Dyspepsia
Gastric upset
Fecal incontinence
Fecal urgency
Flatulence
Malabsorption
Steatorrhea
Contraindications
Pregnancy (category X)
Liver failure
Renal failure and renal insufficiency
Chronic malabsorption syndrome and cholestasis
Other adverse effects
Interferences with absorption of various medications
Increased anticoagulant effects of warfarin (because of reduced vitamin K absorption)
Decreased fat-soluble vitamin absorption (A, D, E and K)
Others

Sympathomimetics (noradrenergics)

Phentermine

As noted in Table 2, there are four sympathomimetic drugs with FDA approval for weight loss: phentermine, diethylpropion, benzphetamine and phendimetrazine; these chemicals mimic norepinephrine action with resultant decrease in food consumption (69, 70). Phentermine is a central adrenergic-mediator which can reduce (suppress) the clearance of serotonin and has received approval as a weight loss drug in a number of countries, including the US-FDA since 1959 (1, 71). This sympathomimetic amine is taken at a dose of 37.5 mg once a day, is approved by the FDA for short-term weight loss (i.e., up to 12 weeks) and is classified as a schedule IV controlled substance in the United States.

Because its chemical structure is similar to amphetamine, some clinicians are hesitant to recommend this drug and it is classified as a narcotic drug in some countries (72, 73). Though relatively inexpensive, it does have an adverse effects profile that includes increase in blood pressure and is contraindicated in pregnancy (category X) and in persons with cardiovascular disease (1). Though not recommended, it is sometimes combined with other sympathomimetic appetite suppressants (74). However, it has recently been combined with topiramate in a combination weight loss drug discussed in the next section.

Diethylpropion (amfepramone)

This noradrenergic chemical has been used as an appetite suppressant for many decades and is FDA-approved for weight loss (short-term) in persons over 16 years of age; it has a structure link with amphetamine and is classified as a Schedule IV controlled drug (75-77). Its beneficial effect for weight loss is seen in someone with a high fat restriction plan and some research suggests it can be helpful in weight reduction for one year or more (78, 79). Adverse effects include dry mouth (the most common side effect), irritability, anxiety, insomnia, dry mouth and constipation; it should not be taken if there is a history of psychosis or pulmonary arterial hypertension (78, 80-83).

Phendimetrazine

This is an appetite suppressant from the morpholine chemicals and classified as a Schedule III drug in the United States since 1970 (84, 85). It has been used in a short-term process (i.e., under 12 weeks) in adults with side effects similar to other sympathomimetic drugs (86-89).

Benzphetamine

This is a schedule III drug FDA approved as a short-term weight loss (under 12 weeks) chemical for persons ≥ 12 years of age; it also has been known and utilized for decades (1-3). Its potential adverse profile is similar to other sympathomimietic amines that includes insomnia, restlessness, gastrointestinal side effects (i.e., nausea, diarrhea, constipation), and increased blood pressure (1-3, 90). It is avoided in persons with cardiovascular heart disease such as cardiac valve disease which can be a side effect as well (1-3). It is also avoided in those with pulmonary hypertension, hyperthyroidism and substance use disorders. Many illicit chemicals have been produced with illicit phenethylamines and this encourages various clinicians to avoid benzphetamine and other Schedule III or IV drugs (91).

Phentermine/topiramate ER

Topiramate is a sulfamate-substituted monosaccharide developed from monosaccharide D-fructose and can be identified as 2,3:4,5-di-O-isopropylidene-β-d-fructopyranose sulfamate (92, 93). It has been used for the management of epilepsy (i.e., partial and generalized seizures) and migraine prophylaxis that includes children and adolescents (92-95). Observations of persons taking the anticonvulsant, topiramate, for epilepsy included that weight loss was one of the results of taking this medication; weight loss may be due to a process of inhibition (selective) of carbonic anhydrase isoforms in mitochondria (93, 96).

Researchers have combined topiramate with the known weight loss sympathomimetic drug, phentermine (see above); this combination resulted in more loss of weight than if using topiramate alone (97-99). The combination of topiramate with phentermine as phentermine/topiramate ER (extended release) was US-FDA approved for long-term management of adult obesity in 2012 (20, 100). This drug is designed to provide immediate (rapid) phentermine release along with extended-release (ER) of topimamate in these combination; 15mg/92mg, 11.25mg/60 mg, 7.5 mg/46 mg and 3.75 mg/23 mg (1).

Studies note that benefits for obese adults taking this combination of phentermine/topiramate ER can include a number of features as listed in Table 5 that includes an average weight loss of 5% to 10% (56, 98, 101-105). Some research concludes that phentermine-topiramate ER and another anti-obesity agent (liraglutide—see below) had the highest chances of reaching 5% weight loss at 52 weeks for overweight or obese adults in comparison to other anti-obesity drugs (orlistat, lorcaserin and naltrexone-bupropion); in this study all these drugs achieved at least 5% weight loss at 52 weeks (106).

Various research notes that phentermine/topiramate ER can have the best weight loss results in adults, versus other anti-obesity drugs (i.e., naltrexone/bupropion, lorcaserin and liraglutide), but also has the highest adverse effect profile as well (107-109). The use of phentermine-topiramate ER has also been shown to be of benefit to reduce binge eating in a small study of persons with binge-eating disorder and bulimia nervosa (110).

Table 5. Potential benefits of phentermine/topiramate ER in adults (56, 98, 101-105)

Weight loss: 5% to 10% on average
Blood pressure: Lower in obese males with hypertension
C-reactive protein: Lower levels
Fibrinogen levels: Better
Glucose levels: Lower
Glucose tolerance: Improved
Lipid levels: Improved
Liver function testing: Improved
Sleep apnea: Improved
Type 2 diabetes mellitus: Improved

The side effect profile of phentermine/topiramate ER is listed in Table 6 (56, 72, 108-114). Further studies are needed in combination drugs to understand if all the known adverse effects of each drug in the combination can occur or if the combination will lessen some of them (56). Also, more extensive research trials are suggested for the use of combination anti-obesity drugs to understand their safety and benefits (1, 15, 16).

Table 6. Side effects profile of phentermine/topiramate ER in adults (partial list) (56, 72, 108-114)

*Due to topiramate
Contraindicated in pregnancy (category X; phentermine)
Abuse
Anxiety
Cognitive dysfunction
Dry mouth
Constipation
Decreased appetite*
Diarrhea*
Dizziness
Dysgeusia*
Fatigue*
Insomnia
Metabolic acidosis (typically mild)
Nausea*
Paresthaesias*
Psychiatric complications
Resting heart rate increase
Teratogenicity
Topiramate level instability
Weight loss*
Others

Naltrexone/bupropion

Another combination product for obesity management in adults is the pairing of 32 mg naltrexone (mu-opioid receptor antagonist) with the antidepressant bupropion (catecholamine reuptake inhibitor) at 360 mg and in 2014 the FDA approved naltrexone SR/bupropion SR for use as an anti-obesity drug for adults (100, 115-117). Using both these chemicals leads to action on the mesolimbic reward pathway as well as the hypothalamic melanocortin pathway that can lower food cravings/overeating in a program that stresses a low-calorie diet with increased exercise (physical activity) (56, 118, 119).

Research notes that adults taking naltrexone SR/bupropion SR do develop 5% weight loss compared to placebo (120, 121). Weight loss and improvement in abnormal eating patterns has also been reported in adults with obesity and binge eating disorder (122). Other parameters (laboratory tests) improved in those on naltrexone SR/bupropion SR with weight loss, such as glucose tolerance and lipid testing (105). Studies have not noted improvement in hepatic steatosis and steatohepatitis in obese adults on this combination—a finding associated with orlistat in some research (123). Even though bupropion has a similar structural design and central nervous system actions as diethylpropion, abuse potential of naltrexone SR/bupropion SR has not been reported in research studies (123, 125).

Some studies note that the weight loss in adults on naltrexone SR/bupropion SR is less than seen with phentermine/topiramate ER, but more than found with orlistat, liraglutide and lorcaserin (107, 124). The completion rates in adults taking naltrexone/bupropion were similar to those taking the anti-obesity drug, lorcaserin but lower than seen with placebo, liraglutide and phentermine/topiramate ER (107). On the other hand, some research on use of naltrexone-bupropion in adults with obesity have shown that it (along with liraglutide) has the lowest rates of discontinuation due to the side effect profile in comparison with other anti-obesity drugs (126).

Adverse side effects

Problems noted with anti-obesity drugs such as naltrexone-bupropion include its potential high cost and potential adverse effects profile on various persons (127, 128). As noted earlier, the combination of different chemicals in one compound presents the person who takes this drug with the potential of side effects from each of the products though how the two chemicals interact in this manner is often unclear or unknown. For example, bupropion has not been associated with increase liver enzymes or liver injury; however, naltrexone can be linked with increase in serum aminotransferase but no overt liver injury but this can be kept in mind by the clinician (57).

Potential adverse effects of naltrexone ER/bupropion ER are listed in Table 7 (72, 102, 116, 129-137). Bupropion is avoided in those with seizure disorders and those taking opioids; it is also avoided in persons undergoing sudden withdrawal from various chemicals/drugs (i.e., anti-epileptics, barbiturates, benzodiazepines, alcohol) (132). Bupropion is traditionally not prescribed for those with a history of anorexia nervosa or bulimia nervosa (132). Though naltrexone/bupropion is approved for obesity in adults, it is also important to understand that both bupropion and naltrexone are prescribed separately for various other indications in pediatric persons (138-146).

Table 7. Potential adverse effects of Naltrexone/bupropion (partial list) (72, 102, 116, 129-137)

Black box warning for suicidality
Seizures (in monotherapy with bupropion: 0.1% under 300 mg/day and 0.4% over 300 mg/day)
Increase in blood pressure
Insomnia
Dizziness
Headache
Gastrointestinal dysfunction
Nausea
Emesis
Constipation
Neuropsychiatric dysfunction
Tic exacerbation
Weight loss
Others

Liraglutide

The glucagon-like peptide (GLP-1) receptor agonist, liraglutide, has been approved in the treatment of type 1 diabetes mellitus and also, at a higher dose (3 mg), for management of obesity in adults (7, 36, 56, 66, 119, 120, 121, 126, 147-153) and recently in adolescents. Other GLP-1 agents, in addition liraglutide, include exenatide, lixisenatide, semaglutide and others (72). These chemicals are polypeptide incretin hormones that induce insulin secretion via gastrointestinal L-cells and also cause appetite suppression increasing a feeling of fullness and/or lowering gastric emptying (147, 149-151). The blood pressure may become lower as well (102).

Liraglutide has high homology (97%) to natural GLP-1; natural GLP-1 would need to be given intravenously due to rapid removal by the enzyme DPP-IV (dipeptidyl-peptidase IV); liraglutide is given subcutaneously at 3 mg per day (1, 119). Some studies noted more weight loss than seen with the now removed lorcaserin but not as much as seen with two other anti-obesity drugs still available: phentermine/topiramate ER and naltrexone/bupropion (107). Glucagon-like peptide 1 receptor agonists can lower glycated hemoglobin along with weight loss and decreased risk for hypoglycemia; they also can ameliorate (reverse) nonalcoholic fatty liver disease (NAFLD) using the Sestrin2-mediated Nrf2/HO-1 pathway (154-156). Liraglutide is used in a program of low caloric intake and increased physical activity (119).

The FDA recently approved liraglutide for the management of obesity in adolescents aged 12 years and older, with a body weight of at least 60 kg. Concerns with utilization of liraglutide in pediatric persons is its administration as an injection drug, its high cost, and the potential side effect profile with gastrointestinal being the most common adverse effects (see Table 8) (72, 107, 147-153). There is a boxed warning on the liraglutide prescribing information about the risk of thyroid c-cell tumors. Adolescents should be monitored for depression, suicidal thoughts, acute gallbladder disease, pancreatic inflammation, kidney impairment, heart rate increase, and hypersensitivity (allergic) reactions.

A potential risk for adults with heart failure has been identified and is undergoing further study (157). It is not recommended for breastfeeding persons at this time (158). Some research notes it has lower rates of discontinuation due to adverse effects than some other anti-obesity medications and is in a discontinuation rate similar to naltrexone-bupropion (126).

Table 8. Potential adverse effects of liraglutide in adults (partial list) (72, 107, 147-153)

Gastrointestinal
*Abdominal pain
*Constipation
*Decreased appetite
*Diarrhea
*Dyspepsia
*Emesis
Gallbladder disease (acute)
*Nausea
Others
Category X drug (contraindicated in pregnancy)
*Dizziness
Fatigue
*Headaches
*Hypoglycemia
*Increased lipase
Increased pulse (over time)
Pancreatitis
Thyroid tumors (warning given)
Others
*≥5%

Current research on glucagon-like peptide (GLP-1) receptor agonists on adolescents with obesity has noted that liraglutide can be helpful in weight reduction in obese adolescents as it has in obese adults (159, 160-163). Another GLP-1 receptor agonist, semaglutide, is being studied for management of obesity and may have more benefit than liraglutide; semaglutide may be given subcutaneously once a week or in one formulation—orally once a day (164, 165).

Other proposed anti-obesity agents

There are a variety of drugs proposed as and under research for being anti-obesity agents; however, they are not FDA-approved for management of obesity in adults (1). A few of these chemicals are briefly considered now as some are utilized by clinicians to manage type 2 diabetes mellitus in youth and adults that leads to variable weight loss as well (Table 9) (1, 166).

Table 9. Miscellaneous, non-FDA approved, anti-obesity medications utilized by clinicians (1)

Alpha-glucosidase inhibitors (acarbose, miglitol)
Metformin
Insulin secretagogues (sitagliptin, vildagliptin and saxagliptin)
SGTL2 inhibitors

Acarbose

As an inhibitor of intestinal alpha-glucoside hydrolase and pancreatic alpha-amylase, acarbose is FDA-approved to manage adults with type 2 diabetes mellitus; there is decreased post-meal blood sugar with delay of absorption of consumed carbohydrates (167-170).

Acarbose is typically started at 25 mg orally three times a day with a maintenance dose of 50 to 100 mg three times a day. Adverse reactions that may occur tend to be gastrointestinal in nature: flatulence, diarrhea and gastrointestinal irritation; if acarbose is added to insulin or other diabetes medications (i.e., sulfonylurea), blood sugar can be lowered to the point of hypoglycemic symptomatology (171).

Acarbose may be beneficial to adult females with the metabolic syndrome and polycystic ovary syndrome with induction of weight loss as well as improvement of cardiovascular markers (epicardial fat thickness, intima-media thickness, C-reactive protein) (168, 172). Acarbose is one of a number of drugs being studied for potential anti-ageing features that will be further evaluated as the 21st century research continues (173). Miglitol is another alpha-glucosidase inhibitor being researched as an anti-obesity medication (174, 175).

Metformin

Identified in 1922 and placed in the biguanide drug classification, metformin has been FDA approved since 1995 for treatment of type 2 diabetes mellitus due to various actions as listed in Table 10; the approval is for those 10 years of age and older (1). Metformin-induced weight loss is a well-known aspect of taking this biguanide and it can be useful for adults and adolescents with obesity, insulin resistance and the metabolic syndrome (176, 177).

Table 10. Actions of metformin for type 2 diabetes mellitus (1)

1.	Liver gluconeogenesis reduction
2.	Cell membrane glucose transport improvement; seen in adipose tissue and skeletal muscles
3.	Improvement insulin uptake/effects in various areas: adipose tissue, liver, muscle

In the 21st century metformin has become the most widely prescribed anti-diabetic drug in the world and is effective in the prevention of type 2 diabetes mellitus in some persons at high risk for this condition; it is also available in immediate-release as well as extended-release forms along with various combination formulations with other antidiabetic drugs (178, 179).

Its mechanism of action remains under study but some research notes its benefits on energy balance and weight include increasing the peptide hormone growth/differentiation factor 15 (GDF15) (179). Metformin can lower HbA1c in association with decrease in weight but no increased risk for low blood sugar (180). It is the first agent prescribed for persons with newly prescribed type 2 diabetes mellitus and is seen in combinations with various hypoglycemic agents such as thiazolidinediones, sodium glucose cotransporter-2 inhibitors, incretin-based drugs, sulfonylureas, and others (178-181).

A study published in 2006 looking at males who were between 9 and 18 years of age noted an average weight loss of 4.35 kg over 6 months on 1 gram of metformin twice a day (182). A weight-inducing dose of metformin for obese youth (10-16 years of age) is 500 mg twice a day;

this can be increased 500 mg weekly up to a maximum of 2 grams a day for those with type 2 diabetes mellitus. In research looking at metformin versus orlistat, weight loss was greater in adult females on orlistat while less android adipose tissue was seen in those on metformin (176).

Also, metformin has been used to help manage adult females with polycystic ovary syndrome having hyperandrogenism and hyperinsulinemia; use of metformin has resulted in reduced androgens, improved menstruation and ovulation enhancement (183-186). Its role as an anti-aging drug continues with exciting research in the 21st century (173, 187, 188).

Adverse side effects

A variety of metformin-induced side effects (see Table 11) may be seen that often are related to the dosage use and typically improve with time. Gastrointestinal adverse effects are often mild and managed with changing the dose (97). Serious side effects may be seen such as lactic acidosis in one in 30,000 that is more common in persons with renal insufficiency and has a 50% mortality rate (53, 178, 183, 189-191). Table 11 lists potential metformin adverse effects and also metformin contraindications (1, 53, 178, 183, 189-191). A product recall was issued by the FDA in 2020 for some metformin products that were contained with the carcinogenic agent, N-nitrosodimethylamine (NDMA) (192).

Table 11. Metformin adverse effects and contraindications (1, 53, 178, 183, 189-191)

A. Adverse effects: Gastrointestinal
1. Abdominal discomfort
2. Diarrhea
3. Flatulence
4. Indigestion
5. Nausea with or without vomiting
6. Vitamin B_{12} malabsorption
B. Adverse effects: Others
1. Lactic acidosis
2. Metformin allergy
C. Contraindications
1. Congestive heart failure
2. Critically ill persons (including hypoxia)
3. Hepatic disease
4. Renal disease (i.e., kidney insufficiency)

SGTL2 inhibitors

SGTL2 [sodium glucose cotransporter-2] inhibitors are another type of medication to manage type 2 diabetes mellitus and they have action on the renal proximal tubule brush border serving as physiologic blockers of renal glucose reabsorption; such action can induce urinary glucose leakage and weight loss (147, 193-195). SGTL2 inhibitors are also called glifozins and include such drugs as canagliflozin, empagliflozin, dapagliflozin and ertugliflozin.

The role of glifozins in adults with type 2 diabetes with or without obesity as well as with or without other anti-obesity medications is being studied and their eventual role in diabetic/obese pediatric patients remains to be determined, if any (196-200). As clinicians have learned over the years of applying pharmacology to obesity, one must be fully aware of potential adverse effects of prescribed and non-prescribed medications. Research studies in adults on glifozins are revealing an increased risk in some for hypoglycemia, diabetic ketoacidosis, fractures, infection (urinary tract and genital), cancer bone fracture, and foot/leg amputation (with 2017 FDA Black Box Warning) (201-203).

DPP-IV inhibitors

Dipeptidyl peptidase-IV (DPP-IV) is a protein (enzyme) that is also known as adenosine deaminase complexing protein 2 (CD26); it is involved with important functions in various areas such as the immune and endocrine systems. Chemicals that inhibit DPP-IV are identified as insulin secretagogues and include such drugs as sitagliptin, vildagliptin and saxagliptin. Research has shown that they are beneficial for the management of type 2 diabetes mellitus and dyslipidemias; the potential for these medications, given orally, for obesity is also under current research (204-207).

Conclusion

The quest to find medications or drugs to manage overweight and obesity has been an intense search in the 20th and 21st centuries (1). In this seeming Herculean task to find safe and effective anti-obesity agents for adults, finding such chemicals for children, has become a Don Quixotean tilting at windmills phenomenon in many situations. Various drugs have come with great expectations but removed from the market usually because of unacceptable potential adverse side effects—as noted in Table 3.

As the third decade of the 21st century unfolds, there are two FDA approved drugs for obesity in children, orlistat and liraglutide, starting at 12 years of age; side effects, often gastrointestinal in nature, limit acceptance by many pediatric persons (1, 2, 15, 57-61). A variety of other FDA-approved drugs are available for adults as noted in Table 2 that include sympathomimetics (*phentermine, diethylpropion, benzphetamine, and phendimetrazine*) and combination drugs (phentermine/topiramate and naltrexone/bupropion) (66). The combination drugs may be used by some clinicians in an off-label or non-FDA approved fashion since each individual drug has been used in the adolescent population for other purposes—as discussed earlier.

Other medications reviewed include acarbose, metformin, SGTL2 inhibitors, and DPP-IV Inhibitors. Metformin was FDA-approved in 1995 for management of type 2 diabetes mellitus but has gained some clinician support for obesity management in adolescents and adults. Type 2 diabetes mellitus is a common co-morbid condition to obesity and various medications used to manage this type of diabetes mellitus have also been found to induce weight loss in obese persons (68). There are many other chemicals under research for potential obesity management as reviewed elsewhere (1).

Clinicians can continuously stress the importance of diet and exercise to all their patients whether of normal or abnormal weight (1, 67). Clinicians caring for children and adolescents should be very careful with regard to the anti-obesity medications they recommend and/or prescribe to their precious patients for obesity management. Clinicians should be cautious with anti-obesity medications used by adults but with little evidence of efficacy as well as safety for the pediatric population. Teach patients and families to be wary of drugs or chemicals available on the internet that may display inaccurate or misleading information (68). Severe adverse effects may occur from over-the-counter herbal products including hepatotoxicity (36).

More medications will arise in the clinician's pharmacopeia but may not be appropriate for children or adolescents due to safety concerns. Clinicians should know the history of the drugs noted in Table 3. Each one has its own story but the conclusion was not to use them in the adult and/or pediatric population. In the pediatric population there remains limited evidence on the safety and efficacy of anti-obesity medications used in adults (26). Also, understanding the transition of healthy weight to unhealthy weight remains in 21st century research (208). Finally, chemicals with the potential of inducing weight loss have been held to high standards for quality and safety - some conclude the standards are too high in contrast to that for chemicals for other disorders (36, 209, 210).

As we enter the third decade of the 21st century, clinicians and society have many challenges to be overcome as we seek to deal with obesity in our children that may begin early in life and is complicated by many factors including inactivity imposed by the 2019-2022 COVID-19 pandemic (211, 212). Clinicians are using more bariatric surgery for those with resistant obesity with its complications including diabetes (213, 214).

Pharmacology for obesity and its complications remains a major goal of research at this time and will remain so as this century continues (214-223). Governments are continuing to be challenged to find policies that can curtail pediatric and adult obesity in the 21st century (224). The challenges are costly and require the highest standards when considering managing obesity in our children. However, our precious children are worth such high standards for their health in the 21st century and beyond (1-3, 225)!

Acknowledgment

This chapter is an updated version of an earlier publication with permission from: Bacopoulou F, Greydanus DE. Pediatric obesity psychopharmacology: Quo Vadis? Int J Disabil Hum Dev 2021;20(4):429-46 (Nova Science Publishers).

References

[1] Greydanus DE, Agana M, Kamboj MK, Shebrain S, Soares N, Eke R, Patel DR. Pediatric obesity: Current concepts. Dis Mon 2018;64(4):98-156.

[2] Greydanus DE, Bricker LA, Feucht C. Pharmacotherapy for obese adolescents. Pediatr Clin North Am 2011;58(1):139-53.

[3] Greydanus DE, Agana MG, Merrick J. Pharmacology for obesity: perspectives of history. Int J Adolesc Med Health 2018 Oct 31:/j/ijamh.ahead-of-print/ijamh-2018-0232/ijamh-2018-0232.xml. doi: 10.1515/ijamh-2018-0232.

[4] Hendricks EJ. Off-label drugs for weight management. Diabetes Metab Syndr Obes 2017;10:223-34.

[5] Bosanquet N. The European Medicines Evaluation Agency. BMJ 1994;308 (6926):430.

[6] Berntgen M, Gourvil A, Pavlovic M, Goettsch W, Eichler HG, Kristensen FB. Improving the contribution of regulatory assessment reports to health technology assessments--a collaboration between the European Medicines Agency and the European network for Health Technology Assessment. Value Health 2014;17(5):634-41.

[7] Wilding JPH. Medication use for the treatment of diabetes in obese individuals. Diabetologia 2018;61(2):265-72.
[8] Verhaegen AA, Van Gaal LF. Drug-induced obesity and its metabolic consequences: a review with a focus on mechanisms and possible therapeutic options. J Endocrinol Invest 2017;40(11):1165-74.
[9] Greydanus DE, Calles JL Jr., Patel DR, Nazeer A, Merrick J, eds. Clinical aspects of psychopharmacology in childhood and adolescence, Second edition, New York: Nova Science, 2017.
[10] Musil R, Obermeier M, Russ P, Hamerle M. Weight gain and antipsychotics: a drug safety review. Expert Opin Drug Saf 2015;14(1):73-96.
[11] Ryan DH, Bray GA. Pharmacologic treatment options for obesity: what is old is new again. Curr Hypertens Rep 2013;15(3):182-9.
[12] Shettar V, Patel S, Kidambi S. Epidemiology of obesity and pharmacologic treatment options. Nutr Clin Pract 2017;32(4):441-62.
[13] Rodríquez JE, Campbell KM. Past, present and future of pharmacologic therapy in obesity. Prim Care 2016;43(1):61-7.
[14] Kim S. Drugs to treat obesity: do they work? Postgrad Med J 2016;92(1089):401-6.
[15] Greydanus DE, Feucht C, Patel DR. Pharmacology for obese adolescents. Int J Child Health Hum Dev 2008;1(4):385-94.
[16] Mead E, Atkinson G, Richter B, Metzendorf MI, Baur L, Finer N, Corpeleijn E, O'Malley C, Ells LJ. Drug interventions for the treatment of obesity in children and adolescents. Cochrane Database Syst Rev 2016;11:CD012436.
[17] Yanovski SZ, Yanovski JA: Obesity. N Engl J Med 2002;346(8):591-602.
[18] White B, Jamieson L, Clifford S, Shield JP, Christie D, Smith F, Wong IC, Viner RM. Adolescent experiences of anti-obesity drugs. Clin Obes 2015;5(3):116-26.
[19] Barlow SE and the Expert Committee. Expert committee recommendations regarding prevention, assessment, and treatment of child and adolescent overweight and obesity: Summary report. Pediatrics 2007;120 (Suppl 4):S164-92.
[20] Khorassani FE, Misher A, Garris S. Past and present antiobesity agents: focus on monoamine modulators. Am J Health Syst Pharm 2015;72(9):697-706.
[21] Velazquez A, Apovian CM. Pharmacological management of obesity. Minerva Endocrinol 2018;43(3):356-66.
[22] Saunders KH, Shukla AP, Igel LI, Kumar RB, Aronne LJ. Pharmacotherapy for Obesity. Endocrinol Metab Clin North Am 2016;45(3):521-38.
[23] Barrea L, Pugliese G, Muscogiuri G, Laudisio D, Colao A, Savastano S. New-generation anti-obesity drugs: naltrexone/bupropion and liraglutide. An update for endocrinologists and nutritionists. Minerva Endocrinol 2020;45(2):127-37.
[24] Rebello CJ, Greenway FL. Obesity medications in development. Expert Opin Investig Drugs 2020;29(1):63-71.
[25] Islam MT, Ali ES, Mubarak MS. Anti-obesity effect of plant diterpenes and their derivatives: A review. Phytother Res 2020;34(6):1216-25.
[26] Gadde KM, Atkins KD. The limits and challenges of antiobesity pharmacotherapy. Expert Opin Pharmacother 2020;21(11):1319-28.
[27] Maier J, Mayer FP, Brandt SD, Sitte HH. DARK classics in chemical neuroscience: Aminorex analogues. ACS Chem Neurosci. 2018;9(10):2484-502.
[28] Kim DD, Krishnarajah J, Lillioja S, et al. Efficacy and safety of beloranib for weight loss in obese adults: a randomized controlled trial. Diabetes Obes Metab 2015;17(6):566-72.
[29] Machovec KA, Ames WA. Primum Non Nocere. J Cardiothorac Vasc Anesth 2019;33(7):1930-1.
[30] de Simone G, Mancusi C. Primum non nocere. J Hum Hypertens 2020;34(8):547-50.
[31] Greenway FL, Ryan DH, Bray GA, Rood JC, Tucker EW, Smith SR. Pharmaceutical cost savings of treating obesity with weight loss medications. Obes Res 1999;7(6):523-31.
[32] Ioannides-Demos LL, Proietto J, Tonkin AM, et al. Safety of drug therapies used for weight loss and treatment of obesity. Drug Saf 2006;29(4):277-302.
[33] Surapaneni P, Vinales KL, Najib MQ, Chaliki HP. Valvular heart disease with the use of fenfluramine-phentermine. Tex Heart Inst J 2011;38(5):581-3.

[34] U.S. Food and Drug Administration. FDA requests the withdrawal of the weight-loss drug Belviq, Belviq XR (lorcaserin) from the market. URL: https://www.fda.gov/drugs/drug-safety-and-availability/fda-requests-withdrawal-weight-loss-drug-belviq-belviq-xr-lorcaserin-market.

[35] LiverTox. Clinical and research information on drug-induced liver injury. Bethesda, MD: National Institute of Diabetes and Digestive and Kidney Diseases, 2012–. Lorcaserin 2020 Jun 5.

[36] LiverTox. Clinical and research information on drug-induced liver injury. Bethesda, MD: National Institute of Diabetes and Digestive and Kidney Diseases, 2012–. Weight loss agents 2020 Jun 5.

[37] Kumar R, Ryan D. Lorcaserin departs, leaving more questions than answers. Obesity (Silver Spring) 2020;28(7):1167. doi: 10.1002/oby.22789.

[38] Sharretts J, Galescu O, Gomatam S, Andraca-Carrera E, Hampp C, Yanoff L. Cancer risk associated with lorcaserin - The FDA's review of the CAMELLIA-TIMI 61 Trial. N Engl J Med 2020;383(11):1000-2.

[39] Ahmad SR. Adverse drug event monitoring at the Food and Drug Administration. J Gen Inter Med 2003;18:57–60.

[40] Yen M, Ewald MB. Toxicity of weight loss agents. J Med Toxicol 2012;8(2):145-52.

[41] Yau WP, Mitchell AA, Lin KJ. Use of decongestants during pregnancy and the risk of birth defects. Am J Epidemiol 2013;178(2):198-208.

[42] Pagotto U, Pasquali R. Fighting obesity and associated risk factors by antagonizing cannabinoid type 1 receptors. Lancet 2005; 365:1363-4.

[43] Pi-Sunyer FX, Arrone LJ, Heshmati HM. Effect of rimonabant, a cannabinoid-1-receptor blocker on weight and cardiometabolic risk factors in overweight or obese patients. JAMA 2006;295:761-75.

[44] Siebenhofer A, Jeitler K, Horvath K. Long-term effects of weight-reducing drugs in people with hypertension. Cochrane Data Syst Rev 2016;3:CD007654.

[45] Venhuis BJ, Zwaagstra ME, Keizers PH. Dose-to-dose variations with single packages of counterfeit medicines and adulterated dietary supplements as a potential source of false negatives and inaccurate health risk assessments. J Pharm Biomed Anal 2014;89:158-65.

[46] Sibutramine for obesity. Med Lett Dr Ther 1998;40:32.

[47] Bansal AB, Al Khalili Y. Orlistat. In: StatPearls. Treasure Island, FL: StatPearls Publishing, 2020 Jan–.

[48] Heck AM, Yanovski JA, Calis KA. Orlistat, a new lipase inhibitor for the management of obesity. Pharmacotherapy 2000;20(3):270-9.

[49] Orlistat for obesity. Med Lett Drugs Ther 1999;41:55.

[50] Orlistat OTC for weight loss. Med Lett Drugs Ther 2007;49:49.

[51] Anderson JW: Low-dose orlistat effects on body weight of mildly to moderately overweight individuals: a 16 week, double-blind, placebo-controlled trial. Ann Pharmacother 2006;40(10):1717-23.

[52] Maahs D, de Serna DG, Kolotkin RL. Randomized, double-blind, placebo- controlled trial of orlistat for weight loss in adolescents. Endocr Pract 2006;12:18-28.

[53] Dunican KC, Desilets AR, Montalbano JK. Pharmacotherapeutic options for overweight adolescents. Ann Pharmacother 2007;41:1445-55.

[54] McDuffie JR, Calis KA, Uwaifo GI. Efficacy of orlistat as an adjunct to behavioral treatment in overweight African American and Caucasian adolescents with obesity-related co-morbid conditions. J Pediatr Endocrinol Metab 2004; 17:307-19.

[55] Ali Khan R, Kapur P, Jain A. Effect of orlistat on periostin, adiponectin, inflammatory markers and ultrasound grades of fatty liver in obese NAFLD patients. Ther Clin Risk Manag 2017;13:139-49.

[56] Hainer V. Overview of new antiobesity drugs. Expert Opin Pharmacother 2014;15(14):1975-8.

[57] LiverTox. Clinical and research information on drug-induced liver injury. Bethesda, MD: National Institute of Diabetes and Digestive and Kidney Diseases, 2012–. Weight loss agents 2020 Jun 5.

[58] Filippatos TD, Derdemezis CS, Gazi IF, Nakou ES, Mikhailidis DP, Elisaf MS. Orlistat-associated adverse effects and drug interactions: a critical review. Drug Saf 2008;31(1):53-65.

[59] Sall D, Wang J, Rashkin M, Welch M, Droege C, Schauer D. Orlistat-induced fulminant hepatic failure. Clin Obes 2014;4(6):342-7.

[60] Martínez Insfran LA, Alconchel Gago F, Parrilla Paricio P. Fulminant liver failure secondary to submassive hepatic necrosis in a patient treated with Orlistat. A case report. Rev Esp Enferm Dig 2019;111(1):83. doi: 10.17235/reed.2018.5740/2018.
[61] Thurairajah PH, Syn WK, Neil DA, Stell D, Haydon G. Orlistat (Xenical)-induced subacute liver failure. Eur J Gastroenterol Hepatol 2005;17(12):1437-8.
[62] Beyea MM, Garg AX, Weir MA. Does orlistat cause acute kidney injury? Ther Adv Drug Saf 2012;3(2):53-7.
[63] Ahmed MH. Orlistat and calcium oxalate crystalluria: an association that needs consideration. Ren Fail 2010;32(8):1019-21.
[64] Karamadoukis L, Shivashankar GH, Ludeman L, Williams AJ. An unusual complication of treatment with orlistat. Clin Nephrol 2009;71(4):430-2.
[65] Khedr N F, Ebeid AM, Khalil RM. New insights into weight management by orlistat in comparison with cinnamon as a natural lipase inhibitor. Endocrine 2020;67(1):109-16.
[66] Singh AK, Singh R. Pharmacotherapy in obesity: a systematic review and meta-analysis of randomized controlled trials of anti-obesity drugs. Expert Rev Clin Pharmacol 2020;13(1):53-64.
[67] Powell A. Obesity: Pharmacotherapy. FP Essent 2020;492:25-9.
[68] Paccosi S, Cresci B, Pala L, Rotella CM, Parenti A. Obesity therapy: How and why? Curr Med Chem 2020;27(2):174-86.
[69] Bray GA. Drug insight: Appetite suppressants. Nat Clin Pract Gastroenterol Hepatol 2005;2(2):89-95.
[70] Gurevich-Panigraphi T, Panigraphi S, Wiechec E, Los M. Obesity: Pathophysiology and clinical management. Curr Med Chem 2009;16(4):506-21.
[71] Seaton DA, Rose K, Duncan LJ. Current therapeutics. 203. Sustained-action chlorphentermine in the correction of refractory obesity. Practitioner 1964;193:698-702.
[72] Fujioka K. Current and emerging medications for overweight or obesity in people with comorbidities. Diabetes Obes Metab 2015;17(11):1021-32.
[73] No authors listed. Phentermine: an appetite-suppressant amphetamine classified as a narcotic in France. Is a combination with topiramate on the horizon? Prescrire Int 2012;21(130):209.
[74] Hampp C, Kang EM, Borders-Hemphill V. Use of prescription antiobesity drugs in the United States. Pharmacotherapy 2013;33(12):1299-307.
[75] Decina L, Tanyol H. Treatment of obesity with a new anorexiant, diethylpropion, without special stress on diet. NY State J Med 1960;60:2702-5.
[76] No Authors listed. Diethylpropion, an appetite suppressant. Med Lett Drugs Ther 1971;12(25):101-2.
[77] Garcia-Mijares M, Bernardes AM, Silva MT. Diethylpropion produces psychostimulant and reward effects. Pharmacol Biochem Behav 2009;91(4):621-8.
[78] Cercato C, Roizenblatt VA, Leança CC. A randomized double-blind placebo-controlled study of the long term efficacy and safety of diethylpropion in the treatment of obese subjects. Int J Obes (Lond) 2009;33(8):857-65.
[79] Kalyanasundar B, Solorio J, Perez Cl. The efficacy of the appetite suppressant, diethylpropion, is dependent on both when it is given (day vs. night) and under conditions of high fat dietary restriction. Appetite 2016;100:152-61.
[80] Arias HR, Santamaría A, Ali SF. Pharmacological and neurotoxicological actions mediated by bupropion and diethylpropion. Int Rev Neurobiol 2009;88:223-55.
[81] No authors listed. Diethylpropion psychosis. Med J Aust 1970;2(23):1052-3.
[82] Carney MW: Diethylpropion and psychosis. Clin Neuropharmacol 1988;11(2):183-8.
[83] Austin ED, Loyd JE, Phillips JA II. Heritable pulmonary arterial hypertension. GeneReviews. Seattle, WA: University of Washington, 1993-2017.
[84] Phear D. Phenmetrazine in the treatment of obesity. Practitioner 1959;183:62-3.
[85] Cass LJ. Evaluation of phenmetrazine bitartrate as an appetite suppressant. Can Med Assoc J 1961;84:1114-6.
[86] Poindexter A. Appetite suppressant drugs: A controlled clinical comparison of benzphetamine, phenmetrazine, d-amphetamine and placebo. Curr Ther Res Clin Exp 1960;2:354-63.
[87] Evans J. Psychosis and addiction to phenmetrazine (preludin). Lancet 1959;2(7095):152-5.

[88] Hood I, Monforte J, Gault R, Mirchandani H. Fatality from illicit phendimetrazine use. J Toxicol Clin Toxicol 1988;26(3-4):249-55.
[89] Landau D, Jackson J, Gonzalez G. A case of demand ischemia from phendimetrazine. Cases J 2008;1(1):105. doi: 10.1186/1757-1626-1-105.
[90] Simkin B, Wallace L. A controlled clinical trial of benzphetamine (didrex) in the management of obesity. Curr Ther Res Clin Exp 1960;2:33-8.
[91] King LA. New phenethylamines in Europe. Drug Test Anal 2014;6(7-8):808-18.
[92] Bays H. Phentermine, topiramate and their combination for the treatment of adiposopathy ('sick fat') and metabolic disease. Expert Rev Cardiovasc Ther 2010;8(12):1777-8.
[93] Khalil NY, AlRabiah HK, Al Rashoud SS, Bari A, Wani TA. Topiramate: Comprehensive profile. Profiles Drug Subst Excip Relat Methodol 2019;44:333-78.
[94] Mohd-Tahir NA, Li SC. Meta-analyses of newer antiepileptic drugs as adjunct for treatment of focal epilepsy in children. Epilepsy Res 2018;139:113-22.
[95] Kanemura H, Sano F, Tando T, Sugita K, Aihara M. [Effects of topiramate on headache in children with epilepsy]. No To Hattatsu 2015;47(1):18-22. [Japanese]
[96] Verrotti A, Scaparrotta A, Agostinelli S, Di Pillo S, Chiarelli F, Grosso S. Topiramate-induced weight loss: A review. Epilepsy Res 2011;95(3):189-99.
[97] Boland CL, Harris JB, Harris KB. Pharmacological management of obesity in pediatric patients. Ann Pharmacother 2015;49(2):220-32.
[98] Garvey WT, Ryan DH, Look M. Two-year sustained weight loss and metabolic benefits with controlled-release phentermine/topiramate in obese and overweight adults (SEQUEL): A randomized, placebo-controlled, phase 3 extension study. Am J Clin Nutr 2012;95(2):297-308.
[99] Sweeting AN, Tabet E, Caterson ID. Management of obesity and cardiometabolic risk – role of phentermine/extended release topiramate. Diabetes Metab Syndr Obes 2014;7:35-44.
[100] Halpern B, Mancini MC. Safety assessment of combination therapies in the treatment of obesity: Focus on naltrexone/ bupropion and phentermine-topiramate extended release. Expert Opin Drug Saf 2017;16(1):27-39.
[101] Cabrerizo Garcia l, Ramos-Levi A, Moreno Lopera C. Update on pharmacology of obesity: benefits and risks. Nutr Hosp 2013;28(Suppl 5):121-7.
[102] Antza C, Stabouli S, Natsis M, Doundoulakis I, Kotsis V. Obesity-Induced Hypertension: New Insights. Curr Pharm Des 2017;23(31):4620-5.
[103] Shyh G, C Heng-Lai A. New obesity agents: Lorcaserin (Belviq) and phentermine/ topiramate ER (Qsymia). Cardio Rev 2014;22(1):43-50.
[104] Guo F, Garvey WT. Cardiometabolic disease predicts effectiveness of weight-loss therapy to prevent type 2 diabetes: pooled results from Phase III clinical trials assessing phentermine/topiramate extended release. Diabetes Care 2017;40(7):856-62.
[105] Cunningham JW, Wiviott SD. Modern obesity pharmacotherapy: weighing cardiovascular risk and benefit. Clin Cardiol 2014;37(11):693-9.
[106] Khera R, Murad MH, Chandar AK. Association of pharmacological treatments for obesity with weight loss and adverse effects: A systematic review and meta-analysis. JAMA 2016;315(22):2424-34.
[107] Nuffer W, Trujillo JM, Megyeri J. A comparison of new pharmacological agents for the treatment of obesity. Ann Pharmacother 2016;50(5):376-88.
[108] Hainer V, Aldhoon-Hainerová I. Tolerability and safety of the new anti-obesity medications. Drug Saf 2014;37(9):693-702.
[109] Kumar RB, Aronne LJ. Efficacy comparison of medications approved for chronic weight management. Obesity (Silver Spring) 2015;23(Suppl 1):S4-7.
[110] Safer DL, Adler S, Dalai SS, Bentley JP, Toyama H, Pajarito S, Najarian T. A randomized, placebo-controlled crossover trial of phentermine-topiramate ER in patients with binge-eating disorder and bulimia nervosa. Int J Eat Disord. 2020;53(2):266-77.
[111] No authors listed. Topiramate + phentermine. An excessively dangerous appetite-suppressant combination. Prescrire Int 2013;22(136):61-4.
[112] Kelly EM, Tungol AA, Wesolowicz LA. Formulary management of 2 new agents: lorcaserin and phentermine/topiramate for weight loss. J Manag Care Pharm 2013;19(8): 642-54.

[113] Woloshin S, Schwartz LM. The new weight-loss drugs, lorcaserin and phentermine-topiramate: slim pickings? JAMA Intern Med 2014;174(4):615-9.
[114] Alfaris N, Minnick AM, Hopkins CM, Berkowitz RI, Wadden TA. Combination phentermine and topiramate extended release in the management of obesity. Expert Opin Pharmacother 2015;16(8):1263-74.
[115] Ali KF, Shukla AP, Aronne LJ. Bupropion-SR plus naltrexone-SR for the treatment of mild-to-moderate obesity. Expert Rev Clin Pharmacol 2016;9(1):27-34.
[116] No authors listed. Contrave—A combination of bupropion and naltrexone for weight loss. Med Lett Drugs Ther 2014;56(1455):112-4.
[117] Mercer SL. ACS chemical neuroscience molecule spotlight on contrave. ACS Chem Neurosci 2011;2(9):484-6.
[118] Padwal R. Contrave, a bupropion and naltrexone combination therapy for the potential treatment of obesity. Curr Opin Investig Drugs 2009;10(10):1117-25.
[119] Barrea L, Pugliese G, Muscogiuri G, Laudisio D, Colao A, Savastano S. New-generation anti-obesity drugs: naltrexone/bupropion and liraglutide. An update for endocrinologists and nutritionists. Minerva Endocrinol 2020;45(2):127-37.
[120] Khalil H, Ellwood L, Lord H, Fernandez R. Pharmacological treatment for obesity in adults: An umbrella review. Ann Pharmacother 2020;54(7):691-705.
[121] Kim BY, Kang SM, Kang JH, Kim KK, Kim B, Kim SJ, et al.; Committee of Clinical Practice Guidelines, Korean Society for the Study of Obesity (KSSO). Current Long-Term Pharmacotherapies for the Management of Obesity. J Obes Metab Syndr 2020;29(2):99-109.
[122] Carbone EA, Caroleo M, Rania M, Calabrò G, Staltari FA, de Filippis R, et al. An open-label trial on the efficacy and tolerability of naltrexone/bupropion SR for treating altered eating behaviours and weight loss in binge eating disorder. Eat Weight Disord. 2020 Apr 30. doi: 10.1007/s40519-020-00910-x.
[123] Pan CS, Stanley TL. Effect of weight loss medications on hepatic steatosis and steatohepatitis: A systematic review. Front Endocrinol (Lausanne) 2020;11:70. doi: 10.3389/fendo.2020.00070.
[124] Verpeut JL, Bello NT. Drug safety evaluation of naltrexone/bupropion for the treatment of obesity. Expert Opin Drug Saf 2014;13(6):831-41.
[125] Arias HR, Santamaría A, Ali SF. Pharmacological and neurotoxicological actions mediated by bupropion and diethylpropion. Int Rev Neurobiol 2009;88:223-55.
[126] Milano W, De Biasio V, Di Munzio W, Foggia G, Capasso A. Obesity: The new global epidemic pharmacological treatment, opportunities and limits for personalized therapy. Endocr Metab Immune Disord Drug Targets 2020;20(8):1232-43.
[127] Onakpoya IJ, Lee JJ, Mahtani KR, Aronson JK, Heneghan CJ. Naltrexone-bupropion (Mysimba) in management of obesity: A systematic review and meta-analysis of unpublished clinical study reports. Br J Clin Pharmacol 2020;86(4):646-67.
[128] Tak YJ, Lee SY. Anti-obesity drugs: Long-term efficacy and safety: An updated review. World J Mens Health 2020 Mar 9. doi: 10.5534/wjmh.200010.
[129] No authors listed. Naltrexone/bupropion: Contrave (R): naltrexone SR/bupropion SR. Drugs R D 2010;10(1):25-32.
[130] Apovian CM, Aronne L, Rubino D. A randomized, phase 3 trial of naltrexone SR/bupropion SR on weight and obesity-related risk factors (COR-II). Obesity (Silver Springs) 2013;21(5):935-43.
[131] Greig SL, Keating GM. Naltrexone ER/Bupropion ER: A review in obesity management. Drugs 2015;75(11):1269-80.
[132] Yanovski SZ, Yanovski JA. Naltrexone extended-release plus bupropion extended-release for treatment of obesity. JAMA 2015;313(12):1213-4.
[133] Davidson J. Seizures and bupropion: A review. J Clin Psychiatry 1989;50(7):256-61.
[134] Costa R, Oliveira NG, Dinis-Oliveira RJ. Pharmacokinetic and pharmacodynamic of bupropion: Integrative overview of relevant clinical and forensic aspects. Drug Metab Rev 2019;51(3):293-313.
[135] Kriikku P, Ojanperä I. The relationship between bupropion and suicide in post-mortem investigations. Forensic Sci Int 2016;266:343-8.

[136] Wightman DS, Foster VJ, Krishen A, Richard NE, Modell JG. Meta-analysis of suicidality in placebo-controlled clinical trials of adults taking bupropion. Prim Care Companion J Clin Psychiatry 2010;12(5):PCC.09m00894. doi: 10.4088/PCC.09m00894blu.

[137] Shah D, Shah A, Tan X, Sambamoorthi U. Trends in utilization of smoking cessation agents before and after the passage of FDA boxed warning in the United States. Drug Alcohol Depend 2017;177:187-93.

[138] Daviss WB: Bupropion for adolescents with attention-deficit/hyperactivity disorder. J Am Acad Child Adolesc Psychiatry 2001;40:307-14.

[139] Ng QX. A systematic review of the use of bupropion for attention-deficit/hyperactivity disorder in children and adolescents. J Child Adolesc Psychopharmacol 2017;27(2):112-6.

[140] Solhkhah R, Wilens TE, Daly J, Prince JB, Van Patten SL, Biederman J. Bupropion SR for the treatment of substance-abusing outpatient adolescents with attention-deficit/hyperactivity disorder and mood di sorders. J Child Adolesc Psychopharmacol 2005;15(5):777-86.

[141] Kweon K, Kim HW. Effectiveness and safety of bupropion in children and adolescents with depressive disorders: A retrospective chart review. Clin Psychopharmacol Neurosci 2019;17(4):537-41.

[142] Hadland SE, Wharam JF, Schuster MA, Zhang F, Samet JH, Larochelle MR. Trends in receipt of buprenorphine and naltrexone for opioid use disorder among adolescents and young adults, 2001-2014. JAMA Pediatr 2017;171(8):747-55.

[143] Camenga DR, Colon-Rivera HA, Muvvala SB. Medications for maintenance treatment of opioid use disorder in adolescents: A narrative review and assessment of clinical benefits and potential risks. J Stud Alcohol Drugs 2019;80(4):393-402.

[144] Viera A, Bromberg DJ, Whittaker S, Refsland BM, Stanojlović M, Nyhan K, et al. Adherence to and retention in medications for opioid use disorder among adolescents and young adults. Epidemiol Rev 2020 Apr 2:mxaa001. doi: 10.1093/epirev/mxaa001.

[145] Riggs PD, Leon SL, Mikulich SK, Pottle LC. An open trial of bupropion for ADHD in adolescents with substance use disorders and conduct disorder. J Am Acad Child Adolesc Psychiatry 1998;37(12):1271-8.

[146] Huecker MR, Smiley A, Saadabadi A. Bupropion. In: StatPearls. Treasure Island, FL: StatPearls Publishing, 2020 Jan–.

[147] Baretić M, Troskot R. How to fight obesity with antidiabetic drugs: targeting gut or kidney? Minerva Endocrinol 2015;40(1):71-83.

[148] Hocking S, Dear A, Cowley MA. Current and emerging pharmacotherapies in Australia. Obes Res Clin Pract 2017 Aug 14. pii: S1871-403X(17)30065-0. doi: 10.1016/j.orcp.2017.07.002.

[149] Mehta A, Marso SP, Neeland IJ. Liraglutide for weight management: A critical review of the evidence. Obes Sci Pract 2017;3(1):3-14.

[150] Prasad-Reddy L, Isaacs D. A clinical review of GLP-1 receptor agonists: efficacy and safety in diabetes and beyond. Drugs Context 2015 Jul 9:212283. doi: 10.7573/dic.212283.

[151] Konstantinos L, Karavis M, Mastorakos G, et al. New molecular targets for the pharmacotherapy of obesity. In: De Groot LJ, Chrousos G, Dungan K, Feinfold KR, Grossman A, Hershman JM, eds. Endotext (internet). South Dartmouth, MA: MDText.com, 2000-2015 Apr 8.

[152] Seo YG. Side Effects Associated with liraglutide treatment for obesity as well as diabetes. J Obes Metab Syndr 2020 Oct 19. doi: 10.7570/jomes20059.

[153] Collins L, Costello RA. Glucagon-like peptide-1 receptor agonists. In: StatPearls. Treasure Island, FL: StatPearls Publishing, 2020 Jan–.

[154] Papaetis GS. Liraglutide therapy in a prediabetic state: Rethinking the evidence. Curr Diabetes Rev 2020;16(7):699-715.

[155] Sheahan KH, Wahlberg EA, Gilbert MP. An overview of GLP-1 agonists and recent cardiovascular outcomes trials. Postgrad Med J 2020;96(1133):156-61. doi: 10.1136/postgradmedj-2019-137186.

[156] Han X, Ding C, Zhang G, Pan R, Liu Y, Huang N, Hou N, Han F, Xu W, Sun X. Liraglutide ameliorates obesity-related nonalcoholic fatty liver disease by regulating Sestrin2-mediated Nrf2/HO-1 pathway. Biochem Biophys Res Commun 2020;525(4):895-901.

[157] Seferović PM, Coats AJS, Ponikowski P, Filippatos G, Huelsmann M, Jhund PS, et al. European Society of Cardiology/Heart Failure Association position paper on the role and safety of new glucose lowering drugs in patients with heart failure. Eur J Heart Fail 2020;22(2):196-213.
[158] Drugs and Lactation Database (LactMed) [Internet]. Bethesda, MD: National Library of Medicine, 2006–. Liraglutide 2020 Jan 20.
[159] Kelly AS, Auerbach P, Barrientos-Perez M, Gies I, Hale PM, Marcus C, Mastrandrea LD, Prabhu N, Arslanian S; NN8022-4180 Trial Investigators. A randomized, controlled trial of liraglutide for adolescents with obesity. N Engl J Med 2020;382(22):2117-28.
[160] Danne T, Biester T, Kapitzke K, Jacobsen SH, Jacobsen LV, Petri KCC, et al. Liraglutide in an adolescent population with obesity: A randomized, double-blind, placebo-controlled 5-week trial to assess safety, tolerability, and pharmacokinetics of liraglutide in adolescents aged 12-17 years. J Pediatr 2017;181:146-53.
[161] Chao AM, Wadden TA, Berkowitz RI. The safety of pharmacologic treatment for pediatric obesity. Expert Opin Drug Saf 2018;17(4):379-85. doi: 10.1080/14740338.2018.1437143.
[162] Maljaei MB, Bahreini A. Liraglutide for adolescents with obesity. N Engl J Med 2020;383(12):1193. doi: 10.1056/NEJMc2023284.
[163] Kelishadi R. Liraglutide for management of adolescent obesity. Nat Rev Endocrinol 2020;16(8):405-6.
[164] Lin CH, Shao L, Zhang YM, Tu YJ, Zhang Y, Tomlinson B, Chan P, Liu Z. An evaluation of liraglutide including its efficacy and safety for the treatment of obesity. Expert Opin Pharmacother 2020;21(3):275-85.
[165] Capehorn MS, Catarig AM, Furberg JK, Janez A, Price HC, Tadayon S, Vergès B, Marre M. Efficacy and safety of once-weekly semaglutide 1.0mg vs once-daily liraglutide 1.2mg as add-on to 1-3 oral antidiabetic drugs in subjects with type 2 diabetes (SUSTAIN 10). Diabetes Metab 2020;46(2):100-109.
[166] Fleischman A, Rhodes ET. Management of type 2 diabetes and prediabetes in children and adolescents. Adolesc Med 2017;28(2):406-22.
[167] McIver LA, Tripp J. Acarbose. In: StatPearls. Treasure Island, FL: StatPearls Publishing, 2020 Jan–.
[168] Khalili N, Safavipour A. Evaluation of the effects of acarbose on weight and metabolic, inflammatory, and cardiovascular markers in patients with obesity and overweight. Int J Prev Med 2020;11:140. doi: 10.4103/ijpvm.IJPVM_229_19.
[169] Smith DL Jr, Orlandella RM, Allison DB, Norian LA. Diabetes medications as potential calorie restriction mimetics-a focus on the alpha-glucosidase inhibitor acarbose. Geroscience 2020 Oct 2. doi: 10.1007/s11357-020-00278-x.
[170] Vos RC, van Avendonk MJ, Jansen H, et al. Insulin monotherapy compared with the addition of oral glucose-lowering agents to insulin for people with type 2 diabetes already on insulin therapy and inadequate glycaemic control. Cochrane Database Syst Rev 2016;9:CD006992.
[171] Derosa G, Maffioli P. Efficacy and safety profile evaluation of acarbose along and in association with other antidiabetic drugs: A systematic review. Clin Ther 2012;34(6):1221-36.
[172] Zhang YY, Hou LQ, Zhao TY. Effects of acarbose on polycystic ovary syndrome: a meta-analysis. Exp Clin Endocrinol Diabetes 2014;122(6):373-8.
[173] Partridge L, Fuentealba M, Kennedy BK. The quest to slow ageing through drug discovery. Nat Rev Drug Discov 2020;19(8):513-532.
[174] Sugimoto S, Nakajima H, Kosaka K. Review: miglitol has potential as a therapeutic drug against obesity. Nutr Metab (Lond) 2015;12:51.doi: 10.1186/s12986-015-0048-8.
[175] LiverTox. Clinical and research information on drug-induced liver injury. Bethesda, MD: National Institute of Diabetes and Digestive and Kidney Diseases, 2012–. Miglitol 2020 Jan 21.
[176] Kujawska-Luczak M, Musialik K, Szulińska M. The effect of orlistat versus metformin on body composition and insulin resistance in obese premenopausal women: 3-month randomized prospective open-label study. Arch Med Sci 2017;13(4):725-31.
[177] Freemark M: Pharmacotherapy of childhood obesity: an evidence-based, conceptual approach. Diabetes Care 2007;30:395-402.

[178] Corcoran C, Jacobs TF. Metformin. In: StatPearls. Treasure Island, FL: StatPearls Publishing, 2020 Jan–.
[179] Coll AP, Chen M, Taskar P, Rimmington D, Patel S, Tadross JA, et al. GDF15 mediates the effects of metformin on body weight and energy balance. Nature 2020;578(7795):444-8.
[180] Schernthaner G, Schernthaner GH. The right place for metformin today. Diabetes Res Clin Pract 2020;159:107946. doi: 10.1016/j.diabres.2019.107946.
[181] LiverTox. Clinical and research information on drug-induced liver injury. Bethesda, MD: National Institute of Diabetes and Digestive and Kidney Diseases, 2012–. Metformin 2020 Jan 21.
[182] Srinivasan S, Ambler GR, Baur LA. Randomized, controlled trial of metformin for obesity and insulin resistance in children and adolescents: Improvement in body composition and fasting insulin. J Clin Endocrinol Metabol 2006;91(6):2074-80.
[183] Nestler JE. Metformin for the treatment of polycystic ovary syndrome. N Engl J Med 2008;358 (1):47-54.
[184] Hoppin AG, Katz ES, Kaplan LM. Case 31-2006: A 15-year-old girl with severe obesity. N Engl J Med 2006;355(15):1593-602.
[185] Harborne L, Fleming R, Lyall H. Metformin or antiandrogen in the treatment of hirsutism in polycystic ovary syndrome. J Clin Endocrinol Metabol 2003;88:4116-23.
[186] Zhou L, Cai X, Yang W. The magnitude of weight loss induced by meformin is independently associated with BMI at baseline in newly diagnosed type 2 diabetes: post-hoc analysis from data of a phase IV open-labeled trial. Adv Clin Exp Med 2017 Jun 27. doi: 10.17219/acem/63025e.
[187] Lv Z, Guo Y. Metformin and its benefits for various diseases. Front Endocrinol (Lausanne) 2020;11:191. doi: 10.3389/fendo.2020.00191.
[188] Piskovatska V, Storey KB, Vaiserman AM, Lushchak O. The use of metformin to increase the human healthspan. Adv Exp Med Biol 2020;1260:319-32.
[189] Webb E, Viner R: Should metformin be prescribed to overweight adolescents in whom dietary/behavioural modifications have not helped? Arch Dis Child 2006;91:793-4.
[190] Flory JH, Hennessy S, Bailey CJ, Inzucchi SE. Reports of lactic acidosis attributed to metformin, 2015-2018. Diabetes Care 2020;43(1):244-6.
[191] Corchia A, Wynckel A, Journet J, Moussi Frances J, Skandrani N, Lautrette A, et al. Metformin-related lactic acidosis with acute kidney injury: results of a French observational multicenter study. Clin Toxicol (Phila) 2020;58(5):375-82.
[192] Statement from Janet Woodcock, MD, director of FDA's Center for Drug Evaluation and Research, on impurities found in diabetes drugs outside the US. URL: https://www.fda.gov/news-events/press-announcements/statement-janet-woodcock-md-director-fdas-center-drug-evaluation-and-research-impurities-found.
[193] Steen O, Goldenberg RM. The role of sodium-glucose cotransporter 2 inhibitors in the management of type 2 diabetes. Can J Diabetes 2017;41(5):517-23.
[194] Esquivel MA, Lansang MC. Optimizing diabetes treatment in the presence of obesity. Cleve Clin J Med 2017;84(7 Suppl 1):S22-9.
[195] Gómez Huelgas R. Weight and type 2 diabetes: New recommendations. Med Clin (Barc) 2016;147(Suppl 1):17-21.
[196] Tanaka K, Takahashi H, Katagiri S, Sasaki K, Ohsugi Y, Watanabe K, et al. Combined effect of canagliflozin and exercise training on high-fat diet-fed mice. Am J Physiol Endocrinol Metab 2020;318(4):E492-503.
[197] Sheu WHH, Chan SP, Matawaran BJ, Deerochanawong C, Mithal A, Chan J, et al. Use of SGLT-2 inhibitors in patients with type 2 diabetes mellitus and abdominal obesity: An Asian perspective and expert recommendations. Diabetes Metab J 2020;44(1):11-32.
[198] Iacobellis G, Gra-Menendez S. Effects of dapagliflozin on epicardial fat thickness in patients with type 2 diabetes and obesity. Obesity (Silver Spring) 2020;28(6):1068-74.
[199] Hollander P, Bays HE, Rosenstock J, et al. Coadministration of canagliflozin and phentermine for weight management in overweight and obese individuals without diabetes: a randomized clinical trial. Diabetes Care 2017;40(5):632-9.

[200] Ferreira-Hermosillo A, Molina-Ayala MA, Molina-Guerrero D, Garrido-Mendoza AP, Ramírez-Rentería C, Mendoza Zubieta V, et al. Efficacy of the treatment with dapagliflozin and metformin compared to metformin monotherapy for weight loss in patients with class III obesity: a randomized controlled trial. Trials 2020;21(1):186. doi: 10.1186/s13063-020-4121-x.

[201] Singh M, Kumar A. Risks associated with SGLT2 inhibitors: An overview. Curr Drug Saf 2018;13(2):84-91.

[202] Blevins TC, Farooki A. Bone effects of canagliflozin, a sodium glucose co-transporter 2 inhibitor, in patients with type 2 diabetes mellitus. Postgrad Med 2017;129(1):159-68.

[203] Heymsfield SB, Raji A, Gallo S, Liu J, Pong A, Hannachi H, Terra SG. Efficacy and safety of ertugliflozin in patients with overweight and obesity with type 2 diabetes mellitus. Obesity (Silver Spring) 2020;28(4):724-32.

[204] Li S, Li H, Wang R, Zhang JP. The effect of sitagliptin on obese patients with insulin treatment-induced diabetes mellitus. Eur Rev Med Pharmacol Sci 2017;21(15):3490-5.

[205] Munir KM, Lamos EM. Diabetes type 2 management: what are the differences between DPP-4 inhibitors and how do you choose? Expert Opin Pharmacother 2017;18(9):839-41.

[206] McKillop AM, Stevenson CL, Moran BM, Abdel-Wahab YHA, Flatt PR. Tissue expression of DPP-IV in obesity-diabetes and modulatory effects on peptide regulation of insulin secretion. Peptides 2018;100:165-72.

[207] McCloskey AG, Miskelly MG, Flatt PR, McKillop AM. Pharmacological potential of novel agonists for FFAR4 on islet and enteroendocrine cell function and glucose homeostasis. Eur J Pharm Sci 2020;142:105104. doi: 10.1016/j.ejps.2019.105104.

[208] Dagpo TD, Nolan CJ, Delghingaro-Augusto V. Exploring therapeutic targets to reverse or prevent the transition from metabolically healthy to unhealthy obesity. Cells 2020;9(7):1596. doi: 10.3390/cells9071596.

[209] Li X, Bello NT. Anorectic state of obesity medications in the United States. Are leaner times ahead? Expert Opin Pharmacother 2020;21(2):167-172.

[210] Halpern B, Mancini MC. Should the same safety scrutiny of antiobesity medications be applied to other chronic usage drugs? Obesity (Silver Spring) 2020;28(7):1171-2.

[211] Pereyra I, Gómez A, Jaramillo K, Ferreira A. Birth weight, weight gain, an obesity among children in Uruguay; A prospective study since birth. Rev Paul Pediatr 2021;39:e2019088.

[212] Robinson E, Boyland E, Chisholm A, Harrold J, Maloney NG, Marty L, et al. Obesity, eating behavior and physical activity during COVID-19 lockdown: A study of UK adults. Appetite 2021;156:104853.

[213] Zenno A, Nadler EP. Surgical treatment of type 2 diabetes mellitus in youth. Adv Exp Med Biol 2021;1307:321-30.

[214] Guimarães M, Pereira SS, Monteiro MP. From entero-endocrine cell biology to surgical interventional therapies for type 2 diabetes. Adv Exp Med Biol 2021;1307:273-97.

[215] Maselli DB, Camilleri M. Effects of GLP-1 and its analogs on gastric physiology in diabetes mellitus and obesity. Adv Exp Med Biol 2021;1307:171-92.

[216] Gökçay Canpolat A, Şahin M. Glucose lowering treatment modalities of type 2 diabetes mellitus. Adv Exp Med Biol 2021;1307:7-27.

[217] Tchang BG, Saunders KH, Igel LI. Best practices in the management of overweight and obesity. Med Clin North Am 2021;105(1):149-74.

[218] Yu Y, Zhang YH, Liu L, Yu LL, Li JP, Rao JA, et al. Bioinformatics analysis of candidate genes and potential therapeutic drugs targeting adipose tissue in obesity. Adipocyte 2022;11(1):1-10.

[219] Spezani R, Mandarim-de-Lacerda CA. The current significance and prospects for the use of dual receptor agonism GLP-1/Glucagon. Life Sci 2022; 288:120188.

[220] Vohra MS, Benchoula K, Serpell CJ, Hwa WE. AgRP/NPY and POMC neurons in the arcuate nucleus and their potential role in treatment of obesity. Eur J Pharmacol 2022;915:174611.

[221] Sun Q, Gong T, Liu M, Ren S, Yang H, Zeng S, et al. Shikonin, a naphthalene ingredient: Therapeutic actions, pharmacokinetics, toxicology, clinical trials and pharmaceutical researches. Phytomedicine 2022;94:153805.

[222] de Moraes Arnoso BJ, Magliaccio FM, de Araújo CA, de Andrade Soares R, Santos IB, de Bem GF, et al. Açaí seed extract (ASE) rich in proanthocyanidins improves cardiovascular remodeling by increasing antioxidant response in obese high-fat diet-fed mice. Chem Biol Interact 2022;351:109721.
[223] Wang L, Wang B, Gasek NS, Zhou Y, Cohn RL, Martin DE, et al. Targeting $p21^{Cip1}$ highly expressing cells in adipose tissue alleviates insulin resistance in obesity. Cell Metab 2022;34(1):75-89.
[224] Arons A, Pomeranz J, Hamad R. Identifying novel predictors of state legislative action to address obesity. J Public Health Manag Pract 2021;27(1):E9-18.
[225] The Lancet Diabetes Endocrinology. Childhood obesity: A growing pandemic. Lancet Diabetes Endocrinol 2022;10(1):1.

Chapter 12

Malnutrition

Dilip R. Patel*, MD, MBA, MPH, Alison Agnetta, MD and Mahesh Shrestha, MD

Department of Pediatric and Adolescent Medicine, Western Michigan University Homer Stryker MD School of Medicine, Kalamazoo, Michigan, United States of America

Abstract

Food insecurity and malnutrition remain significant public health problems in the developing countries. Malnutrition affects an estimated 900 million peoples worldwide with long term adverse health and economic consequences both at individual and societal levels. Although progress has been made with effective treatment and preventive interventions, the overall burden of malnutrition remains significant. This chapter reviews key aspects of prevalence, clinical features, and intervention strategies for malnutrition.

Introduction

Food insecurity and malnutrition are significant concerns worldwide. Food security is defined as "access by all people at all time to sufficient food in terms of quality, quantity and diversity for an active and healthy life without risk of loss of such access" (1-5). Food security thus comprises three dimensions, namely availability, access, and utilization (see Table 1) (1-3).

The spectrum of malnutrition ranges from undernutrition (see Table 2) at one end to obesity at the other end (3-9). Measurement of the mid-upper arm circumference (MUAC) has also been validated as a means for assessing for severe acute malnutrition (SAM), and in some settings, such as those where age is difficult to determine or where a large number of individuals need to be evaluated. When using MUAC, a measurement of <11.5 cm diameter is an independent factor for inpatient treatment and has the additional benefit of usefulness as a marker for hospital discharge as well. The Food and Agriculture Organization measure of

* ***Correspondence:*** Chair and Professor Dilip R Patel, MD, MBA, MPH Department of Pediatric and Adolescent Medicine, Western Michigan University Homer Stryker M.D. School of Medicine, 1000 Oakland Drive, Kalamazoo, MI 49008 United States. Email: dilip.patel@med.wmich.edu.

In: Behavioral Pediatrics II
Editors: Donald E. Greydanus, Dilip R. Patel, Ahsan Nazeer et al.
ISBN: 979-8-88697-019-7

malnourishment refers to "number of persons who are assumed to be unable to meet daily calorie requirements necessary for light activities" (1).

An estimated 900 million people worldwide are reported to be undernourished, of whom 97% live in developing countries (2-5). About 16% of infants in developing countries are born low birth weight. Forty two percent of pregnant women and 47% of children younger than 5 years of age have been reported to have anemia; 1 billion people worldwide have iron deficiency anemia; 2 billion have zinc deficiency and 100-400 million have vitamin A deficiency (10-12). Malnutrition can have wide ranging adverse impact for the individual and society. Major consequences of chronic undernutrition are listed in Table 3 (13).

Table 1. Three dimensions of food security

Dimension	Comments
Availability	Refers to market level supply of food and is generally a reflection of economic conditions of production and trade
Access	Refers to household level ability to purchase food as well as equity of food distribution within household
Utilization	Refers to appropriate use of food in the presence of availability and access

Table 2. Spectrum of undernutrition

Category	Definition or comments
Underweight	Weight that is ≤ 2 SD for age
Stunting	Height that is ≤ 2 SD for age Reflects chronic undernutrition
Wasting	Weight that is ≤ 2 SD for height for age Reflects acute malnutrition
Micronutrient deficiencies	Major deficiencies are for vitamin A, iron, zinc, iodine, and folic acid

Table 3. Major consequences of chronic undernutrition

Consequence	Comments
Premature death	35% of child mortality result from undernutrition Vitamin A deficiency account for 0.6 million deaths per year Zinc deficiency account for 0.4 million deaths per year
Overutilization of health care resources	Low birth weight infant need increased use of neonatal servies Malnourished infants and children more prone to illnesses need more medical care Long term effects in development of diabetes mellitus and cardiovascular diseases
Loss of productivity during adult life	Reduced cognitive abilities and educational achievement result in reduced economic and work productivity in adult years
Effects of future generations	Deficit maternal nutrition result in adverse consequences on future generations

Clinical features of malnutrition

The clinical features of nonedamatous malnutrition or marasmus include failure to gain weight, weight loss leasing to emaciation (2, 3, 12). The infant or child is irritable. Child with edematous malnutrition presents with lethargy, apathy and edema. Infants and children with malnutrition show a number of signs affecting many systems. In kwashiorkar the face is described as moon face whereas in marasmus simian facies is noted. The skin may be shiny, edematous and dry. Follicular hyperkeratosis, hyper or hypopigmentation are common. Nail plates are thin and soft with fissuring or ridges.

Table 4. Major organ system effects of malnutrition

System	Main effects
Cardiovascular	Reduced cardiac output and stroke volume in marasmus with increasingly tenuous fluid balance in cases of edematous malnutrition. Risk of heart failure due to volume overload
Hepatic	Reduced protein synthesis; reduced metabolic clearance of toxins; reduced gluconeogenesis with increased risk for hypoglycemia
Gastrointestinal	Mucosal atrophy with loss of nutrient membrane transporters and decreased capacity for absorption; decreased intestinal motility with risk for bacterial overgrowth
Endocrine	Hypoinsulinemia with resultant glucose intolerance; elevated cortisol
Metabolic	Compensatory reduction in metabolic rate; reduced capacity for temperature regulation
Immunologic	Atrophy of thymus; impaired cellular immunity; decreased production of IgA

Table 5. Causes, manifestations, management and prevention of the major micronutrient deficiencies

Nutrient	Essential for the production or function of	Causes of deficiency	Manifestations of isolated deficiency	Management and prevention
Iron	Hemoglobin Various enzymes Myoglobin	Poor diet Elevated needs (e.g., while pregnant, in early childhood) Chronic loss from parasite infections (e.g., hookworms, schistosomiasis, whipworm)	Anemia and fatigue Impaired cognitive development Reduced growth and physical strength	Foods richer in iron and with fewer absorption inhibitors Iron-fortified weaning foods Low-dose supplements in childhood and pregnancy Cooking in iron pots
Iodine	Thyroid hormone	Except where seafood or salt fortified with iodine is readily available, most diets, worldwide, are deficient	Goiter, hypothyroidism, constipation Growth retardation Endemic cretinism	Iodine supplement Fortified salt Seafood
Vitamin A	Eyes Immune system	Diets poor in vegetables and animal products	Night blindness, xerophthalmia Immune deficiency Increased childhood illness, early death Contributes to development of anemia	More dark green leafy vegetables, animal products Fortification of oils and fats Regular supplementation
Zinc	Many enzymes Immune system	Diets poor in animal products Diets based on refined cereals (e.g., white bread, pasta, polished rice)	Immune deficiency Acrodermatitis Increased childhood illness, early death Complications in pregnancy, childbirth	Zinc treatment for diarrhea and severe malnutrition Improved diet

Adapted Müller O, Krawinkel M. Malnutrition and health in developing countries. CMAJ 2005;173(3):279-86.

Oral mucosa shows angular stomatitis, cheilitis and glossitis. Children have dull, sparse and brittle hair with patchy bands of light and normal color. Abdomen is distended and hepatomegaly or ascites can be present. Cardiovascular manifestations include hypotension, reduced cardiac output and small vessel vasculopathy. Neurologic manifestations include developmental delay, impaired cognition and depressed deep tendon reflexes.

A more severe form of malnutrition is known as marasmic-kwashiorkor and results from severe deficiency of all dietary nutrients. It may be precipitated when marasmus is complicated by overwhelming infection or acutely worsened protein deficiency with a resulting loss of metabolic adaptation. Mixed marasmic-kwashiorkor involves systemic derangement of organ systems and carries a high potential for morbidity and mortality. Sepsis and severe dehydration often complicate the picture and must be addressed concurrently. Effects on organ systems are outlined in Table 4.

The severity of malnutrition becomes pertinent in relation to treatment modalities, with moderate malnutrition (z-scores <-2 to -3 for both wasting and stunting) often amenable to outpatient or community based management. By contrast, severe malnutrition (z-scores less than -3 or any score in the presence of symmetrical edema) is most often managed in an inpatient setting, although recent studies have indicated that a subset of these patients may also be managed at home.

Causes, manifestations and management of major micronutrient deficiencies are summarized in table 5 (2, 4, 11).

Principles of treatment of moderate-to-severe acute malnutrition

Treatment of infants and children with malnutrition generally progresses through gradually progressive phases (14-24). The initial treatment usually lasts for the first week followed by rehabilitation of 2-6 weeks and additional 4-6 weeks of final follow-up phase.

During the initial stabilization phase, dehydration is corrected and appropriate antibiotic treatment is started if indicated. Oral feeding is started with WHO F75 diet (75 kcal/100 ml) followed gradually by WHO F100 diet (100 kcal/100 ml). Twelve smaller feedings are gradually transitioned to about 8 feedings/24 hours. Ready to use therapeutic foods (RUTFs) can also be used. RUTF is an oil-based paste which is a mixture of powdered milk, peanuts, sugar, vitamins and minerals.

Table 6. Consequences of hypophosphatemia

Weakness
Rhabdomyolysis
Hypotension
Cardiorespiratory failure
Cardiac arrhythmias
Seizures
Coma
Hemolysis
Thrombocytosis
Leukocyte dysfunction
Death

As the feedings are tolerated, they can be switched to ad lib and during later phase of rehabilitation, environmental stimulation is integrated in the treatment regimen. Infants and children with severe acute malnutrition without complications are treated in the community setting and those with complications need treatment in the healthcare facility.

Refeeding syndrome is a potential complication during initial phase of nutritional rehabilitation in malnourished infants and children. Refeednig syndrome is characterized by development of severe hypophosphatemia and its consequences (see Table 6) (25-27).

Infants and children at risk for refeeding syndrome require careful management and general principles of management are as follows as described by Mehanna and colleagues (26):

- Identify patients at risk for refeeding syndrome
- Check potassium, calcium, phosphate and magnesium
- Administer thiamine 200-300 mg daily orally, vitamin B high potency 1-2 tablets 3 times daily, multivitamin or trace supplements once daily
- Start feeding 0.0418 MJ/kg/day (If the patient is severely malnourished or if intake is negligible for $\geq$ 2 weeks, start feeding at a maximum of 0.0209 MJ/kg/day)
- Slowly increase feeding over next 7 days
- Rehydrate carefully and supplement and/or correct levels of potassium, phosphate, calcium and magnesium
- Monitor potassium, phosphate, calcium and magnesium for first 2 weeks and amend treatment as appropriate.

Patients with severe acute malnutrition with complications need treatment in a healthcare facility. These include patients with bilateral pitting sever edema, significant loss weight, anorexia, associated infections, severe anemia or severe dehydration.

Once the child displays improved responsiveness and decreased edema, the rehabilitation phase follows, lasting 4-6 weeks. During this phase a higher caloric concentration formula, WHO F100 (100 kcal and 2.9 g protein per 100 ml), is used, with the intent of recovery of weight loss. The feeds are gradually increased according to a prescribed regimen and weight gain often exceeds 10g/kg/day during this phase. In less severe malnutrition, ready to use therapeutic foods (RUTFs), which are an oil-based paste of powdered milk, peanuts, sugar, vitamins, and minerals, may be used instead of the formula food source. Iron and micronutrient supplementation may be judiciously continued throughout this period. Recovery is generally defined as achieving 90% of the median weight-for-height and is an appropriate endpoint for discharge criteria from inpatient setting.

Social dimension of malnutrition

While the effects of malnutrition are medical in nature, the cause of it is often social in origin and reflects the presence of such things as political instability, ineffective agricultural practices, disproportionate resource distribution, drought, poor sanitation, lack of education, poor access to healthcare, and high burden of underlying chronic disease (27).

Within societies where poor nutrition is prevalent, certain populations (women and children) are generally considered to be at further increased risk. Once thought to be in large part due to "pro-male bias in food consumption," this seems not to be the case once adjusted for energy usage and body composition. However, women and children remain at higher risk due to the added physiological demands of pregnancy, lactation, childhood growth and skeletal maturation.

While a woman, at baseline, requires less caloric energy than her male counterpart, she still requires the same quantity of daily micronutrients (or greater quantities, as in the case of iron). This means that to ensure adequate intake of micronutrients she must either consume greater quantities of food, or food that is richer in micronutrient concentration—both general impossibilities in already nutritionally deficient societies. Moreover, during pregnancy and lactation, her nutritional needs increase even further, with caloric consumption rising by 300-500 kcals per day and micronutrient needs going up some times as high as 40% above her previous state (27).

Add into the equation that in many developing countries motherhood begins in the teenage years, before maternal physical development has been completed, pregnancy essentially places the maternal and fetal bodies at odds with each other in the competition to obtain enough nutrition to sustain development. In this manner, the problem of malnutrition becomes cyclic in nature, with the undernutrition of the mother being passed on to the offspring in the form of low birth weight, intrauterine growth restriction, neonatal mortality, and subsequent childhood malnutrition (6). The end result is to place vast segments of a society's upcoming generation at risk for increased infection, growth retardation, impaired cognitive function and school performance, impaired work productivity, and increased risk of overall mortality.

Prevention

Public health and population based interventions can effective in prevention and treatment of malnutrition (27-30). Some of such key interventions for undernutrition include:

- Promotion of breast feeding for all infants. For mothers with HIV/AIDS breast feeding is recommended for first six months in developing countries with rapid weaning at six months.
- Adequate and timely complementary feeding, starting at six months of age
- Promotion of personal hygiene and sanitation practices
- Giving micronutrient supplements to pregnant women, infants, and children
- Deworming of mothers and infected children
- Fortifying commonly consumed food with micronutrients and minerals
- Presumptive treatment of malaria for pregnant women in endemic regions

Prevention efforts should focus on interventions during pregnancy and first two years of life. The adverse effects of malnutrition on brain development to fetus and during first two years are potentially irreversible. Large scale public health efforts can be effective. Supplement of folic acid in pregnancy has been successful in preventing neural tube defects. Two thirds of people in the developing world now have access to iodized salt that has improved care significantly for iodine deficiency and anemia that affect 3.5 billion people. About 450 million children a year receive Vitamin A capsules, reducing blindness and childhood mortality.

Conclusion

Food insecurity and malnutrition are persistent problems in developing world affecting millions of people (31-36). The long term consequences of malnutrition are significant both at individual and societal levels. Although effective treatment and prevention interventions have made significant impact in reducing the burden of malnutrition, enormous challenges still remain to meet the needs of populations worldwide.

References

[1] Food and Agriculture Organization of the United Nations. The state of food security and nutrition in the world 2018. Rome: Food Agriculture Organization United Nations, 2018. URL: http://www.fao.org/state-of-food-security-nutrition/en/.

[2] Abrams S, Brabin BJ, Coulter JBS. Nutrition-associated disease. In: Farrar J, Hotez PJ, Junghanss T, Kang G, Lallo D, White N, eds. Manson's tropical diseases, 23rd edition. Philadelphia, PA: Elsevier, 2014:1151-67.

[3] Pinstrup-Andersen P, Burger S, Habicht JP, Peterson K. Protein-energy malnutrition. In: Jamison DT, Mosley WH, Measham AR, Bobadilla JL, eds. Disease control priorities in developing countries, 2nd ed. Oxford: Oxford University Press, 1993:391-420.

[4] Levin HM, Pollitt E, Galloway R, McGuire J. Micronutrient deficiency disorders. In: Jamison DT, Mosley WH, Measham AR, Bobadilla JL, eds. Disease control priorities in developing countries, 2nd ed. Oxford: Oxford University Press, 1993:421-51.

[5] World Health Organization. World health report. Geneva: WHO, 2004.

[6] World Health Organization and the United Nations Children's Fund: WHO child growth standards and the identification of severe acute malnutrition in infants and children. URL: www.who.int/nutrition/publications/severemalnutrition/9789241598163/en/index.html 2009.

[7] Word Health Organization. Informal consultation to review current literature on severe malnutrition. Gevena: WHO, 2005.

[8] Behrman JHR, Alderman H, Hoddinott J. Hunger and malnutrition. In: Lomborg B, ed. Global crises, global solutions. Cambridge: Cambridge University Press, 2004.

[9] Black RE, Allen LH, Bhutta ZA, Caulfield LE, de Onis M, Ezzati M et al. Maternal and child undernutrition: Global and regional exposures and health consequences. Lancet 2008;371:243-60.

[10] Rice AL, Sacco L, Hyder A, Black RE. Malnutrition as an underlying cause of childhood deaths associated with infectious diseases in developing countries. Bull World Health Organ 2000;78:1207-21.

[11] Black R. Micronutrient deficiency – An underlying cause for morbidity and mortality. Bull World Health Organ 2003;81:79.

[12] Grover Z, Ee LC. Protein energy malnutrition. Pediatr Clin North Am 2009;56:1055-68.

[13] Collins S, Dent N, Binns P, Bahwere P, Sadler K, Hallam A. Management of severe acute malnutrition in children. Lancet 2006;368:1992-2000.

[14] Collins S. Treating severe acute malnutrition seriously. Arch Dis Child 2007;92:453-61.

[15] World Health Organization, United Nations Children's Fund. Joint statement on the management of acute diarrhea. Geneva: WHO, 2004.

[16] World Health Organization. Management of the child with a serious infection or severe malnutrition. Guidelines for care at the first-referral level in developing countries. Geneva: WHO, 2000.

[17] World Health Organization. Management of severe malnutrition: a manual for physicians and other senior health workers. Geneva: WHO, 1999.

[18] Bhan MK, Bhandari N, Bahl R. Management of the severely malnourished child: perspective from developing countries. BMJ 2003;326:146-51.

[19] Centers for Disease Control and Prevention (CDC) Micronutrient facts. URL: https://www.cdc.gov/nutrition/micronutrient-malnutrition/micronutrients/index.html.

[20] World Health Organization (WHO). Malnutrition. URL: https://www.who.int/news-room/fact-sheets/detail/malnutrition.
[21] UNICEF Position paper: Ready-to-use therapeutic food (RUTF) for children with severe acute malnutrition, 2013. URL:https://www.unicef.org/media/files/Position_Paper_Ready-to-use_therapeutic_food_for_children_with_severe_acute_malnutrition__June_2013.pdf.
[22] World Food Programme: Technical specifications for ready-to-use supplmentary food (RUSF), 2016. URL:https://documents.wfp.org/stellent/groups/public/documents/manual_guide_proced/wfp251131.pdf.
[23] World Health Organiztion Guideline: Updates on the management of severe acute malnutrition in infants and children, 2013. URL: https://apps.who.int/iris/bitstream/handle/10665/95584/9789241506328_eng.pdf?ua=1.
[24] World Health Organization. Technical note: Supplmentary foods for the management of moderate acute malnutrition in infants and children 6-59 months. Geneva: WHO, 2012. URL: https://apps.who.int/iris/bitstream/handle/10665/75836/9789241504423_eng.pdf?sequence=1&isAllowed=y.
[25] Fuentebella J, Kerner JA. Refeeding syndrome. Pediatr Clin North Am 2009;56:1201-10.
[26] Mehanna HM, Moledina J, Travis J. Refeeding syndrome: What it is and how to prevent and treat it. BMJ 2008;336:1495-8.
[27] RAO Corporate Document Repository. The state of food insecurity in the world 2000. URL: http://www.fao.org/docrep/X8200E/x8200e04.htm#TopOfPage.
[28] Manary MJ, Sandige HL. Management of acute moderate and severe childhood malnutrition. BMJ 2008;337:1227-30.
[29] Nemer L, Gelban H, Jha P; Commission on Macroeconomics and Health. The evidence base for interventions to reduce malnutrition in children under five and school-age children in low- and middle-income countries. CMH working paper no WG5:11. Geneva: World Health Organization, 2001.
[30] Collins S, Sadler K, Dent N, Khara T, Guerrero S, Myatt M, et al. Key issues in the success of community-based management of severe malnutrition. Food Nutr Bull 2006;27(Suppl 3):S49-82.
[31] World Bank: Repositioning nutrition as central to development: a strategy for large-scale action. Washington, DC: World Bank, 2006.
[32] Betebo B, Eiaio T, Alemseged F, Massa D. Housefold food insecurity and its association with nutritional status of children 6-59 months of age in East Badawacho District, South Ethiopia. J Environ Public Health 2017;2017:6373595. doi: 10.1155/2017/6373595.
[33] Isanaka S, Kodish SR, Berthé F, Alley I, Nackers F, Hanson KE, et al. Outpatient treatment of severe acute malnutrition: response to treatment with a reduced schedule of therapeutic food distribution. Am J Clin Nutr 2017;105(5):1191-7.
[34] Platts-Mills JA, Taniuchi M, Uddin MJ, Sobuz SU, Mahfuz M, Gaffar SA, et al. Association between enteropathogens and malnutrition in children aged 6-23 months in Bangladesh: A case-control study. Am J Clin Nutr 2017;105(5):1132-8.
[35] Shankar B, Agrawal S, Beaudreault AR, Avula L, Martorell R, Osendarp S. Dietary and nutritional change in India: implications for strategies, policies, and interventions. Ann NY Acad Sci 2017;1395(1):49-59.
[36] Power M, Uphoff E, Kelly B, Pickett KE. Food insecurity and mental health: An analysis of routine primary care data of pregnant women in the Born in Bradford cohort. J Epidemiol Commun Health 2017;71(4):324-8. doi: 10.1136/jech-2016-207799.

Chapter 13

Anorexia nervosa in adolescence: International perspectives on medical and psychological assessment and management

Lyubov Matytsina-Quinlan[1,*], MD, PhD,
Donald E Greydanus[2], MD, DrHC(Athens),
Irina V. Babenko-Sorocopud[3], MD and Laura Gwatkin[4], MD
[1]Liverpool University Hospitals NHS Foundation Trust, England, United Kingdom, [2]Department of Pediatric and Adolescent Medicine, Western Michigan University Homer Stryker MD School of Medicine, Kalamazoo, Michigan, United States of America, [3]Reproductive Health of Pediatric, Adolescent and Youth Department, Donetsk Regional Centre of Maternal and Childhood Care, Donetsk, Ukraine and [4]CT4 ACCS, Aneurin Bevan Health Board, Nevill Hall Hospital, Abergavenny, Wales, United Kingdom

Abstract

Eating disorders are .complex biopsychosocial disorders that include anorexia nervosa and bulimia nervosa. This discussion considers both of these disorders with the emphasis on anorexia nervosa and its effects on adolescent females. Concepts of epidemiology, etiology, differential diagnosis, and management are considered. Particular emphasis is given to gynecologic and psychologic effects of anorexia and their management. Clinicians including those involved in adolescent gynecology can be very beneficial to these patients if the condition is recognized early and comprehensive, team-based care is provided.

Introduction

In modern gynecological literature information about anorexia nervosa is often presented in a limited fashion. In the meantime, in the overwhelming majority of cases of menstrual disorders, the first and only concern of the patient with anorexia nervosa may be menstrual dysfunction (i.e., hypomenstrual syndrome, secondary amenorrhea, delay of sexual development or primary amenorrhea).

---

* ***Correspondence:*** Email: lquinlan@nhs.net.

In: Behavioral Pediatrics II
Editors: Donald E. Greydanus, Dilip R. Patel, Ahsan Nazeer et al.
ISBN: 979-8-88697-019-7

Anorexia nervosa

Anorexia nervosa (AN) represents pathologic behavior characterized by deliberate weight loss initiated and maintained by the patient (1). The clinical presentations include loss of weight due to food avoidance, concern that food intake "makes them look fat", and use of various means to avoid weight gain such as inducing vomiting, consuming laxatives or diuretics, and/or establishing a pattern of excessive physical exercises. These all result in somatic and endocrine disorders that can lead to amenorrhea as a result of hypothalamic-pituitary-ovarian system dysfunction. If the disease begins in pre-pubertal period, sexual development is delayed or halted.

Lack of information and awareness in primary care regarding features of AN may often lead to a delayed or even missed diagnosis, especially at the initial stages of the disease. It results in misleading etiology and pathogenesis of sexual system dysfunction. Without the correct diagnosis teenage girls, who comprise the majority of patients with AN, do not receive the necessary psychological help and counseling. Instead, they may be simply prescribed an oral contraceptive to regulate their periods. Hence, etiological factors promoting the occurrence of the disease remain unknown, complicating the choices of adequate treatment therapy.

Anorexia nervosa syndrome was described for the first time by English physician Richard Morton (1637-1698) in 1689 (2). He noted a clinical variant of progressive weight loss and loss of appetite with suppression of digestive function which developed without features of fever, coughing or shortness of breath. In cachectic stages these patients reminded him of “skeletons draped in their own skin”. He named this condition “nervous consumption” (2).

In 1789 the French physician Naudeau described a disease in which the main feature was the patients’ unusual disgust for food. Systematic studying of clinical presentation of AN began from works of French physician E. Charles Lasègue (1816-1883) in 1873 and English physician Sir William Gull (1816-1890) in 1873 (2). Gull was the physician for Queen Victoria (1819-1901) and named this disease “nervous anorexia” (anorexia nervosa); this term was thus established in the English, German and Russian literature. In translation from German (Kylin,1973) patients with anorexia nervosa were also described as having “a passion for exhaustion (2).”

Epidemiology and etiology

AN is a rare disease and is found mainly in adolescent girls (3); out of 10 patients only one is male (4). According to modern figures 1% of adolescent girls have anorexia nervosa (5,6). AN typically presents during the teenage years, making up 40% of all cases (7,8). However, it can be found in children before 11 years of age, as well as adults (9). For the latter two groups the prognosis of the disease is more pessimistic.

The role of genetic predisposition is considered to be highly significant and thus, the role of genetics should not be underestimated (10,11). Concordance rates differ significantly across monozygotic and dizygotic twin pairs for defined self-reported anorexia and bulimia nervosa (BN) (12). With a family history of AN, the risk of developing this disorder increases eight-fold. Genetic and environmental factors account for 74% and 26% respectively in AN syndrome (13). Among relatives having AN, a bulimic component is common; however, there is a comorbid association with affective disorders that are inherited independently.

From a gynecologist's viewpoint one can speculate that AN occurs more often than it is diagnosed, as gynecologists may not gather statistical data about these patients at the early stages of the disease. Also, cases which do not reach cachectic states remain undiagnosed.

In the United States the prevalence of AN is estimated at approximately 1% (14). Among females, there are different prevalence rates given in American reports, with up to 26% of the female subjects having abnormal eating attitudes (15). Lucas and colleagues reported a longitudinal general population-based survey from 1935-1989 in USA, which noted that adolescents and young female from 15 to 24 years old were the most vulnerable group for AN (16).

Recent researchers have shown that the frequency of this disease has remained stable during the last four decades; there are reports in the United States of 145/100,000 females in 1988 and 113/100,000 in 1991 (16). This disease is more common among populations of European origin (>95%). Among females in Western countries, the percentage of abnormal eating attitudes ranged from 8.3% in Germany to 26% in the USA (17). A population-based study of AN in the United Kingdom found that the prevalence of AN among adolescent females aged 15 to 19 years was 0.1% (18).

In recent years a tendency of gradual increase in the number of patients suffering with AN is observed (17). "Anorexia explosion" in the population is explained by the change of the role of a woman in the society, perception of beauty, and strengthening of aesthetic values in adolescent culture including photo models, movie stars, celebrities, and even Barbie dolls (19). While in the developed countries the fashion for slender figures is remaining, one of the woman's merits is plumpness in the developing world. It is noted that the majority of girls in the West who consider themselves plump are afraid of getting plumper (boys usually do not have such fears). Many high school girls diet from time to time in order to become thinner. Even though such self-restrictions in food can be very severe, true eating disorders are much rarer (20).

AN is found more frequently in teenagers of high income families (21). People from less privileged background seldom suffer with AN. Many adolescent girls suffering with AN had obesity in prepubertal and earlier childhood years; as a result of this obesity they were at risk of being bullied. Most often the predispositions for developing AN include a broken family in conjunction with dependent and immature personality of the patient. Competition between brothers and sisters for their parents' attention is typical of such cases. It is thought that these eating disorders are connected with initial feeling of fear and immaturity in the psychosexual area, which is accompanied by rejection of sexual or social interactions. Anorexia nervosa can be an etiological factor of menstrual cycle disorder (MCD) and one of the manifestations of psychodynamic disorders represents a stress-syndrome. Patients are unable to adapt to difficult situations and cope with life stresses; therefore, it requires psychological therapy (*vida infra*).

Etiologic factors

Since the symptoms of anorexia often become apparent in the pubertal age, a hypothesis is formed that this state is caused by a girl turning into a woman. Because of the fears that might be associated with such transformation, she tries to conceal the manifestations of puberty (i.e., breast development, changes in bodily proportions, commencement of menses), which are accompanied by considerable body weight loss through food restriction. Constant preoccupation with body weight gives a girl an opportunity to avoid social and sexual interactions, as well as potential conflicts with parents. At the same time, teenagers of the older age group (17-18 years) have the conflicts of identity formation. They refrain from transition to independent life (for example, acquisition of a profession or starting a family).

Biological causes of AN are studied insufficiently (22). However, it is considered that the start of illness may be favored by abnormal albumin and lipid metabolism, which are related to fasting states. Some authors suggest that with patients suffering with AN, the senses of hunger, cold, and tiredness are blunted, which may have biological predisposition in development of eating disorders; other researchers believe these disorders are inherited (12,13,22).

Mortality

Mortality rates of AN patients fluctuates considerably ranging from 1.8% to 14.1% (23). The causes of death of such patients often are due to cardiovascular complications or as a result of suicide. Decreased myocardial thickness of the left ventricle can be revealed by radiological imaging. Electrocardiogram (ECG) may show sinus bradycardia, ST segment elevation, flattening of the T wave, lowered voltage of QRS complex and right axis deviation. Though some of these enumerated changes may not have precise clinical significance, prolonged QT interval does increase the risk of life-threatening arrhythmias and sudden cardiac events including death (24). The risk of heart decompensation is the highest during the first two weeks of fasting, as in this period the compromised myocardium is sometimes unable to accommodate the increased metabolic demands.

Sufficient differences in statistical data can be explained by including the patients with diseases of different complexity into the study group (20). Frequency of complete recovery can be estimated at 43%, whereas 36% of patients with AN improve, 20% develop chronic eating disorders and 5% die (25).

Clinical symptoms

Exhaustion with weight loss to 36-40 kg at an average height of 163-172 cm is a wide-spread occurrence among patients suffering with AN who can present with a body mass index (BMI) $\leq$ 17.5 kg/m2 (25). This considerable loss of the body weight is caused by restrictions in the food calorie content and exclusion of carbohydrates from the diet. Chronic states of albumin deficiency may develop which can be manifested by joint swelling. Abusing diuretics may cause dehydration while laxative abuse leads to profuse diarrhea and in severe situations, hypokalemia.

The patient does not feel anxious regarding her deteriorating state, whereas the parents are increasingly concerned. Often teenage girls cook meals for the family while starving themselves, which does not raise much suspicion about their state. A painful verdict of being curvy or plump and aspiration to grow thin usually does not carry obtrusive behavior in AN patients. Fixations on losing weight and having a slim figure do not contradict the internal aims, and thus are not accompanied by anxiety. Only in rare cases AN is combined with neurosis of an obtrusive state, and then typical obtrusiveness of such patients can be revealed.

Behavioral features that are typical in AN patients include obsession with calorie counting, provoking of vomiting after meals, excessive physical exercise and laxative use. Many changes in personality and behavior in AN are consequences of starvation and malnutrition. These involve fixed thoughts about food, slow and thorough chewing, depression, fatigability, decreased sexual activity as well as libido, social isolation, and worsening of cognitive functions (20).

Patients suffering with AN can cook refined dishes for others, make food reserves and create unusual rituals accompanying eating. This resembles behavioral features of obsessive-compulsive personality disorder and such actions are often not limited to meals. As a rule, patients suffering with AN keep their feeding habits in secret and refuse joint meals. An attempt to reveal these problems are decisively repulsed. Very often they wear clothes of larger sizes in order to conceal their skinniness.

AN represents a number of disorders associated with substantial psychological morbidity (20). Patients with suicidal ideations are of great concern and suicide is the most common reason of death in such patients. Risk of self-harm usually grows during the period of weight gain, which can be accompanied by aggravation of their emotional state (23). Therefore, these patients require special clinical attention during this period.

Anorexia can alternate with bulimic episodes, during which a patient binges on food that leads to feelings of guilt as well as anxiety, thus provoking vomiting. This type of behavior is more attributed to impulsive, less constrained people. It is possible to hypothesize that bulimia plays a role of a compensatory mechanism boarding on the edge of being life threatening.

On clinical examination the following signs can be found: cold extremities; peripheral cyanosis; thin downy hair (fluff) on the back and face; bradycardia of 40-55 beats per minute; hypotension 90/66 mmHg, and hypothermia (22). The metabolism is slowing down while the disease is in progress, which affects tissue composition. Furthermore, some dystrophic changes of internal organs may develop.

Diagnostic criteria

Diagnostic criteria for anorexia nervosa have often been based on the well-known guidelines of the American Psychiatric Association's diagnostic and statistical manual of mental disorders (DSM). The Fifth edition of this manual was published in 2013 and is essentially the same as the DSM-IV version with a few exceptions (23). Amenorrhea has been eliminated in the DSM-5 as a requirement for the diagnosis of anorexia nervosa in females. Also, Criterion A (first criteria) emphasizes restricting calorie intake and removed the word "refusal" with reference to weight maintenance; this was accomplished because it is very challenging to clearly assess patient's intent in this regard (23). The concept of the patient being at a significantly low body weight with reference to their developmental stage was expanded. Criterion B now includes the concept of regular or persistent behavior interring with weight gain in addition to the previously included weight gain fear (23).

Clinical effects of anorexia nervosa

One of the first clinical problems that patients with anorexia may present to a gynecologist is menstrual function disorder (MFD). Weight loss of 10% or more can lead to MFD and include secondary amenorrhea or oligoamenorrhea (27). However, the majority of the patients have amenorrhea as the first symptom when there is no significant weight deficit yet expressed. Moreover, the restoration of body weight back to normal is not always accompanied by return of normal menstrual function and does not always correlate to the degree of weight loss or cachexia.

MFD in anorexia nervosa reflects the leading role of hypothalamic disorders and hypothalamic-pituitary-ovarian axis dysfunction in the pathophysiology of MFD in patients suffering with AN. Current theory suggests that amenorrhea combined with malnutrition represents a functional hypothalamic amenorrhea due to dysfunctional secretion of gonadotropin releasing hormone (GnRH). Disorders of reproductive function in AN serve as the body's defensive mechanism in the circumstances of nutritional deficiency and psychological changes. Reproductive system changes in AN are characterized by central inhibition of GnRH secretion, abrupt decrease of gonadotrophic function of the pituitary gland, inhibition of folliculogenesis and synthesis of steroid hormones in the ovaries (especially estradiol). Decreased levels of estrogen lead to progressive involution changes in target-organs, such as hypoplasia of the uterus and breasts, inhibition of proliferative changes in the endometrium and halted menstrual function (28).

Forty percent of patients suffering with AN have decreased vasopressin secretion, similar to those with diabetes insipidus. This disorder is neurogenic in nature; as with vasopressin injection, urine concentration increases. With increase in body weight, the secretion of vasopressin goes back to normal.

Hormonal changes include increase in growth hormone (GH) level and also in cortisol concentration in blood plasma as well as a decrease in free thyroxine (T_4). Progesterone level is monotonously low and corresponds to the basal level of first phase of menstrual cycle. Levels of testosterone and androstenedione often correspond to the lower limits of normal. The other changes in blood serum are increased levels of cholesterol and carotene. Leukopenia and anemia may also be present while levels of calcium and potassium are decreased.

Osteopenia

Osteopenia is a serious complication of AN (29,30). Decreased osseous tissue density in adolescent girls is caused not only by low levels of progesterone, which accelerates bone regeneration processes, but also by lowering of the insulin-like growth factor 1 (IGF-1) which stimulates collagen synthesis. It is also influenced by parathyroid hormone, which causes decalcification of the bone and regulates calcium content in the blood serum. The process of mineral absorption in the gastrointestinal tract (including calcium) is suppressed in patients provoking vomiting. Patients with hypocalcemia are at risk of osteoporotic ribs and consequent fractures. In contrast to menopausal changes, where the strength of osseous tissue can be stabilized by estrogen supplement therapy and physiotherapy, patients with AN do not benefit from physical exercise, which can only aggravate the demineralization processes (31).

Neuroendocrine and metabolic changes

Starvation resulting in exhaustion causes secondary neuro-endocrine and metabolic changes (22). These changes, in turn, influence the cortical function causing personality changes. A similar vicious circle of psychologic disorders is created by peculiarities of cerebral, metabolic and endocrine functioning in adolescent girls.

An original integration system providing neuro-humoral coordination is the hypothalamus, which functionally is closely related to cerebral cortex, the pituitary gland and lymphoreticular complex structures. The hypothalamus is extremely sensitive to humoral changes, as well as the signals from cerebral cortex. Close interrelations in the hypothalamic-pituitary system lay at the basis of development of vegetative, endocrine, trophic, and psychological disorders.

Alongside with changes in synthesis of testosterone in AN, there are expressed changes of its metabolism. Disorders of albumin metabolism in AN may result in dysproteinemia and disorders of synthesis in globulin fraction in the liver such as binding steroids (i.e., sexual hormone binding globulin [SHBG]). Decrease in SHBG synthesis is associated with deficiency of albumin, and is aggravated by insufficiency of steroid system function. Decrease of SHBG results in increase of biologically active free testosterone; also, the activity of enzymes involved in testosterone metabolism (5-alpha- and 5-beta-reductase) is changed. High levels of free testosterone along with changes in enzyme activity and tissue metabolism probably explain intensification of growth of fluff hair (lanugo) on shoulders, back, and waist in patients suffering with AN.

Slowing of psychosexual development may result from the development of endocrine and asthenic disorders in AN, in addition to increase of intensity and a variety of persuasive phenomena. Occurrence of uncontrollable food binging (bulimia) coincides with the general disinhibition of desires including sexual. Development of AN may coincide with important psychosexual development and establishment of sexual relationships.

Gastrointestinal changes

Disorders of gastrointestinal function become apparent with delayed peristalsis (22). Constipation is also a typical presentation of patients suffering with anorexia. Moreover, these patients may have decreased motility and slow passage of gastric and intestinal contents as well as stomach atrophy. Serious electrolyte disorders can lead to paresis of intestines and intestinal impassability, and also stagnation of gastric contents with gastric distension as well as risk of rupture. Patients who vomit have acidic gastric contents, which damages teeth enamel resulting in their fast destruction. Gastrointestinal complications can also include liver dysfunction (32).

Miscellaneous clinical changes

Chronic starvation can cause cerebral atrophy with reduction of its volume. Muscular weakness is a typical neurological symptom. Increased blood urea nitrogen level is observed in patients with severe dehydration while the glomerular filtration rate is simultaneously reduced. Electrolyte imbalance is most commonly seen in patients with vomiting; the levels of essential minerals (i.e., potassium, calcium, magnesium, and phosphorus) in their bodies are abnormal. Thus, hypovolemia, sodium depletion, hypomagnesemia, and hypophosphatemia are common in AN (32).

Stages of anorexia nervosa development

Based on physical signs and psychological changes the following four stages of AN development can be identified:

- Stage 1 - dysmorphophobic stage, which is characterized by occurrence of over-valued, dysmorphophobic ideas which result in cyclic restrictions in ingestion of food and low mood.
- Stage 2 - dysmorphomanic stage, which is characterized by the presence of active persevering restriction in food ingestion leading to full refusal of meals. The patient engages in excessive physical exercise and may provoke vomiting. Progressive weight loss is accompanied by occurrence of somatic and endocrine disorders as the hypothalamic-pituitary-ovarian (HPO) system is affected. If the disease begins in the prepubertal period, it is manifested by primary amenorrhea or delayed sexual development.
- Stage 3 - cachexic stage develops on the average in two years time from the beginning of the disease. In terms of the patient's mental state, there is a prevalence of asthenoadynamic disorders, whereas alimentary cachexia reveals the somatic manifestation of the disorder.
- Stage 4 - AN reduction stage, which comes after treatment and is characterized by normalization of mental and somatic states.

Laboratory findings

During the second and third stages of AN, the results of full blood count reveal anemia, leukopenia and relative lymphocytosis. On urinalysis, proteinuria may develop at the second and third stages of the disease. On biochemical analysis of blood during the second stage of AN hypoalbuminemia can develop, and at the third stage – there is an increase of cholesterol levels with normal levels of triglycerides. Blood electrolytes show hypokalemia, and in patients provoking vomiting – hypochloremia (32). On fecal analyses for dysbacteriosis there is an increased levels of lactose-negative bacteria at the second and third stages.

On pelvic ultrasound scan (USS) reduction of all uterine dimensions (length, width and anteroposterior measurements) occurs proportionally to progression of AN. On USS cyclic changes in the endometrium (M-echo of 2-4 mm with no reflection of cyclic changes) are not observed. Reduction of the ovaries to the sizes of those in prepubertal period is noted (33).

Endocrine and metabolic disorders are variable but all of them are consequences of starvation. Reduction in luteinizing (LH) and follicle-stimulating hormone (FSH) concentrations are accompanied by amenorrhea; usually amenorrhea is secondary to weight loss, but sometimes it can be primary.

It is interesting to note that in AN, out of all endocrine functions of the body, reproductive system dysfunction develops first and is the last to recover. Having suffered severe AN after clinical recovering and normalization of all endocrine functions, the reproductive system may remain dysfunctional leading to subfertility (34).

Psychological effects

It is determined that AN in childhood and adolescent years can vary in presentation, but could be recognized by the presence of dysmorphophobic ideas combined with obsessive-compulsive and affective disorders. Patients with AN can have dominating monothematic dysmorphophobia with over-valued ideations of obsessive-compulsive nature and depressive disorders with clearly expressed triads:

- anorexia nervosa syndrome with dominating bulimia, polythematic obsessive-compulsive disorders and affective component in the form of prolonged depressive disorders and short hypomania.
- anorexia nervosa syndrome with dominating bulimia combined with vomitophobia of obsessive-compulsive nature and with expressed catatonic-like stereotypes, cenesthopathy and body-focused delusions with delirious depersonalization.

There can be the presence of certain premorbid disposition characterized by combination of schizoid, hysterical, epileptoid and agitated personality features; these are particularly atypical for patients with anorexia nervosa developing in childhood and during adolescence. The syndrome of AN in childhood and adolescence is heterogeneous in nosological nature. In patients presenting during this period, AN is seen almost with identical frequency in those with accentuated personality and schizophrenia (35).

During adolescence patients with AN may exhibit pathologically proceeding crises characterized by premorbid perfectionism as well as hysterical and perturbed features. The syndrome of anorexia nervosa may develop as perturbed depression with dominating monothematic dysmorphophobia accompanied by active weight loss, obsessive-compulsive and phobic disorders, cenesthopathy, and asthenic symptoms.

Differential diagnosis

In a patient's history with suspicion for AN, it is necessary to gather detailed information about changes in body weight, diet peculiarities and physical exercise (30,36). It is also essential to make a note of any weight loss in the past few months and/or failure of expected physiological body weight gain during adolescence (37).

Manifestations of malnutrition may be identified on the physical examination (22). It is important to weigh patients and measure their height. Body mass index (BMI) here generally has only relative significance. The patient's age and constitution must be taken into account. As a rule, there are some changes of vitally important functions such as bradycardia at rest as well as hypotension and hypothermia; as a rule, AN patients have cold extremities.

Patients can complain of poor tolerance of cold environment and cold weather. Orthostatic hypotension is typical of patients with AN. Dry skin, thinning of body hair (lanugo type), hypotrophy or complete atrophy of mammary glands, and enlargement of submaxillary as well as parotid salivary glands are noted in AN. Lymph nodes, however, are not enlarged. Normal dieting differs from AN by absence of amenorrhea and overvalued ideas about excessive weight.

Body weight loss can be a consequence not only of psychiatric, but also somatic disorders, such as hyperthyroidism, adrenal insufficiency or diabetes mellitus. That is why an endocrinologist's consultation can be helpful.

In hysterical anorexia the patients refuse meals in a categorical manner in order to draw attention, instead of secretly disposing of food. Artificially provoked vomiting is followed by involuntary episodes of vomiting after some time. There is no severe lethargy due to starvation, as the patients may still eat secretly or let somebody persuade them to take food. More often hysterical anorexia is a consequence of psychologically provoked attacks of severe vomiting (i.e., after family conflicts, death of a relative, others). Here, vomiting is a signal for action: "Pay attention to me!" In order to prevent vomiting, patients begin to restrict their meals and fear of vomiting (vomitophobia) and therefore fear of eating develops. Hysterical anorexia may be resolved after psychotherapeutic treatment.

In severe depression the differentiation between the two conditions (i.e., mood disorder and eating disorder) can be challenging, because there are no psychological features particular to AN. There are typical vegetative symptoms. Appetite decreases abruptly, for example, as a consequence of feeling worthless or having inappropriate guilt; this patient considers herself unworthy of meals or money which can be spent on it. This can be a defining symptom in AN.

Cachexia in Simmonds disease is notable, due to the exhaustion, which is connected with an abrupt drop in appetite. These patients do not fear to become fat. Languor, passivity, weakness, fatigability and hypodynamia all progress quickly out of clinical symptoms. In pituitary cachexia, insulin tolerance falls abruptly. A gastroenterologist's consultation is necessary to check for inflammatory bowel diseases, malignant neoplasms, chronic infections, and congenital or acquired metabolic disorders.

Depressive and obsessive symptoms would be related to corresponding psychiatric disorders. However, such peculiar features can be a distinctive feature of AN such as weight loss of more than 15% of normal or weight loss initiated by the patient from food restrictions. A fear of getting fat and a distorted notion of one's own body, and also, systematic endocrine disorders of HPO axis usually indicate a correct diagnosis.

Electroencephalogram (EEG) analysis displays abnormal features in patient and control groups. A stable organized α-rhythm is registered in adolescent girls with AN. Paroxysmal activity on EEG could be a feature of diencephalic trunk dysfunction. In AN, patients with underlying schizophrenia, desynchronized EEG is often seen with low amplitude and increase of β-activity index. It reflects intensification of excitability in the cerebral cortex.

EEG desynchronization most often occurs in patients suffering with schizophrenia whose anorexia nervosa is combined with episodes of bulimia and vomitomania. β-activity in this group of patients is more intense than in the group with schizophrenia alone. According to these findings, the connection between EEG abnormalities and patients' mental health has been established.

Management of anorexia nervosa in adolescent girls

Subcategorization of somatic and psychiatric treatment compromises a holistic approach to patient care. That is why in the department of child and adolescent gynecology in Donetsk Regional Centre of Maternity and Child Care (DRCMCC) in the Ukraine, there is no such separation in treatment approach, which helps to achieve better results in AN therapy.

The first step is to convince the patient and the relatives of the necessity of treatment and give a detailed explanation regarding the treatment as well as the condition itself. It may be very time-consuming and require much effort as the patients usually underestimate the seriousness of their condition. Nevertheless, it is essential to gain consent and persuade these patients to comply, as otherwise the treatment would not be of any benefit. Almost always, except in early stages of AN when weight loss is not significant, hospitalization is required. The treatment in the hospital begins with restoration of body weight including full nourishment. It must also incorporate restoration of normal eating habits including portion size and calorie intake, often managed by a dietician and a psychiatric occupational therapist.

From our experience of dealing with AN patients, the most important information given to patient is regarding adipose tissue functions in the body, its physiological correlation with height and weight, and its relation to a natural female figure, as well as importance in reproductive function. The emphasis is on the significance of a multidisciplinary approach to patients with AN, because the psychological aspect of their disorder is equally as important as the associated gynecological or other medical problems (5, 22,37).

Usually a method of positive reinforcement is used. For example, if during a week the patient gains weight, then she is 'rewarded' with additional independence (i.e., meeting with friends, leaving the hospital floor or unit). It is very important that patients define a 'prize' themselves. After the weight begins to increase (i.e., 500 grams a week at an additional 3500-7000 kcal per week), family and personal psychotherapy starts; this is beneficial for improving social skills, assistance with formation of mature personality and development of independence.

Medical management (method of Ukraine)

Taking into account the severity of this patient's somatic state, this person receives intravenous administration of 10% glucose (from 200 to 400 ml) with addition of insulin from 2 to 6 units (10 infusions maximum). The patients can be prescribed vitamin therapy that includes intramuscular injections of vitamins B_1, B_6, C (i.e., 5-15 injections), and oral multivitamins. Since anemia is a common complication of malnutrition in AN, ferrous sulfate or ferrous fumarate preparations are often given in an age-adjusted dose and also intramuscular injection of vitamin B_{12}.

For normalization of cardiovascular activity, clinicians in the Ukraine and other countries use various drug mixtures such as cardiomin (aminophylline) and panangin (i.e., potassium and magnesium asparaginat) as well as intramuscular ATP (adenosine triphosphate). The majority of patients with secondary gastritis and colitis can be prescribed spasmolytics (i.e., hyoscine butylbromide), antacids and adsorbent preparations. For persistent constipations lactulose is often beneficial.

For prophylaxis and treatment of osteoporosis and regulation of osseous metabolism calcitriol is recommended since it has a beneficial effect based on it being the most active metabolite of vitamin D (1,25 dihydroxycholecalciferol). The course of treatment lasts from 3-6 months. The treatment must start with a minimum dose to monitor calcium levels in blood (i.e., serum electrolytes, bone profile) weekly. The preparation dose can be increased by 0.25 mcg. When the minimum therapeutic dose is reached, calcium levels are checked in 3-5 weeks. The main mechanisms of action of calcitriol and alfacalcidol (1,25-hydroxycholecolciferol) are in noted in Table 1.

Table 1. Mechanisms of action for calcitriol and alfacalcidol

• increase of calcium and phosphorus absorption in the GI tract; • increase of calcium reabsorption in kidneys; • correction of bone mineralization and osteoblastic stimulation; • decrease of parathyroid hormone levels in blood.
Main effects: • restoration of positive calcium balance; • decreased risk of fractures; • reduction of musculoskeletal pain; • improvement in neuro-muscular conductivity and reduction in manifestation of chronic fatigue syndrome.

Psychopharmacologic management

In terms of management of eating behavior, several mediators are involved. For instance, serotonin (monoamine neurotransmitter) causes the feeling of satiety, which is why high levels of serotonin lead to ceased ingestion and desire of food. Duration of food consumption is regulated by hormones, such as cholecystokinin. Adrenergic substances can enhance as well as suppress food cravings depending on the individual body state. Opioid and dopaminergic substances stimulate enjoyment of the meals.

There are no published clinical research trials using pharmacologic agents for eating disorders in children and adolescents (38). Thus, clinicians often use their personal experience in this area. From the first days of treatment psychotropic medications (the initial dose of which is dependent on the severity of weight loss) may be prescribed alongside with the above mentioned therapy and a thorough regime of observation and nutrition. Olanzapine has been shown to be effective in treating some aspects of AN, including helping to increase the body mass index and reduce obsessions (40).

In order to prevent social isolation and phobia of eating, benzodiazepines (diazepam from 2,5 to 10 mg; phenazepam from 0.5 to 1.5 mg/day) are used; attention to potential side effects must be given by clinicians. In order to prevent anxiety and deactualization of dysmorphophobia disorders, Ukrainian clinicians may use a benzamide (benzoic acid derivative), such as sulpiride (an antipsychotic agent---initial dose of 20-100 mg/day) as long as the somatic state is improving. As an atypical antipsychotic, it acts as anti-anxiolytic and helps to improve insomnia. In one of the author's (LM) experience, sulpiride has an antiemetic effect which is particularly important for bulimic patients.

The patients who suffer from persistent vomiting may benefit from combination of antipsychotics, such as piperazine phenothiazine (perphenazine) with another phenothiazine (chlorpromazine), in which the antiemetic effect of these preparations is shown to be of benefit. The combination of a butyrophenone (haloperidol) and a phenothiazine (trifluoperazine) could also be used. Other antipsychotics may be used, as atypical types; however, they are not United States Food and Drug Administration (FDA) approved for anorexia nervosa in adolescents and should be used with caution as well as with clear understanding of potential side effects (40,41).

If patients exhibit symptoms of delirious dysmorphomania or dysmorphomanic reactions during periods of exacerbation of personal anxiety, they could benefit from treatment with a combination of atypical antipsychotics including risperidone at a dose of 2 mg/day.

If depressive, anxiophobic and obsessive-compulsive phenomena dominate, then the doses of antipsychotics should be gradually increased with careful monitoring for benefit versus adverse effects. The selective serotonin reuptake inhibitor (SSRI), fluoxetine, has been used to manage bulimia in adolescents with bulimia nervosa (38). Also, with bulimic disorders, the psychoactive drugs, benzodiazepines, can be used in microdoses along with selective serotonin reuptake inhibitors (i.e., fluoxetine up to 60 mg/day). Non-hormonal stimulation therapy in the form of cyclical vitamin therapy, biogenic stimulators, and herbal therapy may utilized, though this is not FDA-approved.

In one of the author's (LM) experience, St. John's wort preparation (1 dragee of helarium hypericum contains 255-285 mg of dried extract) has also shown beneficial antidepressant and anxiolytic effects. The preparation is taken as 1 dragee three times daily for 4 to 5 weeks per course. Considering negative stigma attached to the use of antipsychotics and negative attitudes of some patients' parents towards it, St. John's wort may have an advantage. The parents much prefer their children being treated on the outpatient basis with such a herbal preparation, which is perceived to be of a lower toxicity and with fewer side-effects, compared to inpatient care with antipsychotic therapy. Clinicians must understand, however, that this is not FDA-approved for use in management of eating disorders or depression.

Pharmacologic management of gynecologic conditions

The hormonal therapy at the very first stages of AN may be advantageous, because progressive oligomenorrhea can lead to secondary amenorrhea with hypotrophic changes in the sexual and reproductive system; these include decreasing uterus size seen on ultrasound and absence of sufficient proliferative changes in the endometrium. In the case of AN manifesting in young girls prior to menarche and/or with delayed sexual development, hormonal medications should be used with close monitoring of secondary sexual characteristics' development and ultrasound changes of the uterine size, including utero-cervical ratio (UCR) measurements (8).

Hormonal therapy is prescribed with the aim of prophylaxis of secondary hypotrophic changes of the sexual and reproductive system, as well as prophylaxis of reduction in bone density and osteopenia which is associated with AN (42). Small doses of estrogens exhibit stimulating effects on the hypothalamic-pituitary function, improves mood and helps to increase body weight. Clinical experience regarding treating patients with disorders of menstrual cycle with the background of anorexia shows positive effects of small dose estrogen therapy (ethinyl estradiol —0.05 mg) during the first and second stages of AN; this includes the cases of menstrual cycle disorders associated with low BMI. If by the start of treatment, the patient presents with dystrophic changes of the sexual and reproductive systems, management should be started with small doses of estrogens in a continuous two to three months course with ultrasound monitoring.

After two to three courses of ethinyl estradiol, it is recommended to change to transdermal estrogen (0.5 mg once daily trans-dermally for 21 days) (33). With sufficient manifestation of proliferative changes in the endometrium (thickness of endometrium more than 6 mm), it is possible to substitute with cyclical hormonal therapy; this includes progesterone (1% 1.0 ml IM once daily for 7 days, from day 21 to day 28 of menstrual cycle), norethisterone (5 mg once daily for 7 days), or dydrogesterone (10 mg twice daily from day 16 to day 28 of the menstrual cycle).

As it has been already noted, dystrophic changes in the sexual and reproductive system are accompanied by reduction of uterine receptor sensitivity to sex steroids. As a result, the beneficial effects of substitutive hormonal therapy (namely, the rate of proliferative changes in endometrium and size of the uterus) may be inadequate or delayed.

Post-hospitalization therapy

Follow-up is required after hospitalization for AN. Such treatment of AN patients could be undertaken in a pediatric gynecology outpatient setting with involvement of a multidisciplinary approach that includes a psychiatrist, psychologist and occupational therapist (22). Long-term amenorrhea accompanied by dystrophic changes in sexual and reproductive health can lead to infertility. In any patient presenting with amenorrhea, one must exclude AN, treat it accordingly and be able to recognize severe (i.e., prognostically unfavorable) disease stages. In this light prescription of sex steroids may be considered as an attempt to provide prophylaxis of secondary uterine hypertrophy with maintenance of its function.

Psychological therapy

The patient's goal should be to reach normal weight which is maintained for six months. The basis of outpatient treatment consists of psychotherapy; this is directed to the patient's psychological support, distraction from persistent thoughts of weight control as well as concerns about her figure, problem-solving techniques, teaching to control food bingeing in provoking situations and development of a healthy as well as well-adapted psycho-emotional environment. Psychotherapy is recommended as often as once per week for up to 20 sessions in six months. Family therapy, which assumes participation of all the family members, is helpful as adjuvant AN therapy.

Predisposing personality traits (especially in premorbid states) and psychogenic factors (which is important as a "disease-start mechanisms") play important roles in the pathogenesis of AN; thus, it is necessary for early prophylaxis. This must start from an early age and should be directed to harmonious development of one's personality as a whole as well as creating a healthy and adaptable psycho-emotional environment.

Even the most trivial psychological problems arising from psychosomatic disorders affect the social activity and may limit self-actualization. Other issues to be addressed include partial or complete loss of coping mechanisms, feeling 'defective' in one way or another and dependence on doctors as well as medications. As a solution to this, change in social role by means of patient involvement in their psychological as well as physical wellbeing may be beneficial. Therefore, a psycho-corrective approach during treatment of AN patients and the rehabilitation of adolescent girls is important to prevent further relapses.

Treatment of AN by psychotherapeutic strategies should be tailored to suit individual personality traits of these adolescent girls. A psychotherapeutic course is recommended continuously for 15 days, then once weekly over the following three months. After a month break, the course is continued for another three months with once weekly sessions. Individual sessions are carried out every two months over 1-2 years.

Group psychotherapy allows for 4 to 5 patients with AN to be present at the session. During psychotherapy different techniques are used, such as neuro-linguistic programming (NLP) and techniques aimed at development of active imagination, symbol drama and creative self-expression therapy. In the symbol drama not only the positive dynamics of food behavior are noted, but also depressive and other symptoms (such as autism or demonstrativeness) may improve in AN patients.

The psychotherapy approach should focus on formation of the patient's personal maturity and development of independence adequate to the patient's age. The treatment should be directed to body weight restoration which could be achieved by cognitive behavioral therapy (CBT). Family psychotherapy is also important to achieve the best results. The combination of "nonspecific" and "specific" treatment with psychotherapy enables developing and establishing a stable as well as desirable style of food behavior in those with stable improvement.

Bulimia nervosa

Bulimia nervosa (BN) diagnostic criteria is essentially the same in DSM-5 (2013) as it was in DSM-IV (1994)---except that the 2013 edition cuts down the minimal frequency of binge eating and related behaviors ("compensatory" behaviors) to once a week (versus a minimum of twice weekly in DSM-IV) (23). BN could manifest in combination with depressive mood and low self-esteem. More than 80% of these patients induce vomiting and may abuse laxatives or diuretics in order to prevent food digestion and consequent absorption into their gastrointestinal systems (22). In order to stop the weight gain, these patients often diet and engage in excessive physical exercise, which can lead to exhaustion. However, in most cases, this is ineffective as the majority of patients with BN have normal or slightly raised BMI.

Patients with bulimia, unlike those having anorexia nervosa, are more impulsive and not only in terms of food binging, but also in the use of medications and alcohol. They are more prone to suicidal attempts and are less selective in sexual relationship as well as exhibiting other attributes of personal dissatisfaction. It is often difficult to differentiate between symptoms and behaviors in AN and BN. About 40% of patients with AN also have bulimic episodes. There are two subtypes of BN, those with vomiting and those without vomiting. Table 2 outlines diagnostic criteria for bulimia nervosa.

Table 2. Diagnostic criteria of bulimia nervosa

Repeated episodes of binging with the following features: • Ingestion of large volume of food for the fixed time interval (for example, for 2 hours) which would exceed the recommended daily calorific intake • Feeling of losing self-control during meals, for example, inability to control how much and what one has eaten • Self-provoked vomiting • Overuse of laxatives, diuretics • Periods of fasting/ starvation • Excessive physical exercise • Episodes on average recur at least once a week in 3 months • Feeling of guilt, depression, social isolation, anxiety, suicidal ideations • Distorted body image influences self-esteem • Does not necessarily arise with episodes of anorexia nervosa

Conclusion

Medical clinicians (i.e., pediatricians, adolescent medicine specialists, pediatric and adolescent gynecologists, family doctors) should be able to recognize the features of AN at first contact with adolescent girls even on outpatient basis. Discussing the features of these patients' diet and desirable body weight is essential in order to get to the bottom of their perception of self, ideal weight, and the ways they are utilizing to achieve it.

It is important to educate parents and young children about physiological body changes in the pre- and pubertal periods, marked by characteristically plump appearance. Furthermore, it is necessary to make sure these patients understand the role of body weight in normal pubertal development on other organs and functions in the body. This may aid to resist harmful illusions of desire to weigh as much (i.e., as little) as a model from a fashion magazine.

The patients in the high-risk groups for AN must be asked the following questions: "Do you feel you have any problems related to eating habits?", and "Do you have any concerns about your weight? If so, do you feel these are excessive?"

The importance of body image in the media should not be underestimated as it influences young girls in the way they want to look, which can lead to development of food disorders. Care should also be taken by medical staff when recommending adolescent girls lose some weight.

In spite of the fact that gynecologists and other clinicians are not able to influence existing risk factors for anorexia nervosa, early recognition of the disease and prompt treatment considerably improve the outcome. Adequate awareness of eating disorders in primary care and the ability to involve these patients in their treatment plans are extremely important for prevention of serious and hazardous complications of anorexia nervosa. Management is a combination of astute attention to medical and psychological complications of this complex condition that can be challenged by various issues of resistance, COVID-19 pandemic of 2019-2022 and others (22,37,38,43-60).

Acknowledgements

This chapter is an updated and revised version of Matytsina L, Greydanus DE, Babenko-Sorocopud IV, Matytsina L. Anorexia nervosa in adolescence: Current concepts of medical and psychological assessment and management. Int J Child Adolesc Health 2014;7(3):167-81.

References

[1] Hebebrand J, Casper R, Treasure J, Schweiger J. Need to revise the diagnostic criteria for anorexia nervosa. J Neural Transm 2004;111(7):827-40.
[2] Pearce JMS. Richard Morton: Origins of anorexia nervosa. Eur Neurol 2004;(52):191-2.
[3] Reijonen JH, Pratt HD, Patel DR, Greydanus DE. Eating disorders in the adolescent population: an overview. J Adolesc Res 2003;18(3):209-22.
[4] Treasure J, Claudino AM, Zucker N. Eating disorders. Lancet 2010;375(9714):583– 93.
[5] Matytsina LA. Importance of diagnose and treatment of psycho emotional disorders in adolescent girls with amenorrhea (clinical case analysis). Ukrainian Medical Almanac 2001;4(3):114-8.
[6] Hoek HW. Incidence, prevalence and mortality of anorexia nervosa and other eating disorders. Curr Opin Psychiatry 2006;19(4):389–94.
[7] Gowers S, Bryant-Waugh R. Management of child and adolescent eating disorders: the current evidence base and future directions. J Child Psychol Psychiatr 2004;45(1):63–83.
[8] Matytsina LA, Babenko-Sorocopud IV. Anorexia nervosa in adolescent girl (clinical lecture)-- medico-social family problems. Women's Health 2003;8(4):120-7.
[9] Pratt HD, Phillips EL, Greydanus DE, Patel DR. Eating disorders in the adolescent population: future directions. J Adolesc Res 2003;18(3):297-317.
[10] Wade TD, Bulik CM, Neale M, Kendler KS. Anorexia nervosa and major depression: shared genetic and environmental risk factors. Am J Psychiatr 2000;157(3):469–71.
[11] Watts AG, Sanchez-Watts G, Kelly AB. Distinct patterns of neuropeptide gene expression in the lateral hypothalamic area and arcuate nucleus are associated with dehydration-induced anorexia. J Neurosci 1999;19(14):6111-21.
[12] Kortegaard LS, Hoerder K, Joergensen J, Gillberg C, Kyvik KO. A preliminary population-based twin study of self-reported eating disorder. Psychol Med 2001; 31(2):361-5.
[13] Klump KL, Miller KB, Keel PK, McGue M, Iocono WG. Genetic and environmental influences on anorexia nervosa syndromes in a population–based twin sample. Psychol Med 2001;31(4):737-40.
[14] Hoek HW. The distribution of eating disorders. In: Brownell KD, Fairburn CG, eds. Eating disorders and obesity: a comprehensive handbook. New York: Guilford, 1995;207-11.
[15] Graber JA, Tyrka AR, Brooks-Gunn J. How similar are correlates of different subclinical eating problems and bulimia nervosa? J Child Psychol Psychiatr 2003;44:262-73.
[16] Lucas AR, Crowson CS, O'Fallon WM, Melton LJ 3rd. The ups and downs of anorexia nervosa. Int J Eat Disord 1999;26:397-405.
[17] Makino M, Tsuboi K, Dennerstein L. Prevalence of eating disorders: A comparison of western and non-western countries. MedGenMed 2004;6(3):49.
[18] Rooney B, McLelland L, Crisp AH, Sedgwick PM. The incidence and prevalence of anorexia nervosa in three suburban health districts in south west London, UK. Int J Eat Disord 1995;18:299-307.
[19] Gray R. The performance identities of Lady Gaga. Jefferson, NC: McFarland, 2012:33–51.
[20] Thomas JJ, Vartanian LR, Brownell KD. The relationship between eating disorder not otherwise specified (EDNOS) and officially recognized eating disorders: meta-analysis and implications for DSM. Psychol Bull 2009;135(3):407–33.

[21] Lindberg L, Hjern A. Risk factors for anorexia nervosa: A national cohort study. Int J Eat Disord 2003;34(4):397–408.

[22] Vinch J, Reddy VN. Eating disorders. In: Greydanus DE, Patel DR, Pratt HD, Calles JL Jr, Merrick J, eds. Behavioral pediatrics, 4th edition. New York: Nova Biomedical, 2015:353-71.

[23] Strober M, Freeman R, Morrell W. The long-term course of severe anorexia nervosa in adolescents: Survival analysis of recovery, relapse, outcome predictors over 10-15 years in a prospective study. Int J Eat Dis 1997;22(4):339–60.

[24] Esposito C, Bellotti N, Fasoli G, Foschi A, Plati AR, Dal Canton A. Hyperkalemia-induced ECG abnormalities in patients with reduced renal function. Clin Nephrol 2004; 62(6):465–8.

[25] Eating disorders: Anorexia and bulimia nervosa. In: Collier J, Longmore M, Amarakone K. Oxford handbook of clinical specialties. Oxford: Oxford University Press, 2006:348-9.

[26] American Psychiatric Association. Diagnostic and Statistical Manual of Mental Disorders, 5th ed (DSM-5). Washington, DC: American Psychiatric Association, 2013:338-50.

[27] Golden NH, Jacobson MS, Schebendach, J, Solanto MV, Hertz SM, Shenker IR. Resumption of menses in anorexia nervosa Arch Pediatr Adolesc Med 1997;151(1):16-21.

[28] Matytsina LA, Babenko-Sorocopud IV. Case of secondary amenorrhea in adolescent girl with anorexia nervosa. Women's Health 2003;4(16):87-91.

[29] Brooks ER, Ogden BW, Cavalier DS. Compromised bone density 11.4 years after diagnosis of anorexia nervosa. J Womens Health 1998;7:567-74.

[30] McAnarney ER, Greydanus DE, Campanella VA, Hoekelman RA. Rib fractures and anorexua nervosa. J Adolesc Health Care 1983;2(1):40-3.

[31] Patel DR, Greydanus DE, Pratt HD. Eating disorders in adolescent athletes. J Adolesc Res 2003;18(3):280-96.

[32] Mitchella JE, Crowb S. Medical complications of anorexia nervosa and bulimia nervosa. Curr Opin Psychiatry 2006;19:438–43.

[33] Matytsina LA. Primary amenorrhea in adolescent girls: definition, prevalence, classification. Paediatr Obstet Gynecol;2001(4):140-2.

[34] Loucks AB. Energy availability and infertility. Curr Opin Endocrinol Diabetes Obes 2007;14(6):470–4.

[35] Rosenvinge JH, Martinussen M, Ostensen E. The comorbidity of eating disorders and personality disorders: a meta-analytic review of studies published between 1983 and 1998. Eat Weight Disord 2000;5(2):52–61.

[36] Greydanus D, Patel D, Pratt H. Female athlete triad part I. Southwest Mich Med J 2004;1(1):28-31.

[37] Patel DR, Pratt HD, Greydanus DE. Treatment of adolescents with anorexia nervosa J Adolesc Res 2003;18(3):244-60.

[38] Golden NH, Attia E. Psychopharmacology of eating disorders in children and adolescents. Pediatr Clin North Am 2011;58(1):121-38.

[39] Bissada H, Tasca GA, Barber AM, Bradwejn J. Olanzapine in the treatment of low body weight and obsessive thinking in women with anorexia nervosa: A randomized, double-blind, placebo-controlled trial. Am J Psychiatry 2008;165(10):1281–8.

[40] Greydanus DE, Calles Jr J, Patel DR, Nazeer A, Merrick J, eds. Clinical aspects of psychopharmacology in childhood and adolescence, 2nd Ed.. New York: Nova Biomedical, 2017.

[41] Nazeer A, Calles JL. Schizophrenia. In: Greydanus DE, Patel DR, Omar HA, Feucht C, Merrick J, eds. Adolescent medicine: Pharmacotherapeutics in general, mental and sexual health. Berlin: Walter de Gruyter, 2012:269-81.

[42] Gordon CM, Grace E, Emans SJ. Effects of oral dehydroepiandrosterone on bone density in young women with anorexia nervosa. J Bone Miner Res 1999;14:136-45.

[43] Golden NH. Eating disorders: Anorexia nervosa and bulimia nervosa in the adolescent. In: Greydanus DE, Patel DR, Pratt HD, eds. Essential adolescent medicine. New York: McGraw-Hill Medical, 2006:635-50.

[44] Mitchell JE, Roerig J, Steffen K. Biological therapies for eating disorders. Int J Eat Dis 2013;46(5):470-7.

[45] Moukhaiber S, Piette C, Triffaux JM. Starving to death: the paradox of anorexia nervoxa. Rev Med Liege 2016;71(11):495-51. [French]

[46] Fox JR, Dean M, Whittlesea A. The experience of caring for or living with an individual with an eating disorder: A meta-synthesis of qualitative studies. Clin Psychol Psychother 2017;24(1):103-25.

[47] Fox JR, Whittlesea A. Accommodation of symptoms in anorexia nervosa: a qualitative study. Clin Psychol Psychother 2017;24(2):488-500.

[48] Munro C, Randell L, Lawrie SM. An integrative bio-psycho-social theory of anorexia nervosa. Clin Psychol Psychother 2017;24(1):1-21.

[49] Monteleone AM, Castellini G, Volpe U, Ricca V, Lelli L, Monteleone P, et al. Neuroendocrinology and brain imaging of reward in eating disorders: a possible key to the treatment of anorexia nervosa and bulimia nervosa. Prog Neuropsychopharmacol Biol Psychiatry 2017 Mar 1. pii: S0278-5846(16)30488-2. doi: 10.1016/j.pnpbp.2017.02.020.

[50] Treasure J, Cardi V. Anorexia nervosa, theory and treatment: where are we 35 years on from Hilde Bruch's foundation lecture? Eur Eat Disord Rev 2017;25(3):139-47.

[51] Haripersad YV, Kannegiesser-Bailey M, Morton K, Skeldon S, Shipton N, Edwards K, et al. Outbreak of anorexia nervosa admissions during the COVID-19 pandemic. Arch Dis Child 2021;106(3):e15.

[52] Muratore AF, Attia E. Current therapeutic approaches to anorexia nervosa: State of the art. Clin Ther 2021;43(1):85-94.

[53] Smith S, Woodside DB. Characterizing treatment-resistant anorexia nervosa. Front Psychiatry 2021;11:542206.

[54] Bou Khalil R. Targeting all psychopathological dimensions in the treatment of anorexia nervosa. Encephale 2021;47(1):79-81.

[55] Meule A, Schrambke D, Furst Loredo A, Schlegl S, Naab S, Voderholzer U. Inpatient treatment of anorexia nervosa in adolescents: A 1-year follow-up study. Eur Eat Disord Rev 2021;29(2):165-77.

[56] Himmerich H, Kan C, Au K, Treasure J. Pharmacological treatment of eating disorders, comorbid mental health problems, malnutrition and physical health consequences. Pharmacol Ther 2021;217:107667.

[57] Ehrlich S, Tam FI. Editorial: Refeeding in anorexia nervosa: Quo vadis? J Am Acad Child Adolesc Psychiatry 2021;60(5):566-7.

[58] Hiney-Saunders K, Ousley L, Caw J, Cassinelli E, Waller G. Effectiveness of treatment for adolescents and adults with anorexia nervosa in a routine residential setting. Eat Disord 2021;29(1):103-17.

[59] Williams R, Smith M, Wright D. Anorexia: a literature review of young people's experiences of hospital treatment. Nurs Child Young People 2021;33(2):10-7.

[60] Greydanus DE, Bacopoulou F, Apostolaki D. Gynecological features of eating disorders. In: Omar HA, Greydanus DE, Patel DR, Merrick J, eds. Pediatric and adolescent sexuality and Gynecology: Principles for the primary care clinician, Second edition. New York: Nova Science, 2021:565-88.

Chapter 14

Gynecological and behavioral features of eating disorders

Donald E. Greydanus[1,*], MD, DrHC (Athens), Flora Bacopoulou[2], MD, IFEPAG, PhD and Despoina Apostolaki[2], MD, IFEPAG

[1]Department of Pediatric and Adolescent Medicine, Western Michigan University Homer Stryker M.D. School of Medicine, Kalamazoo, Michigan, United States of America

[2]Center for Adolescent Medicine and UNESCO Chair on Adolescent Health Care, First Department of Pediatrics, School of Medicine, National and Kapodistrian University of Athens, Aghia Sophia Children's Hospital, Goudi, Athens, Greece

Abstract

Gynecologic features of eating disorders include relationships to puberty, fertility effects, and the low estrogen underpinnings of eventual osteopenia as well as osteoporosis. It is concluded that clinicians should provide judicious observation for potential eating disorders in pubertal females along with prompt management of anorexia nervosa, bulimia nervosa, or other eating disorders that may be arise in children, adolescents and adults.

Introduction

Eating disorders (EDs) in females include anorexia nervosa (AN) with a prevalence of 1.4% (0.1-3.6%) and bulimia nervosa (BN) with a prevalence of 1.9% (0.3-4.6%) (1-3). Eating disorders may occur less commonly in males but are not considered in this treatise (2, 3). This discussion (see Table 1) considers various gynecologic features or complications of these eating disorders (i.e., anorexia and bulimia nervosa) in adolescent females. The potential inter-relationship between eating disorders and puberty is now considered as well as genetic influences and potential effects of abuse.

* *Correspondence:* Professor Donald E Greydanus, MD, DrHC (Athens), Founding Chair, Department of Pediatric and Adolescent Medicine, Western Michigan University Homer Stryker MD School of Medicine, 1000 Oakland Drive, D48G, Kalamazoo, MI 49008-1284, United States. Email: Donald.greydanus@med.wmich.edu.

In: Behavioral Pediatrics II
Editors: Donald E. Greydanus, Dilip R. Patel, Ahsan Nazeer et al.
ISBN: 979-8-88697-019-7

Table 1. Outline of discussion

- Eating disorders and puberty
  1. Physical changes of puberty
  2. Reactions to puberty
  3. Genetic influences
  4. Eating disorders and abuse
- Eating disorders and associated gynecologic effects
  1. Amenorrhea
  2. Fertility and pregnancy
  3. Bone loss, osteopenia and amenorrhea
  4. Sexual dysfunction
- Gynecologic Evaluation
  1. History
  2. Physical examination
  3. Management
- Conclusions

Eating disorders and puberty

During puberty, several psychosocial and biological events take place; indeed, puberty is considered a significant risk period for the development of eating disorders in girls (4, 5). Studies exploring rates of eating disorders in children versus adolescents show significantly increased prevalence of all forms of eating disorders in individuals in mid-late adolescence as compared to pre-adolescence. In addition, studies examining rates of eating disorders by pubertal status and timing show that girls who are at more advanced stages of pubertal development demonstrate increased rates of EDs (4). Also, eating disorders can have effects on growth and puberty such as growth restriction and pubertal delay (6).

Physical changes of puberty

The onset of puberty in *Homo sapiens* leads to classic changes in physical characteristics, sexual maturation, body composition alterations and heightened body (skeletal) growth (7). In over 8 out of 10 girls, breast development is the first clinical indication of puberty that typically occurs between 8 and 13 years of age (7, 8). In the classic Tanner stage of maturation (sexual maturity rating; SMR) from 1 (pre-pubertal stage) to 5 (adult stage), SMR 2 in females or Tanner breast stage 2 was noted at estimated mean age of 10.88 years in a 1991 study and 9.86 years in a 2006 study (9). Menarche or age of menstruation initiation is typically two years after thelarche and was noted at 13.42 years in the 1991 group of females as well as 13.13 years in the 2006 group (9).

Recent data from girls in low and middle-income countries notes that pooled mean age estimates of Tanner stage (breast stage) 2 was 10.4 years (9.2-11.6 with 95% CI) for normal girls, 10.2 years (9.3 to 11.4 years) for thin girls, and 8.4 years (6.8 to 10.0 years) for overweight girls based on body mass index (BMI) (10). In another study, menarche occurred at 13.0 years of age and SMR or Tanner Breast stage 5 occurred at 15.8 years of age (11).

The classic growth in puberty involves peak height velocity that is typically at age 12 years in females after thelarche versus age 14 years in boys (7). Lean body mass (i.e., mainly muscle mass) starts to increase in early puberty for girls (as well as boys) while increase in fat mass is classic for females in the later pubertal stages; however, overweight/obese conditions can result in earlier fat mass accumulation and earlier onset of puberty as well as increased height versus same-age peers due to increased leptin and androgen levels (7, 12, 13).

Reactions to puberty

Such dramatic changes to girls and boys during puberty induces a variety of emotional reactions that may stimulate an eating disorder in some teenagers. Mean body fat as part of overall weight can rise from 8% in childhood to over 22% in puberty; as early pubertal girls can have increased height as well as weight, in contrast to same-age male peers, concerns about appearance may arise that can be exacerbated by peer-teasing and underlying anxiety/depression that puberty can worsen in some teenagers (7, 8, 14).

Some girls learn that an anorexic approach to food may result in transient improvement in anxiety that research relates to lowered serotonin (14). Though such teasing may contribute to the development of an eating disorder in some youth, major life stresses are known to trigger eating disorders in some while difficulties with sexuality are known to stimulate the beginning of anorexia nervosa in some as well (15). The role of sexuality and sexual activity initiation in the development of eating disorders remains under study (15-21). The role of hormonal variations in puberty can influence some with eating disorder formation or influence, as noted by research describing increased testosterone with menstrual irregularities and acne in some females with bulimia (22).

Genetic influences

Links of depression and/or anxiety in some pubertal females with eating disorders remain under study, but seems to be, in part, linked to genetic as well as psychosocial factors (16, 17). Some data confirm that associations between early pubertal timing and key disordered eating symptoms are due to genetic rather than environmental risk factors (23, 24).

Findings from twin studies provide support for a role of genetic factors in increased risk for eating disorders in girls. Genetic influences appear to become "activated" during the pubertal period and may increase phenotypic risk for the disorders in girls (25-27). Dramatic increases in genetic effects that have been observed across adolescence are also attributed to estrogen activation during puberty. These changes are not present in boys, providing further, indirect support for pubertal hormone influences on risk for eating disorders in girls (27-29).

Eating disorders and abuse

Various factors can influence puberty as well as the development of eating disorders and menstrual dysfunction in complex ways; these include abuse in various forms such as bullying, physical abuse, sexual abuse and others (30, 31). In a national study of women in the United States, a history of sexual assault was significantly increased in those with bulimia nervosa

(32). Other research has linked sexual abuse with development of eating disorders in females as well (33-40).

Eating disorders and associated gynecologic effects

This article now considers gynecologic effects of eating disorders that includes amenorrhea, fertility/pregnancy, and osteopenia/osteoporosis with amenorrhea.

Amenorrhea

A classic gynecologic effect of anorexia nervosa (AN) with malnutrition is functional amenorrhea. Amenorrhea is often classified as either *primary* (i.e., absence of menarche by age 15 years or thereafter) or *secondary* (i.e., absence of menses for more than three months in girls or women who previously had regular menstrual cycles or six months in girls or women who had irregular menses) (41). A diagnostic criterion for anorexia nervosa in women in the American Psychiatric Association's 2000 "Diagnostic and statistical manual of mental disorders, Fourth Edition, Text Revision (DSM-IV TR)" was three cycles or more of secondary amenorrhea; it also noted that primary amenorrhea with weight loss and body-image alteration was representative of an EDNOS (eating disorder not otherwise specified) (42).

In the 2013 "Diagnostic and statistical manual of mental disorders-5th edition (DSM-5)," amenorrhea has been removed as a criterion for anorexia nervosa because its use was never validated, the DSM-5 also excluded males, premenarchal females, and adolescents who remain eumenorrheic despite low body weight (3). However, amenorrhea is still considered as a frequent occurrence in patients with AN and appears to be an indicator of physiological dysfunction (3, 43, 44). If present, amenorrhea is usually a consequence of the weight loss, but in a minority of individuals it may actually precede the weight loss; also, in prepubertal females, menarche may be delayed (45, 46). Some females with anorexia nervosa and amenorrhea relate that it is a "pleasant" issue that allows them to avoid the potential unpleasantness (aches, pains, others) of menstruation and a sense of being "more clean" or "more pure" without such bleeding.

In patients with anorexia nervosa, secretion of gonadotropin releasing hormone is reduced followed by decreased secretion of gonadotropins, which ultimately prevents ovulation and causes functional hypothalamic amenorrhea (FHA) as well as reversion to a pre-pubertal state with low serum estradiol concentrations (47). Weight gain usually restores normal menstrual cycles which is considered a physiologic marker for recovery from anorexia nervosa. There are several published methods predicting the weight an anorexic patient needs to attain in order to resume menses (48-51).

Amenorrheic women have lower leptin levels and less body fat than menstruating women of similar weight, suggesting that a certain proportion of fat mass is needed to preserve menstrual function (44, 52-54). In addition, weight gain and increases in fat mass lead to increases in leptin levels, associated with a resumption of menses (55).

Menstrual irregularity or amenorrhea occurs in about one half of females with bulimia nervosa as well as low levels of both estradiol and progesterone (56-58). It is uncertain whether such disturbances are related to weight fluctuations, to nutritional deficiencies, or to emotional distress (59, 60).

Functional hypothalamic amenorrhea (FHA) and polycystic ovary syndrome (PCOS) may coexist and as patients recover, manifestations of PCOS may emerge, including irregular menses. Women that are normoandrogenic with PCOS morphology and elevated anti-müllerian hormone (AMH) levels are at high risk for hyperandrogenic PCOS when hypothalamic function normalizes (61). Furthermore, one study suggested that women with FHA and underlying PCOS had higher BMI, bone mineral density (BMD), luteinizing hormone (LH) as well as testosterone concentrations, and incidence of hyperandrogenism compared with women with FHA; they also exhibited increased hyperandrogenism and irregular menses with weight gain. However, they seemed to be at similar risk for developing osteopenia and osteoporosis (62).

Fertility and Pregnancy

Fertility dysfunction may occur in females with anorexia nervosa due to various factors, including severe malnourishment, amenorrhea and rejection of sexual behavior; however, clinicians should instruct even such malnourished females that they can ovulate and become pregnant (63-66). Such pregnancies may not be planned partially due to the belief of some females with eating disorders that pregnancy is not possible and thus, contraception is not needed with sexual activity. In one study, the rate of unplanned pregnancy and abortion was higher in women with anorexia nervosa compared to women with no eating disorder: 50 versus 19 percent and 24 versus 15 percent respectively (67).

Pregnancy in anorexia nervosa is associated with a greater incidence of complications including miscarriages, premature birth, smaller head circumference, and low-birth-weight infants, especially if the disease is active (68-76). The exact risks vary in different studies and many variables can complicate these outcomes such as overall weight gain, substance use or abuse during pregnancy and many others. For example, relative to unexposed women, women with anorexia nervosa had, on average, a lower body weight but a higher rate of weight gain subsequently; also, women with bulimia nervosa had a higher body weight but a lower rate of weight gain (77).

It is noted that patients with anorexia nervosa may conceal their eating disorder when seeking treatment for infertility (63). One study of 66 women treated in an infertility clinic revealed that 7.6% had anorexia nervosa or bulimia nervosa; among infertile women with amenorrhea or oligomenorrhea, 58% had eating disorders (78). In a longitudinal prospective birth cohort of 14,663 women, those with anorexia nervosa (OR 1.6, 95% CI 1.1-2.5; $P<0.021$) and women with AN & BN (OR 1.9, 95% CI 1.1-3.4; $P<0.020$) were more likely to have seen a doctor for lifetime fertility problems, and women with AN & BN were also more likely to take longer than 6 months to conceive (OR 1.9, 95% CI 1.0-3.5; $P<0.04$), and to have conceived the current pregnancy with fertility treatment (79).

Unplanned pregnancies were more common in the AN group compared with the general population. All eating disorder groups more frequently experienced negative feelings upon discovering their pregnancy, which remained higher in the AN & BN group at 18 weeks of gestation (79). Although it is possible for amenorrheic women to conceive by inducing ovulation, the presence of active anorexia nervosa is commonly felt to be a contraindication for this type of infertility treatment.

Contraception should be offered by the clinician caring for a sexually active female (adolescent or adult) who has an eating disorder. Also, a pregnant female with a history of eating disorders (active disease or past history) should be followed carefully during the pregnancy; her offspring should be followed carefully as well. Ultrasound measurements of ovaries and uteri in children with anorexia nervosa reveal organs smaller than expected for age while ovarian follicles typically are not seen; this is comparable to that seen in adult females with anorexia nervosa (80, 81). As the person's weight increases, there is also an increase in growth of the uterus and ovaries with menarche typically seen with maturity indicated by appropriate organ size. The accepted weight of the patient can be linked to that which allows menstruation---typically a BMI of 20; however, overt eating patterns may be more important for menstruation with normal ovarian functioning than body mass index per se (82-85). This discussion now considers issues of bone mineral loss, osteopenia and amenorrhea.

Bone mineral loss, osteopenia, and amenorrhea

A classic feature of chronic anorexia with malnutrition is bone mass loss and the failure to accrue normal bone mass (86-88). While in adults, markers of bone resorption are increased and markers of bone formation are decreased, adolescents with anorexia nervosa present with reduction of both bone resorption and formation (89, 90). In one study of 130 young female outpatients with anorexia nervosa (mean age 24 years), 92 percent had osteopenia and 38 percent met World Health Organization (WHO) criteria for osteoporosis (91). Furthermore, BMD including microarchitecture is impaired, bone marrow fat is increased and estimated bone strength is diminished (92-95).

In the healthy and normal process, the osseous mineralization reaches its zenith in the teenage years with a complex development requiring healthy nutrition that particularly includes the minerals calcium and phosphorus in addition to the hormonal effects of regular menstrual cycles. Healthy bone mineralization in the female is linked to the overall estrogen levels along with menses-induced cyclic alterations; the cholesterol-derived estrogen becomes impaired with chronic caloric undernourishment. Even limited times of malnutrition due to anorexia can lead to significant reduction in mineral density (as measured in the lumbar spine as well as total-body computations).

Research notes that various factors result in significantly severe mineral loss and these include chronic illness, reduced menarcheal age, and major fatty tissue deprivation (96, 97). Other factors that contribute to bone loss in addition to estradiol deficiency and nutritional deficiencies are growth hormone (GH) resistance, hypercortisolemia and low testosterone (89, 90, 98-100). Abnormalities in hormones involved in appetite regulation, such as oxytocin, leptin and peptide YY (PYY) may also play a role in bone loss in anorexia nervosa (99, 101-103).

The first step for recovery of normal bone metabolism is correcting the energy imbalance, usually by gaining weight, which eventually leads to a resumption of menses. Evidence shows that weight gain causes preferential increases in bone density of the total hip and whole body, whereas menses resumption leads to preferential increases in bone density at the lumbar spine (104). However, despite these improvements in bone density, normalization of bone mass does not always occur (105). Furthermore, reductions in cortical bone density appear not to be rapidly reversed by recovery from anorexia nervosa and females with anorexia nervosa have increased risks for fractures in contrast to other females---up to seven times (106-108).

Estrogen replacement is considered in adolescents and young women with functional hypothalamic amenorrhea as well as low bone density and/or evidence of skeletal fragility who have not had resumption of menses after a reasonable trial of nutritional, psychological, and/or modified exercise intervention (usually 6 to 12 months). Typically, transdermal estradiol (E2) therapy with cyclic oral progestin is used. Indirect evidence from trials in adolescent girls with AN suggests that physiologic doses of transdermal E2 increase bone accrual rates over 18 months (109, 110). Oral contraceptive pills (OCPs) prescription is not recommended as studies underline limited or no benefit on bone mineral density (BMD) (111-113). Research also notes that exogenous replacement of estrogen does not help restore bone density without concomitant weight restoration (91, 104).

Studies reveal that bone mineral turnover may be improved (normalized) and BMD augmented with use of the endogenous steroid hormone, dehydroepiandrosterone (DHEA; androstenolone) (114). Such an effect is essentially similar to that seen from hormone replacement treatment and if one controls for weight gain, the effect is not significant as noted from research (115).

In addition, the use of bisphosphonates has been noted in some studies to reduce resorption of bone along with augmenting BMD in women who are postmenopausal as well as have osteopenia; however, one study in adolescents with anorexia nervosa found no effect of oral alendronate at the lumbar spine compared with controls---there was though some improvement of bone density at the hip (116).

Some research studies have concluded that spinal bone density was augmented in adult females with anorexia after taking the bisphosphonate, risedronate, even though there was no weight normalization (117). However, these studies were small, used different bisphosphonate formulations as well as protocols, and no study examined efficacy as well as safety in patients with functional hypothalamic amenorrhea (FHA)--outside of an eating disorder. Furthermore, because bisphosphonates reside in bone for up to 10 years, there are concerns that even pre-pregnancy administration of bisphosphonates may result in drug mobilization from the maternal skeleton during pregnancy, with transplacental passage that can result in the potential for fetal teratogenicity. Thus, bisphosphonates are not approved nor recommended to manage adolescent females with bone mineral loss found in anorexia nervosa (108).

The use of other experimental therapies (i.e., denosumab, testosterone, and leptin) to improve BMD in adolescents and women with FHA and low bone density in the context of anorexia nervosa, are still under exploration and are not recommended (108).

Sexual dysfunction

Sexual dysfunctions in eating disorder patients, compared to other psychiatric or medical comorbidities, are infrequently considered in research; however, this is gradually changing with more recent studies (19-21, 118-120). Body image distortion and body dissatisfaction are common features in all eating disorders and this relationship with their bodies has been considered as a possible mediator of the sexual dysfunction. Specifically, lower female sexual index scores were correlated with higher shape concerns measured by means of the eating disorder examination in anorexia nervosa (AN), bulimia nervosa (BN) as well as in binge eating disorder (BED) (118-120).

Research has also noted less positive attitudes and pleasure in sexual behavior in those with eating disorders versus control groups in adult research. The severity of sexual dysfunction has been also associated with frequency of binge eating behaviors in AN binge/purging type, BN and BED patients (121, 122). The decrease of sexual interest in AN patients has also been associated with hypogonadism and emaciation while weight restoration has been reported to favor an increase in sexual drive (123-125).

Although anorexic and bulimic patients suffer from relevant sexual dysfunctions, studies suggest different ways of coping with the developmental challenges in sexuality during adolescence with general attitudes to sexuality and dating experiences being more negative in the AN group than in the BN group (104, 126). Research looking at adult females with BN find they have inner conflicts of wishing close sexual partner relationships compromised by worries about being cast aside; also, they may have intense fears of acting in ways that ruin such relationships as well as being embarrassed and uncomfortable during sexual behavior (127, 128).

The number of partners and sexual intercourses has also been considered as a manifestation of multi-impulsivity, and the rates of specific disordered eating behaviors were associated with higher numbers of sex partners in adult research (129). Indeed, BN patients and AN binge/purging type patients reported higher rate of multiple partners compared with AN restricting type patients (122). Other adult research links sexual dysfunction with a history of eating disorders in females (130, 131). The application of such adult research studies to adolescent females with eating disorders remains an interesting and challenging topic. This discussion now considers issues related to the gynecologic evaluation of persons with eating disorders.

Gynecologic evaluation in eating disorder persons

Screening children and youth for potential eating disorders as well as other problematic conditions/disorders is an important aspect of primary care practice; also, if present, hopefully the eating disorder is not well-advanced when identified (132-134). Table 2 outlines eating disorder screening tools that are available. Gynecologic complications of eating disorders should be considered by clinicians caring for pediatric and adolescent persons (2-5, 14, 57, 63, 106). Eating disorders can occur in pre-pubertal persons and having an eating disorder can influence the reproductive processes; this is particularly seen with anorexia nervosa. Comments are now provided with regard to medical history and physical evaluation of those with eating disorders.

Table 2. Eating disorder screening tools (132-135, 139)

• The Eating disorder screening for primary care (ESP)
• SCOFF Questionnaire
• The Eating Attitudes Test (EAT-26)
• The Eating Disorder Examination (EDE)
• The Questionnaire for Eating Disorder Diagnosis (Q-EDD)
• Others

History

Clinicians should ask the parent (s) of the child being evaluated about the diet and eating habits seen in the child. Children and adolescents can be asked a variety of questions in this regard and as noted, a variety of screening tools are available to guide the clinician (see Table 2) (132-135). As queries are made regarding food intake and habits, a careful menstrual history is also taken of adolescent females. As noted, the cascade of events happening in anorexia nervosa typically leads to secondary amenorrhea. In addition, the presence of primary amenorrhea in one who has not had normal weight gain for age or has had overt weight loss may lead the clinician to provide a work-up for anorexia nervosa. Screening for possible abuse (physical, sexual) in the past and/or present is always part of primary care screening that includes screening for eating disorders (18, 30-40). Clinicians should understand that the youth with an eating disorder may seek to keep issues of weight, diet, and desire for thinness hidden from family, friends, and health care professionals.

Points of physical examination

The youth with anorexia nervosa may present to the clinician's office with clothes that hide her thin or wasting-away appearance; some may even water-load to falsely inflate the weight that potentially can lead to hyponatremia-induced seizure activity. If the patient has been diagnosed with anorexia nervosa, various techniques can be employed by the clinician to weigh the person with minimal clothes (as underwear, examination gown), check a urine specific gravity and others. A youth with cachexia may have no or minimal pubertal development with failure to progress along normal Tanner stages, delayed puberty, reduced height and other features of severe malnutrition (6, 8, 132-138).

Table 3 outlines possible physical features that may be seen in anorexia nervosa while Table 4 outlines possible laboratory findings depending on the chronicity and/or extent of malnutrition that may be present (2, 3, 136-140). Radiologic testing, such as abdominal and pelvic ultrasonography, can use very beneficial in pinpointing the cause of existing primary amenorrhea (84, 85, 96).

Table 3. Physical findings in adolescents with eating disorders (139)

- *General*: Impaired linear growth
- *Skin*: sallow appearance, carotenemia, dry skin, brittle hair and nails, appearance of lanugo hair.
- *Eyes*: subconjunctival hemorrhages (appear after retching and vomiting).
- *Mouth and throat*: dry mucosa (from dehydration), palatal and pharyngeal lacerations (from fingers or other objects used to induce vomiting), erosion of the posterior surfaces of teeth.
- *Chest*: prominent ribs.
- *Lungs*: rales from pulmonary edema due to hypoproteinemia (rare).
- *Heart*: bradycardia, hypotension, orthostatic hypotension, and tachycardia, heart rate lability even at rest; gallop rhythms.
- *Abdomen*: scaphoid with wasting of abdominal wall musculature, hypoactive bowel sounds; palpable stool in descending colon.
- *Back*: prominent vertebrae, lanugo; sacral edema.
- *Extremities*: muscle wasting and prominent joints, lacerations on dorsal knuckles (*Russell sign*); dependent edema
- *Neurologic*: slow mentation, cognitive dysfunction, poor short-term memory.

Table 4. Laboratory findings in adolescents with eating disorders (139)

- Signs of bone marrow suppression, including leukopenia and neutropenia
- Anemia, thrombocytopenia
- Decrease in complement levels, especially C_3 and alternative pathway components
- Deficiency of vitamin K dependent clotting factors
- Hypokalemia (especially in those with bulimia nervosa)
- Elevated blood urea nitrogen
- Hypoglycemia
- Hypocalcemia
- Hypomagnesemia
- Hypophosphatemia
- Hypozincemia
- Hypoproteinemia
- Hypoalbuminemia and low pre-albumin
- Decreased antidiuretic hormone
- Hypo-chloremic metabolic alkalosis with vomiting
- Metabolic acidosis (especially with laxative abuse)
- Elevated amylase with normal lipase
- Others

Management

Table 5 lists various management concepts utilized to treat those with eating disorders (3, 47, 51, 64-70, 88, 110, 132, 136-139). A key concept is the prevention of eating disorders that includes helping children, adolescents and adults deal with the message of excessive thinness found on social media (140-144). A key concept of management when anorexia/bulimia nervosa is present is psychotherapy along with proper nutrition correction. Family therapy (family behavioral therapy; FBT) can be helpful to children/teenagers but youth as well as adults should be involved in cognitive behavioral therapy (CBT) or other therapy---such as dialectical behavioral therapy (DBT) or acceptance and commitment therapy (ACT) (137, 145-154).

A variety of psychopharmacologic agents have been used in the overall management of eating disorders. These medications include selective serotonin reuptake inhibitors (SSRIs; fluoxetine), antipsychotic mediations (olanzapine, others), cyproheptadine, and others (see Table 5) (155-158). Fluoxetine is often used in high doses for persons with bulimia nervosa; other antidepressant mediations may be used as well (155-157).

Psychopharmacology for binge eating disorder can utilize antidepressants as well as use of medications that reduce appetite, such as the central nervous system stimulant, lisdexamfetamine (155-157). Research has also suggested that the atypical antipsychotic, olanzapine, may help with those having anorexia nervosa (155-158). Research is also looking at the use of the anticonvulsant, topiramate, as well as the use of the microbiome concept in management of eating disorders (158). Methods of neuromodulation are under study and include repetitive transcranial magnetic stimulation (rTMS) and deep brain stimulation (DBS) (156).

Table 5. Management principles for adolescents with eating disorders (2, 132, 136-139)

- Nutritional support
- Psychotherapy: Cognitive behavioral therapy, family therapy and "third-wave" behavioral therapies: Dialectical behavioral therapy (DBT) as well as Accept and commitment therapy (ACT)
- Hospitalization: Management of severe malnutrition and treatment for life-threatening conditions (i.e., severe electrolyte disturbances, bradycardia, self-injury thoughts/attempts, refeeding syndrome, others
- Osteopenia management: Improve nutrition, monitor with DEXA (dual-energey X-ray absorptiometry
- Psychopharmacology: Selective serotonin reuptake inhibitors (SSRIs; fluoxetine), antipsychotic mediations (olanzapine, others), cyproheptadine, others

Clinicians and eating disorder teams (inpatient and outpatient) seek to help persons with eating disorders learn to establish healthier eating and nutrition habits so they can eat to live in a more healthy manner (159). Depending on the state of malnutrition, various plans have been developed that involve refeeding at a low level and gradually increasing to a more normal caloric intake (160, 161). For example, the malnourished person may be started at 1000 to 1200 calories per day and then increased by 200 calories each day under medical supervision to achieve a more normal diet/caloric intake. Monitoring and correction, if necessary, of various chemical elements (i.e., calcium, phosphorus, potassium, others [see Table 4]) is part of the treatment protocol along with regular weight checks and management of any eating disorder complications that may arise (2, 136, 139, 162). Such complications include death, the refeeding syndrome and others as noted in Table 6 (106, 140, 162-181).

Table 6. Medical complications of eating disorders (partial-list) (also see Table 3)

1. Malnutrition
2. Electrolyte disturbances (hypochloremia; hypokalemia; others-Table 3)
3. Cardiac dysrhythmias (Prolonged QT intervals) due to electrolyte imbalance
4. Hypochloremic metabolic alkalosis (due to purging/emesis & potassium loss)
5. Metabolic acidosis (laxative abuse with bicarbonate loss in stools)
6. Metabolic alkalosis (excessive diuretic use)
7. Ipecac abuse with emetine-toxic effects of myopathy (skeletal;cardiac)
8. Excessive emesis-induced upper gastrointestinal trauma (i.e., Mallory-Weiss tear, rupture of the esophagus or stomach)
9. Chronic emesis-induced dental surface erosion
10. Finger-induced emesis with resultant trauma to the palatal tissues or dorsal knuckle trauma (calluses, scars: Russell sign)
11. Osteropenia/osteoporosis
12. Refeeding syndrome (140, 158-161).
13. Structural brain changes with anorexia nervosa, others
14. Death
15. OTHERS

Osteopenia/osteoporosis

Osteopenia and osteoporosis are respectively identified as BMD less than 1.5 or 2.0 standard deviations below the mean density as per age; this can be recorded as z-scores of less than -1.5 for osteopenia or -2.0 for osteoporosis. As noted, BMD can be measured with DEXA (dual-energy X-ray absorptiometry) and DEXA is not typically utilized until the person has had several months of amenorrhea; thus, it can be done 6 months or more after the LMP (last menstrual period).

Management of a female with osteoporosis/osteopenia with amenorrhea is difficult and challenging. These patients are encouraged to take daily calcium and supplemental vitamin D, although supplementation alone is **not** sufficient to prevent or treat low BMD. Repeat DEXA is typically done every 12 months and physiologic recovery from anorexia may be suggested by restitution of menstruation. Unfortunately, low BMD may not return to normal levels at any time in the future even with management but certainly not unless menstruation recurs.

Therapy seeks to help the patient learn to improve eating habits, improve nutrition, normalize weight and resume menstruation (2, 105, 136, 137, 139). Current research is evaluating use of medications used to manage adult females with osteoporosis with or without a history of fractures; these include transdermal estrogen replacement, estrogen agonist/antagonist (i.e., raloxifene), parathyroid hormone analogs (i.e., teriparatide, abaloparatide), immunologic agents (i.e., denosumab), and others (2, 110-117). The use of bisphosphonates (such as alendronate with and without vitamin D, risedronate, ibandronate) in young females remains in controversy (as noted previously) and research due to identified safety concerns and teratogenicity reports (2, 116, 117, 182-186).

Conclusion

Issues related to puberty are key aspects to the development of eating disorders in adolescent females and important influences on reproductive procedures as well as actions of puberty that may occur. Those with eating disorders may have such severe nutritional dysfunction that reproductive neuroendocrine activity is impaired with delayed puberty (187). Anorexia nervosa is a metabolic-psychiatric disorder involving various central nervous systems including the Ghrelin-AgRP (Agouti-related) neuron nexus among others (188, 189). Structural changes in the brain development of adolescents are noted in those developing anorexia nervosa (190). Studies in epigenetics are adding valuable insights into epigenetic influences on the development of eating disorders (191).

A key potential development is osteopenia in eating disorders due to malnutrition (including low calcium consumption) with reduced estrogen and possible excessive exercise; this can lead to amenorrhea and eventual osteoporosis with various complications including risk of fractures. DEXA screening is recommended for those with amenorrhea for 6 to 12 months. Management of osteopenia/osteoporosis is difficult and prevention with proper nutrition is a key goal of management.

Eating disorders can have a profoundly negative effect on the quality of life of the patient as well as family members (192-195). Research into the pathogenesis and management principles of eating disorders remains important as the 21st century continues and as life stresses continue for these precious persons, stresses that include the catastrophic 2019-2022 COVID-19 pandemic (191, 195-210).

Acknowledgments

Consultation with Vinay N Reddy, MD, MS, MSE (Kalamazoo, Michigan, USA) in the preparation of this manuscript is gratefully acknowledged. This chapter used with permission is updated and revised from: Greydanus DE, Bacopoulou F, Apostolaki D. Gynecological features of eating disorders. In: Omar HA, Greydanus DE, Patel DR, Merrick J, eds. Pediatric and adolescent sexuality and Gynecology: Principles for the primary care clinician, Second edition. New York: Nova Science 2021:565-88.

References

[1] American Psychiatric Association. Diagnostic and statistical manual of mental disorders, Fifth edition. DSM-5. Washington, DC: American Psychiatric Publishing, 2013:329-54.
[2] Mitchison D, Mond J, Bussey K, Griffiths S, Trompeter N, Lonergan A, et al. DSM-5 full syndrome, other specified, and unspecified eating disorders in Australian adolescents: Prevalence and clinical significance. Psychol Med 2020;50(6):981-90.
[3] Hay P. Current approach to eating disorders: A clinical update. Intern Med J 2020;50(1): 24-9.
[4] Klump KL. Puberty as a critical risk period for eating disorders: A review of human and animal studies. Horm Behav 2013;64(2):399-410.
[5] Ma R, Mikhail ME, Fowler N, Culbert KM, Klump KL. The role of puberty and ovarian hormones in the genetic diathesis of eating disorders in females. Child Adolesc Psychiatr Clin North Am 2019;28(4):616-28.
[6] Neale J, Pais SMA, Nicholls D, Chapman S, Hudson LD. What are the effects of restrictive eating disorders on growth and puberty and are effects permanent? A systematic review and meta-analysis. J Adolesc Health 2020;66(2):144-56.
[7] Wheeler MD. Physical changes of puberty. Endocrinol Metab Clin North Am 1991; 20(1):1-14.
[8] Tanner JM. Foetus into man: Physical growth from conception to maturity. London: Open Books, 1978.
[9] Aksglaede L, Sørensen K, Petersen JH, Skakkebaek NE, Juul A. Recent decline in age at breast development: the Copenhagen Puberty Study. Pediatrics 2009;123(5):e932-9.
[10] Moodie JL, Campisi SC, Salena K, Wheatley M, Vandermorris A, Bhutta ZA. Timing of pubertal milestones in low- and middle-income countries: A systematic review and meta-analysis. Adv Nutr 2020 Feb 6. pii: nmaa007. doi: 10.1093/advances/nmaa007.
[11] Brix N, Ernst A, Lauridsen LLB, Parner E, Støvring H, Olsen J, et al. Timing of puberty in boys and girls: A population-based study. Paediatr Perinat Epidemiol 2019;33(1):70-8.
[12] Shalitin S, Kiess W. Putative effects of obesity on linear growth and puberty. Horm Res Paediatr 2017;88(1):101-10.
[13] Li W, Liu Q, Deng X, Chen Y, Liu S, Story M. Association between obesity and puberty timing: A systematic review and metal-analysis. Int J Environ Res Public Health 2017 Oct 24;14(10). pii: E1266. doi: 10.3390/ijerph14101266.
[14] Kaye W. Neurobiology of anorexia and bulimia nervosa. Physiol Behav 2008;94(1):121-35.
[15] Schmidt U, Tiller J, Andrews B, Blanchard M, Treasure J. Is there a specific trauma precipitating onset of anorexia nervosa? Psychol Med 1997;27(3):523-30.
[16] Zehr JL, Culbert KM, Sisk CL, Klump KL. An association of early puberty with disordered and anxiety in a population of undergraduate women and men. Horm Behav 2007;52(4):427-35.
[17] Ackard DM, Peterson CB. Association between puberty and disordered eating, body image, and other psychological variables. Int J Eat Disord 2001;29(2):187-94.
[18] Beumont P, Abraham S, Simson K. The psychosexual histories of adolescent girls and young women with anorexia nervosa. Psychol Med 1981;11(1):131-40.

[19] Mangweth-Matzek B, Rupp CI, Hausmann A, Kemmler G, Biebl W. Menarche, puberty, and first sexual activities in eating-disordered patients as compared with a psychiatric and a nonpsychiatric control group. Int J Eat Disord 2007;40(8):705-10.
[20] Cassioli E, Rossi E, Castellini G, Sensi C, Mancini M, Lelli L, et al. Sexuality, embodiment and attachment style in anorexia nervosa. Eat Weight Disord 2019 Nov 2. doi: 10.1007/s40519-019-00805-6.
[21] Castellini G, Lelli L, Ricca V, Maggi M. Sexuality in eating disorder patients: etiologic factors, sexual dysfunction and identity issues: A systematic review. Horm Mol Biol Clin Investig 2016;25(2):71-90.
[22] Naessén S, Carlström K, Byström B, Pierre Y, Hirschberg A. Effects of an antiandrogenic oral contraceptive on appetite and eating behavior in bulimic women. Psychoneuroendocrinology 2007;32(5):548-54.
[23] Harden KP, Mendle J, Kretsch N. Environmental and genetic pathways between early pubertal timing and dieting in adolescence: distinguishing between objective and subjective timing. Psychol Med 2012;42(1):183-93.
[24] Baker JH, Thornton LM, Bulik CM, Kendler KS, Lichtenstein P. Shared genetic effects between age at menarche and disordered eating. J Adolesc Health 2012;51(5):491-6.
[25] Klump KL, Perkins PS, Alexandra Burt S, McGue M, Iacono WG. Puberty moderates genetic influences on disordered eating. Psychol Med 2007;37(5):627-34.
[26] Culbert KM, Burt SA, McGue M, Iacono WG, Klump KL. Puberty and the genetic diathesis of disordered eating attitudes and behaviors. J Abnorm Psychol 2009;118(4): 788-96.
[27] Klump KL, Burt SA, Spanos A, McGue M, Iacono WG, Wade TD. Age differences in genetic and environmental influences on weight and shape concerns. Int J Eat Disord 2010;43(8):679-88.
[28] Klump KL, Culbert KM, Slane JD, Burt SA, Sisk CL, Nigg JT. The effects of puberty on genetic risk for disordered eating: evidence for a sex difference. Psychol Med 2012;42(3):627-37.
[29] Klump KL, Keel PK, Sisk C, Burt SA. Preliminary evidence that estradiol moderates genetic influences on disordered eating attitudes and behaviors during puberty. Psychol Med 2010;40(10):1745-53.
[30] Noll JG, Trickett PK, Long JD, Negriff S, Susman EJ, Shaley I, et al. Childhood sexual abuse and early timing of puberty. J Adolesc Health 2017;60(1):65-71.
[31] González-Chica DA, Licinio J, Musker M, Wong M, Bowden J, Hay P, et al. Bullying and sexual abuse and their association with harmful behaviours, antidepressant use and health-related quality of life in adulthood: a population-based study in South Australia. BMC Public Health 2019;19(1):26. doi: 10.1186/s12889-018-6367-8.
[32] Dansky BS, Brewerton TD, Kilpatrick DG, O'Neil PM. The National Women's Study: Relationship of victimization and posttraumatic stress disorder to bulimia nervosa. Int J Eat Disord 1997;21:213-28.
[33] Sanci L, Coffey C, Olsson C, Reid S, Carlin JB, Patton G. Childhood sexual abuse and eating disorders in females: Findings from the Victorian Adolescent Health Cohort Study. Arch Pediatr Adolesc Med 2008;162(3):261-67.
[34] Smolak L, Murnen S. Meta-analytic examination of the relationship between child sexual abuse and eating disorders. Int J Eat Disord 2002;31:136-50.
[35] Rai T, Mainali P, Raza A, Rashid J, Rutkofsky I. Exploring the link between emotional child abuse and anorexia nervosa: A psychopathological correlation. Cureus 2019;11(8):e5318. doi: 10.7759/cureus.5318.
[36] Hazzard VM, Bauer KW, Mukherjee B, Miller AL, Sonneville KR. Associations between childhood maltreatment latent classes and eating disorder symptoms in a nationally representative sample of young in adults in the United States. Child Abuse Negl 2019;98:104171. doi: 10.1016/j.chiabu.2019.104171.
[37] Robinson LD, Kelly PJ, Deane FP, Reis SL. Exploring the relationships between eating disorders and mental health in women attending residential substance use treatment. J Dual Diagn 2019;15(4):270-80.
[38] Túry F, Kovács-Tóth B. The role of traumatization in eating disorders. Possible therapeutic modalities with special regard to cognitive behavioural methods. Psychiatr Hung 2019; 34(4):419-25. [Polish]

[39] Opydo-Szymaczek J, Jarząbek-Bielecka G, Kędzia W, Borysewicz-Lewicka M. Child sexual abuse as an etiologic factor of overweight and eating disorders – considerations for primary health care providers. Ginekol Pol 2018;89(1):48-54.
[40] Calugi S, Franchini C, Pivari S, Conti M, El Ghoch M, Dalle Grave R. Anorexia nervoxa and childhood sexual abuse: Treatment outcomes of intensive cognitive behavioural therapy. Psychiatry Res 2018;262:477-81.
[41] Deligeoroglou E, Athanasopoulos N, Tsimaris P, Dimopoulos KD, Vrachnis N, Creatsas G. Evaluation and management of adolescent amenorrhea. Ann NY Acad Sci 2010;1205:23-32.
[42] American Psychiatric Association. Diagnostic and statistical manual of mental disorders, Fourth edition, text revision. Washington, DC: American Psychiatric Association, 2000.
[43] Bravender T, Bryant-Waugh R, Herzog D, Katzman D, Kriepe RD, Lask B, et al; Workgroup for Classification of Eating Disorders in Children and Adolescents. Classification of eating disturbance in children and adolescents: proposed changes for the DSM-V. Eur Eat Disord Rev 2010;18(2):79–89.
[44] Miller KK, Grinspoon S, Gleysteen S, Grieco KA, Ciampa J, Breu J, et al. Preservation of neuroendocrine control of reproductive function despite severe undernutrition. J Clin Endocrinol Metab 2004;89(9):4434–8.
[45] Golden NH, Carlson JL. The pathophysiology of amenorrhea in the adolescent. Ann NY Acad Sci 2008;1135:163-78.
[46] Muñoz T, Argente J. Anorexia nervosa in female adolescents: endocrine and bone mineral density disturbances Eur J Endocrinol 2002;147(3):275-86.
[47] Gordon CM. Clinical practice. Functional hypothalamic amenorrhea. N Engl J Med 2010;363(4):365-71.
[48] Frisch R. Fatness and fertility. Sci Am 1988;258(3):88-95.
[49] Swenne I. Weight requirements for return of menstruation in teenage girls with eating disorders, weight loss and secondary amenorrhea. Acta Paediatr 2004;93(11):1449-55.
[50] Golden NH, Jacobson MS, Schebendach J, Solanto MV, Hertz SM, Shenker IR. Resumption of menses in anorexia nervosa. Arch Pediatr Adolesc Med 1997;151(1):16-21.
[51] Golden NH, Jacobson MS, Sterling WM, Hertz S. Treatment goal weight in adolescents with anorexia nervosa: use of BMI percentiles. Int J Eat Disord 2008;41(4):301-6.
[52] Frisch RE, Mcarthur JW. Menstrual cycles: Fatness as a determinant of minimum weight for height necessary for their maintenance or onset. Science 1974;185:949–51.
[53] Misra M, Miller KK, Kuo K, Griffin K, Stewart V, Hunter E, et al. Secretory dynamics of leptin in adolescent girls with anorexia nervosa and healthy adolescents. Am J Physiol Endocrinol Metab 2005;289(3):373-8.
[54] Misra M, Prabhakaran, Miller KK, Tsai P, Lin A, Lee N, et al. Role of cortisol in menstrual recovery in adolescent girls with anorexia nervosa. Pediatr Res 2006;59:598–603.
[55] Pitts S, Blood E, Divasta A, Gordon CM. Percentage body fat by dual-energy X-ray absorptiometry is associated with menstrual recovery in adolescents with anorexia nervosa. J Adolesc Health 2014;54(6):739-41.
[56] Fairburn C, Cooper P. The clinical features of bulimia nervosa. Br J Psychiat 1984; 144(3):238-46.
[57] Seidenfeld ME, Rickert VI. Impact of anorexia, bulimia and obesity on the gynecologic health of adolescents. Am Fam Physician 2001;64(3):445-50.
[58] Pirke K, Schweiger U, Strowitzki T, Tuschl R, Laessle R, Broocks A, et al. Dieting causes menstrual irregularities in normal weight young women through impairment of episodic luteinizing hormone secretion. Fertil Steril 1989;51(2):263-8.
[59] Gendall KA, Bulik CM, Joyce PR, McIntosh VV, Carter FA. Menstrual cycle irregularity in bulimia nervosa. Associated factors and changes with treatment. J Psychosom Res 2000;49(6):409-15.
[60] Vyver E, Steinegger C, Katzman D.K. Eating disorders and menstrual dysfunction in adolescents. Ann NY Acad Sci 2008;1135:253–64.
[61] Robin G, Gallo C, Catteau-Jonard S, Lefebvre-Maunoury C, Pigny P, Duhamel A, et al. Polycystic ovary-like abnormalities (PCO-L) in women with functional hypothalamic amenorrhea. J Clin Endocrinol Metab 2012;97(11):4236–43.

[62] Sum M, Warren MP. Hypothalamic amenorrhea in young women with underlying polycystic ovary syndrome. Fertil Steril 2009;92(6):2106–8

[63] Katz MG, Vollenhoven B. The reproductive endocrine consequences of anorexia nervosa. BJOG 2000;107(6):707-13.

[64] Wohl ML, Gur E. Pregnancy in anorexia nervosa—an oxymoron that has become reality. Harefuah 2015;154(7):456-9,468. [Hebrew]

[65] Cardwell MS. Eating disorders during pregnancy. Obstet Gynecol Surv 2013;68(4)312-23.

[66] Kiani-Sheikhabadi M, Beigi M, Mohebbi-Dehnavi Z. The relationship between perfectionism and body image with eating disorder in pregnancy. J Educ Health Promot 2019;8:242. doi: 10.4103/jehp.jehp_58_19.

[67] Bulik CM, Hoffman ER, Von Holle A, Torgersen L, Stoltenberg C, Reichborn-Kjennerud T. Unplanned pregnancy in women with anorexia nervosa. Obstet Gynecol 2010; 116(5):1136-40.

[68] Brinch M, Isager T, Tolstrup K. Anorexia nervosa and motherhood: reproductional pattern and mothering behavior of 50 women. Acta Psychiat Scand 1988;77:98-104.

[69] Bulik CM, Sullivan PF, Fear JL, Pickering A, Dawn A, McCullin M. Fertility and reproduction in women with anorexia nervosa: A controlled study. J Clin Psychiatry 1999;60(2):130-5.

[70] Abraham S. Sexuality and reproduction in bulimia nervosa patients over 10 years. J Psychosom Res 1998;44:491-502.

[71] Kouba S, Hallstrom T, Lindholm C, Hirschberg AL. Pregnancy and neonatal outcomes in women with eating disorders. Obstet Gynecol 2005;105(2):255-60.

[72] Martínez-Olcina M, Rubio-Arias JA, Reche-García C, et al. Eating disorders in pregnant and breastfeeding women: A systematic review. Medicina (Kaunas) 2020;56(7):352. Published 2020 Jul 15. doi:10.3390/medicina56070352

[73] Mantel Ä, Lindén Hirschberg A, Stephansson O. Association of maternal eating disorders with pregnancy and neonatal outcomes. JAMA Psychiatry 2019 Nov 20. doi: 10.1001/jama psychiatry.2019.3664.

[74] Eik-Nes TT, Horn J, Strohmaier S, Holmen TL, Micali N, Bjørnelv S. Impact of eating disorders on obstetric outcomes in a large clinical sample: A comparison with the HUNT study. Int J Eat Disord 2018;51(10):1134-43.

[75] Arnold C, Johnson H, Mahon C, Agius M. The effects of eating disorders in pregnancy on mother and baby: a review. Psychiatr Danub 2019;31(Suppl 3):615-8.

[76] Charbonneau KD, Seabrook JA. Adverse birth outcomes associated with types of eating disorders: A review. Can J Diet Pract Res 2019;80(3):131-6.

[77] Micali N, De Stavola B, dos-Santos-Silva I, Steenweg-de Graaff J, Jansen PW, Jaddoe VW, et al. Perinatal outcomes and gestational weight gain in women with eating disorders: a population-based cohort study. BJOG 2012;119(12):1493-502.

[78] Stewart DE, Robinson E, Goldbloom DS, Wright C. Infertility and eating disorders. Am J Obstet Gynecol 1990;163(4 Pt 1):1196-9.

[79] Easter A, Treasure J, Micali N. Fertility and prenatal attitudes towards pregnancy in women with eating disorders: Results from the Avon Longitudinal Study of Parents and Children. BJOG 2011;118(12):1491-8.

[80] Lai KY, dr Bruyn R, Lask B, Bryant-Waugh R, Hankins M. Use of pelvic ultrasound to monitor ovarian and uterine maturity in childhood onset anorexia. Arch Dis Child 1994; 71:228-31.

[81] Kraeft JJ, Uppot RN, Heffess AM. Imaging findings in eating disorders. AJR Am J Roentgenol 2013;200(4):328-35.

[82] Mason HD, Key A, Allan R, Lask B. Pelvic ultra-sonography in anorexia nervosa: what the clinician should ask the radiologist and how to use the information provided. Eur Eat Disord Rev 2007;15:35–41.

[83] Allan R, Sharma R, Sangani B, Hugo P, Frampton I, Mason H, Lask B. Predicting the weight gain required for recovery from anorexia nervosa with pelvic ultrasonography: an evidence-based approach. Eur Eat Disord Rev 2010;18:43–8.

[84] Key A, Mason H, Allan R, Lask B. Restoration of ovarian and uterine maturity in adolescents with anorexia nervosa. Int J Eat Disord 2002;32(3):319-25.

[85] Andolf E, Theander S, Aspenberg P. Changes in ultrasound appearance of the internal female genital organs during treatment for eating disorders. Eur J Obstet Gynecol Reprod Biol 1997;73(1):49-53.
[86] Legroux I, Cortet B. Factors influencing bone loss in anorexia nervosa: assessment and therapeutic options. RMD Open 2019;5(2):e001009. doi: 10.1136/rmdopen-2019-001009.
[87] Steinman J, Shibli-Rahhal A. Anorexia nervosa and osteoporosis: Pathophysiology and treatment. J Bone Metab 2019;26(3):133-43.
[88] Fazeli PK. Low bone mineral density in anorexia nervosa: Treatments and challenges. Clin Rev Bone Miner Metab 2019;17(2):65-76.
[89] Misra M, Miller KK, Bjornson J, Hackman A, Aggarwal A, Chung J, et al. Alterations in growth hormone secretory dynamics in adolescent girls with anorexia nervosa and effects on bone metabolism. J Clin Endocrinol Metab 2003;88(12):5615-23.
[90] Soyka LA, Misra M, Frenchman A, Miller KK, Grinspoon S, Schoenfeld DA, et al. Abnormal bone mineral accrual in adolescent girls with anorexia nervosa. J Clin Endocrinol Metab 2002;87(9):4177-85.
[91] Grinspoon S, Thomas E, Pitts S, Gross E, Mickley D, Miller K, et al. Prevalence and predictive factors for regional osteopenia in women with anorexia nervosa. Ann Intern Med 2000;133:790-4.
[92] Bredella MA, Misra M, Miller KK, Madisch I, Sarwar A, Cheung A, et al. Distal radius in adolescent girls with anorexia nervosa: trabecular structure analysis with high-resolution flat-panel volume CT. Radiology 2008;249(3):938-46.
[93] Bredella MA, Fazeli PK, Miller KK, Misra M, Torriani M, Thomas BJ, et al. Increased bone marrow fat in anorexia nervosa. J Clin Endocrinol Metab 2009;94(6):2129-36.
[94] Bachmann KN, Fazeli PK, Lawson EA, Russell BM, Riccio AD, Meenaghan E, et al. Comparison of hip geometry, strength, and estimated fracture risk in women with anorexia nervosa and overweight/obese women. J Clin Endocrinol Metab 2014;99(12):4664-73.
[95] Singhal V, Tulsiani S, Campoverde KJ, Mitchell DM, Slattery M, Schorr M, et al. Impaired bone strength estimates at the distal tibia and its determinants in adolescents with anorexia nervosa. Bone 2018;106:61-8.
[96] Jagielska G, Wolanczyk T, Komender J, Tomaszewicz-Libidzic C, Przedlacki J, Ostrowski K. Bone mineral density in adolescent girls with anorexia nervosa: A cross-sectional study. Eur Child Adolesc Psychiatry 2002;22(2):57-62.
[97] Legroux-Gerot I, Vignau J, D'Herbonnez M, Collier F, Marchandise X, Duquesnoy B, et al. Evaluation of bone loss and its mechanisms in anorexia nervosa. Calcif Tissue Int 2007;81(3):174-82.
[98] Miller KK, Lawson EA, Mathur V, Wexler TL, Meenaghan E, Misra M, et al. Androgens in women with anorexia nervosa and normal-weight women with hypothalamic amenorrhea. J Clin Endocrinol Metab 2007;92(4):1334-9.
[99] Lawson EA, Miller KK, Bredella MA, Phan C, Misra M, Meenaghan E, et al. Hormone predictors of abnormal bone microarchitecture in women with anorexia nervosa. Bone 2010;46(2):458-63.
[100] Lawson EA, Donoho D, Miller KK, Misra M, Meenaghan E, Lydecker J, et al. Hypercortisolemia is associated with severity of bone loss and depression in hypothalamic amenorrhea and anorexia nervosa. J Clin Endocrinol Metab 2009;94(12):4710-6.
[101] Lawson EA, Donoho DA, Blum JI, Meenaghan EM, Misra M, Herzog DB, et al. Decreased nocturnal oxytocin levels in anorexia nervosa are associated with low bone mineral density and fat mass. J Clin Psychiatry 2011;72(11):1546-51.
[102] Schorr M, Marengi DA, Pulumo RL, Yu E, Eddy KT, Klibanski A, et al. Oxytocin and its relationship to body composition, bone mineral density, and hip geometry across the weight spectrum. J Clin Endocrinol Metab 2017;102(8):2814-24.
[103] Utz AL, Lawson EA, Misra M, Mickley D, Gleysteen S, Herzog DB, et al. Peptide YY (PYY) levels and bone mineral density (BMD) in women with anorexia nervosa. Bone 2008;43(1):135-9.
[104] Miller KK, Lee EE, Lawson EA, Misra M, Minihan J, Grinspoon SK, et al. Determinants of skeletal loss and recovery in anorexia nervosa. J Clin Endocrinol Metab 2006;91(8):2931-37.
[105] Misra M, Prabhakaran R, Miller KK, Goldstein MA, Mickley D, Clauss L, et al. Weight gain and restoration of menses as predictors of bone mineral density change in adolescent girls with anorexia nervosa-1. J Clin Endocrinol Metab 2008;93(4):1231-7.

[106] Katzman DK. Medical complications in adolescents with anorexia nervosa: A review of the literature. In J Eat Disord 2005;37:52-9.
[107] Vestergaard P, Emborg C, Støving RK, Hagen C, Mosekilde L, Brixen K. Fractures in patients with anorexia nervosa, bulimia nervosa, and other eating disorders: A nationwide register study. Int J Eat Disord 2002;32(3):301-8.
[108] Rigotti NA, Neer RM, Skates SJ, Herzog DB, Nussbaum SR. The clinical course of osteoporosis in anorexia nervosa. A longitudinal study of cortical bone mass. JAMA 1991;265(9):1133-8
[109] Misra M, Katzman D, Miller KK, Mendes N, Snelgrove D, Russell M, et al. Physiologic estrogen replacement increases bone density in adolescent girls with anorexia nervosa. J Bone Miner Res 2011;26(10):2430-8.
[110] Gordon CM, Ackerman KE, Berga SL, Kaplan JR, Mastorakos G, Misra M, et al. Functional hypothalamic amenorrhea: An Endocrine Society clinical practice guideline. J Clin Endocrinol Metab 2017;102(5):1413–39.
[111] Warren MP, Brooks-Gunn J, Fox RP, Holderness CC, Hyle EP, Hamilton WG, et al. Persistent osteopenia in ballet dancers with amenorrhea and delayed menarche despite hormone therapy: a longitudinal study. Fertil Steril 2003;80(2):398–404.
[112] Cobb KL, Bachrach LK, Sowers M, Nieves J, Greendale GA, Kent KK, et al. The effect of oral contraceptives on bone mass and stress fractures in female runners. Med Sci Sports Exerc 2007;39(9):1464–73.
[113] Strokosch GR, Friedman AJ, Wu SC, Kamin M. Effects of an oral contraceptive (norgestimate/ethinyl estradiol) on bone mineral density in adolescent females with anorexia nervosa: a double-blind, placebo-controlled study. J Adolesc Health 2006;39(6):819-27.
[114] Gordon CM, Grace E, Emans SJ, Goodman E, Crawford MH, LeBoff MS. Changes in bone turnover markers and menstrual function after short-term oral DHEA in young women with anorexia nervosa. J Bone Miner Res 1999;14(1):136-45.
[115] Gordon CM, Grace E, Emans SJ, Feldman HA, Goodman E, Becker KA, et al. Effects of oral dehydroepiandrosterone on bone density in young women with anorexia nervosa: A randomized trial J Clin Endocrinol Metab 2002;87(11):4935-41.
[116] Golden NH, Iglesias EA, Jacobson MS, Carey D, Meyer W, Schebendach J, et al. Alendronate for the treatment of osteopenia in anorexia nervosa: a randomized, double-blind, placebo-controlled trial. J Clin Endocrinol Metab 2005;90(6):3179-85.
[117] Miller KK, Grieco KA, Mulder J, Grinspoon S, Mickley D, Yehezkel R, et al. Effects of risedronate on bone density in anorexia nervosa. J Clin Endocrinol Metab 2004; 89(8):3903-6.
[118] Piontek A, Szeja J, Błachut M, Badura-Brzoza K. Sexual problems in the patients with psychiatric disorders. Wiad Lek 2019;72(10):1984-8.
[119] Towe M, La J, El-Khatib F, Roberts N, Yafi FA, Rubin R. Diet and female sexual health. Sex Med Rev 2019 Oct 25. pii: S2050-0521(19)30098-8. doi: 10.1016/j.sxmr.2019.08.004.
[120] Maier S, Spiegelberg J, van Zutphen L, Zeeck A, Tebartz van Elst L, Hartmann A, et al. Neurobiological signature of intimacy in anorexia nervosa. Eur Eat Disord Rev 2019; 27(3):315-22.
[121] Castellini G, Mannucci E, Mazzei C, Lo Sauro C, Faravelli C, Rotella CM, et al. Sexual function in obese women with and without binge eating disorder. J Sex Med 2010;7:3969–78.
[122] Castellini G, Lelli L, Lo Sauro C, Fioravanti G, Vignozzi L, Maggi M, et al. Anorectic and bulimic patients suffer from relevant sexual dysfunctions. J Sex Med 2012;9:2590–9.
[123] Tuiten A, Panhuysen G, Everaerd W, Koppeschaar H, Krabbe P, Zelissen P. The paradoxical nature of sexuality in anorexia nervosa. J Sex Marital Ther 1993;19:259–75.
[124] Rothschild BS, Fagan P, Woodall C, Andersen AE. Sexual functioning of female eating disordered patients. Int J Eat Disord 1991;10:389–94.
[125] Meguerditchian C, Samuelian-Massat C, Valéro R, Begu-Le Corroller A, Fromont I, Mancini J, et al. The impact of weight normalization on quality of recovery in anorexia nervosa. J Am Coll Nutr 2009;28:397–404.
[126] Ruuska J, Kaltiala-Heino R, Koivisto AM, Rantanen P. Puberty, sexual development and eating disorders in adolescent outpatients. Eur Child Adolesc Psychiatry 2003;12(5):214-20.

[127] Schembri C, Evans L. Adverse relationship processes: The attempts of women with bulimia nervosa symptoms to fit the perceived ideals of intimate partners. Eur Eat Disord Rev 2008;16(1):59-66.
[128] Kaltiala-Heino R, Rissanen A, Rimpelä M, Rantanen P. Bulimia and impulsive behaviour in middle adolescence. Psychother Psychosom 2003;72:26–33.
[129] Ackard DM, Fedio G, Neumark-Sztainer D, Britt HR. Factors associated with disordered eating among sexually active adolescent males: gender and number of sexual partners. Psychosom Med 2008;70:232–8.
[130] Dunkley CR, Gorzalka BB, Brotto LA. Associations between sexual function and disordered eating among undergraduate women: An emphasis on sexual pain and distress. J Sex Marital Ther 2020;46(1):18-34.
[131] Carter FA, Carter JD, Luty SE, Jordan J, McIntosh VV, Bartram AF, et al. What is worse for your sex life: Starving, being depressed, or a new baby? Int J Eat Disord 2007; 40(7):664-7.
[132] Lenton-Brym T, Rodrigues A, Johnson N, Couturier J, Toulany A. A scoping review of the role of primary care providers and primary care-based interventions in the treatment of pediatric eating disorders. Eat Disord 2020;28(1):47-66.
[133] Maguen S, Hebenstreit C, Li Y, Dinh JV, Donalson R, Dalton S, et al. Screen for disordered eating: Improving the accuracy of eating disorder screening in primary care. Gen Hosp Psychiatry 2018;50:20-5.
[134] Klein DA, Paradise SL, Landis CA. Screening and counseling adolescents and young adults: A framework for comprehensive care. Am Fam Physician 2020;101(3):147-58.
[135] Kutz AM, Marsh AG, Gunderson CG, Maguen S, Masheb RM. Eating disorder screening: a systemic review and meta-analysis of diagnostic test characteristics of SCOFF. J Gen Intern Med 2019 Nov 8. doi: 10.1007/s11606-019-05478-6.
[136] Sigman GS. Eating disorders in children and adolescents. Pediatr Clin North Am 2003;50:1139–77.
[137] Campbell K, Peebles R. Eating disorders in children and adolescents: State of the art review. Pediatrics 2014;134:582-92.
[138] Tanner J, Davies P. Clinical longitudinal standards for height and height velocity for North American children. J Pediatr 1985;107(3):317-29.
[139] Vinch J, Reddy VN. Eating disorders. In: Greydanus DE, Patel DR, Pratt HD, Calles Jr JL, Nazeer A, Merrick J, eds. Behavioral pediatrics, 4th edition. New York: Nova Biomedical, 2015:353-71.
[140] Ghaddar R, Chartrand J, Benomar A, Jamoulle O, Taddeo D, Frappier JY, et al. Excessive laboratory monitoring to prevent adolescent's refeeding syndrome: Opportunities for enhancement. Eat Weight Disord 2019 Jun 5. doi: 10.1007/s40519-019-00723-7.
[141] Bauer S, Bilić S, Reetz C, Ozer F, Becker K, Eschenbeck H, et al. Efficacy and cost-effectiveness of Internet-based selective eating disorder prevention: study protocol for a randomized controlled trial within the ProHead Consortium. Trials 2019;20(1):91. doi: 10.1186/s13063-018-3161-y.
[142] Saul JS, Rodgers RF. Adolescent eating disorder risk and online world. Child Adolesc Psychiatr Clin North Am 2018;27(2):221-8.
[143] Wade TD, Wilksch SM. Internet eating disorder prevention. Curr Opin Psychiatry 2018;31(6):456-61.
[144] Bauer S, Kindermann SS, Moessner M. Prevention of eating disorder: A review. Z Kinder Jugendpsychiatr Psychother 2017;45(5):403-13. [German]
[145] de Jong M, Spinhoven P, Korrelboom K, Deen M, van der Meer I, Danner UN et al. Effectiveness of enhanced cognitive behavior therapy for eating disorders: A randomized controlled trial. Int J Eat Disord 2020 Feb 10. doi: 10.1002/eat.23239.
[146] Agras WS. Cognitive behavior therapy for the eating disorders. Psychiatr Clin North Am 2019;42(2):169-79.
[147] Marzola E, Porliod A, Panero M, De-Bacco C, Abbate-Daga G. Affective temperaments and eating psychopathology in anorexia nervosa: Which role for anxious and depressive traits. J Affect Disord 2020;266:374-80.
[148] Le Grange D, Gorrell S, Hughes EK, Accurso EC, Yeo M, Pradel M, et al. Delivery of family-based treatment for adolescent anorexia nervosa in a public health care setting: Research versus non-research specialty care. Front Psychiatry 2020;10:1001. doi: 10.3389/fpsyt.2019.01001.

[149] Dalle Grave R, Eckhardt S, Calugi S, Le Grange D. A conceptual comparison of family-based treatment and enhanced cognitive behavior therapy in the treatment of adolescents with eating disorders. J Eat Disord 2019;7:42. doi: 10.1186/s40337-019-0275-x.

[150] Wade S, Byrne S, Allen K. Enhanced cognitive behavioral therapy for eating disorders adopted for a group setting. Int J Eat Disord 2017;50(8):863-72.

[151] Chand SP, Kuckel DP, Huecker MR. Cognitive behavior therapy (CBT). In: StatPearls. Treasure Island (FL): StatPearls Publishing; June 9, 2020.

[152] Peterson CM, Van Diest AMK, Mara CA, Matthews A. Dialectical behavioral therapy skills group as an adjunct to family-based therapy in adolescents with restrictive eating disorders. Eat Disord 2019;23:1-13.

[153] Reilly EE, Orloff NC, Luo T, Berner LA, Brown TA, Claudat K, et al. Dialectical behavioral therapy for the treatment of adolescent eating disorders: a review of existing work and proposed future directions. Eat Disord 2020;28(2):122-141.

[154] Saito E, Tebbett-Mock AA, McGee M. Dialectical behavior therapy decreases depressive symptoms among adolescents in an acute-care inpatient unit. J Child Adolesc Psychopharmacol 2020 Feb 11. doi: 10.1089/cap.2019.0149.

[155] Crow SJ. Pharmacologic treatment of eating disorders. Psychiatr Clin North Am 2019;42(2):253-62.

[156] Davis LE, Attia E. Recent advances in therapies for eating disorders. F1000Res 2019 Sep 26;8. pii: F1000 Faculty Rev-1693. doi: 10.12688/f1000research.19847.1.

[157] Bello NT, Yeomans BL. Safety of pharmacotherapy options for bulimia nervosa and binge eating disorder. Expert Opin Drug Saf 2018;17(1):17-23.

[158] Himmerich H, Treasure J. Psychopharmacological advances in eating disorders. Expert Rev Clin Pharmacol 2018;11(1):95-108.

[159] McMaster CM, Wade T, Franklin J, Hart S. A review of treatment manuals for adults with an eating disorder: nutritional content and consistency with current dietetic evidence. Eat Weight Disord 2020 Jan 30. doi: 10.1007/s40519-020-00850-6.

[160] Couturier J, Isserlin L, Norris M, Spettigue W, Brouwers M, Kimber M, et al. Canadian practice guidelines for the treatment of children and adolescents with eating disorders. J Eat Disord 2020;8:4. doi: 10.1186/s40337-020-0277-8.

[161] Espel-Huynh H, Thompson-Brenner H, Boswell JF, Zhang F, Juarascio AS. Lowe MR. Development and validation of a progress monitoring tool tailored for use in intensive eating disorder treatment. Eur Eat Disord Rev 2020;28(2):223-36.

[162] Ernest S, Kuntz HM. Emergency department management of eating disorder complications in pediatric patients. Pediatr Emerg Med Pract 2020;17(2):1-16.

[163] Edakubo S, Fushimi K. Mortality and risk assessment for anorexia nervosa in acute-care hospitals: a nationwide administrative database analysis. BMC Psychiatry 2020;20(1):19. doi: 10.1186/s12888-020-2433-8.

[164] Suokas JT, Suvisaari JM, Gissler M, Löfman R, Linna MS, Raevuori A, et al. Mortality in eating disorders: a follow-up study of adult eating disorder patients treated in tertiary care, 1995-2010. Psychiatry Res 2013;210(3):1101-6.

[165] Suokas JT, Suvisaari JM, Grainger M, Raevuori A, Gissler M, Haukka J. Suicide attempts and mortality in eating disorders: a follow-up study of eating disorder patients. Gen Hosp Psychiatry 2014;36(3):355-7.

[166] Fichter MM, Quadflieg N. Mortality in eating disorders – results of a large prospective clinical longitudinal study. Int J Eat Disord 2016;49(4):391-401.

[167] Friedli N, Stanga Z, Sobotka L, Culkin A, Kondrup J, Laviano A, et al. Revisting the refeeding syndrome: Results of a systematic review. Nutrition 2017;35:151-60.

[168] Friedli N, Odermatt J, Reber E, Schuetz P, Stanga Z. Refeeding syndrome: update and clinical advice for prevention, diagnosis and treatment. Curr Opin Gastroenterol 2020; 36(2):136-40.

[169] Boot R, Koekkoek KWAC, van Zanten ARH. Refeeding syndrome: relevance for the critically ill patient. Curr Opin Crit Care 2018;24(2):235-40.

[170] Peebles R, Sieke EH. Medical complications of eating disorders in youth. Child Adolesc Psychiatr Clin North Am 2019;28(4):593-615.

[171] Gibson D, Workman C, Mehler PS. Medical complications of anorexia nervosa and bulimia nervosa. Psychiatr Clin North Am 2019;42(2):263-74.

[172] Mehler PS, Brown C. Anorexia nervosa – medical complications. J Eat Disord 2015;3:11. doi: 10.1186/s40337-015-0040-8.

[173] Brown C, Mehler PS. Medical complications of anorexia nervosa and their treatments: an update on some critical aspects. Eat Weight Disord 2015;20(4):419-25.

[174] Westmoreland P, Krantz MJ, Mehler PS. Medical complications of anorexia nervosa and bulimia. Am J Med 2016;129(1):30-7.

[175] Trent SA, Moreira ME, Colwell CB, Mehler PS. ED management of patients with eating disorders. Am J Emerg Med 2013;31(5):859-65.

[176] Giovinazzo S, Sukkar SG, Rosa GM, Zappi A, Bezante GP, Balbi M, et al. Anorexia nervosa and heart disease: a systematic review. Eat Weight Disord 2019;24(2):199-207.

[177] Farasat M, Watters A, Bendelow T, Schuller J, Mehler PS, Krantz MJ. Long-term cardiac arrhythmia and chronotropic evaluation in patients with severe anorexia nervosa (LACE-AN): A pilot study. J Cardiovasc Electrophysiol 2020;31(2):432-9.

[178] Sachs KV, Harnke B, Mehler PS, Krantz MJ. Cardiovascular complications of anorexia nervosa: A systematic review. Int J Eat Disord 2016;49(3):238-48.

[179] Antonelli JR, Seltzer R. Oral and physical manifestations of anorexia and bulimia nervosa. Tex Dent J 2016;133(9):528-35.

[180] Lourenço M, Azevedo Á, Brandão I, Gomes PS. Orofacial manifestations in outpatients with anorexia nervosa and bulimia nervosa focusing on the vomiting behavior. Clin Oral Investig 2018;22(5):1915-22.

[181] Bassiouny MA. Oral health considerations in anorexia and bulimia nervosa. 1. Symptomatology and diagnosis. Gen Dent 2017;65(4):34-40.

[182] Sokal A, Elefant E, Leturcq T, Beghin D, Mariette S, Seror R. Pregnancy and newborn outcomes after exposure to bisphosphonates: A case-control study. Osteoporos Int 2019;30(1):221-9.

[183] Stathopoulos IP, Liakou CG, Katsalira A, Trovas G, Lyritis GG, Papaioannou NA, et al. The use of bisphosphonates in women prior to or during pregnancy and lactation. Hormones (Athens) 2011;10(4):280-91.

[184] Sølling ASK, Harsløf T, Landahl B. Current status of bone-forming therapies for the management of osteoporosis. Drugs Aging 2019;36(7):625-38.

[185] Biver E, Ferrari S. Osteoporosis. Rev Med Suisse 2020;16(676-7):78-80. [French]

[186] Carbone LD, Gonzalez B, Miskevics S, Ray C, Etingen B, Guihan M, et al. Association of bisphosphonate therapy with incident of lower extremity fractures in persons with spinal cord injuries or disorders. Arch Phys Med Rehabil 2020;101(4):633-641.

[187] Ojeda SR, Lomniczi A. Puberty in 2013: Unravelling the mystery of puberty. Nat Rev Endocrinol 2014;10(2):67-9.

[188] Méquinion M, Foldi CJ, Andrews ZB. The ghrelin-AgRP neuron nexus in anorexia nervosa: implications for metabolic and behavioral adaptations. Front Nutr 2020;6:190. Published 2020 Jan 9. doi:10.3389/fnut.2019.00190.

[189] Watson HJ, Yilmaz Z, Thornton LM, Hübel C, Coleman JRI, Gaspar HA, et al. Genome-wide association study identifies eight risk loci and implicates metabo-psychiatric origins for anorexia nervosa. Nat Genet 2019;51(8):1207-14.

[190] Olivo G, Gaudio S, Schiöth HB. Brain and cognitive development in adolescents with anorexia nervosa: A systematic review of fMRI studies. Nutrients 2019;11(8):1907. Published 2019 Aug 15. doi:10.3390/nu11081907.

[191] Booij L, Steiger H. Applying epigenetic science to the understanding of eating disorders: a promising paradigm for research and practice [published online ahead of print, 2020 Jun 22]. Curr Opin Psychiatry 2020;10.1097/YCO.0000000000000632.

[192] Jenkins PE, Hoste RR, Doyle AC, Eddy K, Crosby RD, Hill L, et al. Health-related quality of life among adolescents with eating disorders. J Psychosom Res 2014;76(1):1-5.

[193] Ágh T, Kovács G, Supina D, Pawaskar M, Herman BK, Vokó Z, et al. A systematic review of the health-quality of life and economic burdens of anorexia nervosa, bulimia nervosa, and binge eating disorder. Eat Weight Disord 2016;21(3):353-64.

[194] Fjermestad KW, Rø AE, Espeland KE, Halvorsen MS, Halvorsen IM. "Do I exist in this world, really, or is it just her?" Youths' perspectives of living with a sibling with anorexia nervosa. Eat Disord 2020;28(1):80-95.

[195] Hauck C, Cook B, Ellrott T. Food addiction, eating addiction and eating disorders. Proc Nutr Soc 2020;79(1):103-12.

[196] Hardin SL, Thornton LM, Munn-Chernoff MA, Baker JH. Premenstrual symptoms as a marker of ovarian hormone sensitivity in eating disorders. Int J Eat Disord 2020;53(2):296-301.

[197] Hart LM, Wade T. Identifying research priorities in eating disorders: A Delphi study building consensus across clinicians, researchers, consumers, and careers in Australia. Int J Eat Disord 2020;53(1):31-40.

[198] Ortiz SN, Espel-Huynh HM, Felonis C, Scharff A. Qualitative perceptions of and preferences for the research process among patients with eating disorders. Int J Eat Disord 2020;53(1):41-51.

[199] Skøt L, Mejldal A, Guala MM, Støving RK, Ascone L, Stenager E, Lichtenstein MB, Mellentin AI. Eating disorders and subsequent risk of substance use disorders involving illicit drugs: a Danish nationwide register-based cohort study. Soc Psychiatry Psychiatr Epidemiol 2022 Jan 5. doi: 10.1007/s00127-021-02201-x.

[200] Castellini G, Rossi E, Ricca V. Are There Common Pathways for Eating Disorders and Female Sexual Dysfunction? J Sex Med 2022;19(1):8-11.

[201] Cetik S, Acikgoz A, Yildiz BO. Investigation of taste function and eating behavior in women with polycystic ovary syndrome. Appetite 2022;168:105776.

[202] Gröbner EM, Zeiler M, Fischmeister FPS, Kollndorfer K, Schmelz S, Schneider A, et al. The effects of probiotics administration on the gut microbiome in adolescents with anorexia nervosa-A study protocol for a longitudinal, double-blind, randomized, placebo-controlled trial. Eur Eat Disord Rev 2022;30(1):61-74.

[203] Dunn CP, Riley JB, Hawkins KB, Tercyak KP. Factors associated with disordered eating behavior among adolescent girls: Screening and education. J Prim Care Community Health 2022;13:21501319211062673.

[204] Doersam AF, Moser J, Throm J, Weiss M, Zipfel S, Micali N, et al. Maternal eating disorder severity is associated with increased latency of foetal auditory event-related brain responses. Eur Eat Disord Rev 2022;30(1):75-81.

[205] Fergerson AK, Brausch AM. Resilience mediates the relationship Between PTSD symptoms and disordered eating in college women who have experienced sexual victimization. J Interpers Violence 2022;37(1-2):NP1013-NP1030.

[206] Weissman RS, Klump KL, Rose J. Conducting eating disorders research in the time of COVID-19: A survey of researchers in the field. Int J Eat Disord 2020;53(7):1171-81.

[207] Weissman RS, Bauer S, Thomas JJ. Access to evidence-based care for eating disorders during the COVID-19 crisis. Int J Eat Disord 2020;53(5):369-76.

[208] Zipfel S, Schmidt U, Giel KE. The hidden burden of eating disorders during the COVID-19 pandemic. Lancet Psychiatry 2022;9(1):9-11.

[209] Toulany A, Kurdyak P, Guttmann A, Stukel TA, Fu L, Strauss R, et al. Acute care visits for eating disorders among children and adolescents after the onset of the COVID-19 pandemic. J Adolesc Health 2022;70(1):4247.

[210] Schulte EM, Kral TVE, Allison KC. A cross-sectional examination of reported changes to weight, eating, and activity behaviors during the COVID-19 pandemic among United States adults with food addiction. Appetite 2022;168:105740.

Section four: Acknowledgements

About the editors

Donald E Greydanus, MD, DrHC(Athens), FAAP, FIAP(Hon) is Professor and Founding Chair of the Department of Pediatric and Adolescent Medicine at the Western Michigan University Homer Stryker MD School of Medicine (WMED), Kalamazoo, Michigan, USA. He is also Clinical Professor of Pediatrics and Human Development at Michigan State University College of Human Medicine (East Lansing, Michigan, USA). Received the Mayo Clinic Distinguished Alumnus designation in 2017 from the Mayo Clinic Graduate School of Medicine, Rochester, Minnesota, USA.

Received the 1995 American Academy of Pediatrics' Adele D. Hofmann Award for "Distinquished Contributions in Adolescent Health", the 2000 Mayo Clinic Pediatrics Honored Alumnus Award for "National Contributions to the field of Pediatrics," and the 2003 William B Weil, Jr, MD Endowed Distinguished Pediatric Faculty Award from Michigan State University College of Medicine for "National and international recognition as well as exemplary scholarship in pediatrics." Received the 2004 Charles R Drew School of Medicine (Los Angeles, CA) Stellar Award for contributions to pediatric resident education and awarded an honorary membership in the Indian Academy of Pediatrics—an honor granted to only a few pediatricians outside of India. Was the 2007-2010 Visiting Professor of Pediatrics at Athens University, Athens, Greece and received the Michigan State University College of Human Medicine Outstanding Community Faculty Award in 2008. In 2010 he received the title of Doctor Honoris Causa from the University of Athens (Greece) as a "distinguished scientist who through outstanding work has bestowed praise and credit on the field of adolescent medicine (Ephebiatrics)." In 2010 he received the Outstanding Achievement in Adolescent Medicine Award from the Society for Adolescent Medicine "as a leading force in the field of adolescent medicine and health." In 2014 he was selected by the American Medical Association as AMA nominee for the ACGME Pediatrics Residency Review Committee (RRC) in Chicago, Illinois, USA. Past Chair of the National Conference and Exhibition Planning Group (Committee on Scientific Meetings) of the American Academy of Pediatrics and member of the Pediatric Academic Societies' (SPR/PAS) Planning Committee (1998 to Present). In 2011 elected to The Alpha Omega Alpha Honor Society (Faculty member) at Michigan State University College of Human Medicine, East Lansing, Michigan. Former member of the Appeals Committee for the Pediatrics' Residency Review Committee (RRC) of the Accreditation Council for Graduate Medical Education (Chicago, IL) in both adolescent medicine and general pediatrics. Numerous publications in pediatric and adolescent health as well as lectureships in many countries on adolescent health. Email: donald.greydanus@med.wmich.edu

Dilip R Patel, MD, FAAP, FSAM, FAACPDM, FACSM, is Professor and Chair, Department of Pediatric and Adolescent Medicine, Western Michigan University Homer

Stryker MD School of Medicine, Kalamazoo, Michigan, United States. Dr Patel has subspecialty training and interests in neurodevelopmental disabilities, developmental-behavioral pediatrics, adolescent medicine and sports medicine. He has subspecialty training and interests in neurodevelopmental disabilities, developmental-behavioral pediatrics, adolescent medicine and sports medicine. Dr Patel also has interests and holds certifications in healthcare quality and healthcare management. He is a Vanguard Member of the American College of Physican Executives. Dr Patel has received many professional awards including the Adele Hoffmann Visiting Professor Award of the Society for Adolescent Medicine, and the William Weil Endowed Distinguished Pediatric Faculty Award of the Michigan State University College of Human Medicine. He is an elected fellow of the American Academy of Cerebral Palsy and Developmental Medicine as well as the American College of Sports Medicine. He has served on numerous national committees including the editorial board of American Academy of Pediatrics Developmental-Behavioral Pediatrics PREP Program. Dr Patel has published extensively and presented at numerous national and international professional and academic events. E-mail: dilip.patel@med.wmich.edu.

Ahsan Nazeer, MD, is the division chief of Child and Adolescent Mental Health Services at Sidra Medicine. He is leading an effort to improve access to psychiatric care for children and adolescents in Qatar, clinical and education services within the Division and working to broaden psychiatric awareness particularly in the area of prevention. Dr Nazeer joined Sidra Medicine in January of 2017. Before then, he was an Associate Professor of Child and Adolescent Psychiatry at Michigan State University and then at Western Michigan University, Homer Stryker M.D School of Medicine, Kalamazoo, Michigan, United States.

Dr Nazeer went to medical school at Rawalpindi Medical College, Rawalpindi, Pakistan. He completed his psychiatry residency training at Kalamazoo Center for Medical Studies and fellowship in child and adolescent psychiatry from The University of Michigan, Ann Arbor. Dr Nazeer is certified by American Board of Psychiatry and Neurology (ABPN) in both adult and child and adolescent psychiatry.

Author of numerous articles and co-editor of two books, Dr Nazeer's research endeavors have focused on pediatric psychopharmacology and severe psychiatric disorders in youth. He is currently the co-principal investigator on a SIRF grant examining the Neurogenomics model of children with ADHD. Also, Dr. Nazeer is the PI and co-lead PI of numerous research studies ranging from investigating the validity of the rating scales to genetic underpinnings of ADHD and autism. Email: anazeer@sidra.org

Roger A Apple, PhD, is a licensed psychologist and Chief, Division of Pediatric Psychology, Director of the Autism Center and Associate Professor, Department of Pediatric and Adolescent Medicine, Western Michigan University, Homer Styker MD School of Medicine, Kalamazoo, Michigan, USA. He trained with Helen D Pratt, PhD. He has published numerous articles in pediatric psychology. Email: roger.apple@med.wmich.edu

Joav Merrick, MD, MMedSci, DMSc, born and educated in Denmark is professor of pediatrics, child health and human development, Division of Pediatrics, Hadassah Hebrew University Medical Center, Mt Scopus Campus, Jerusalem, Israel and Kentucky Children's Hospital, University of Kentucky, Lexington, Kentucky United States and professor of public health at the Center for Healthy Development, School of Public Health, Georgia State University, Atlanta, United States, the medical director of the Health Services, Division for Intellectual and Developmental Disabilities, Ministry of Social Affairs and Social Services, Jerusalem, the founder and director of the National Institute of Child Health and Human Development in Israel.

Numerous publications in the field of pediatrics, child health and human development, rehabilitation, intellectual disability, disability, health, welfare, abuse, advocacy, quality of life and prevention. Received the Peter Sabroe Child Award for outstanding work on behalf of Danish Children in 1985 and the International LEGO-Prize ("The Children's Nobel Prize") for an extraordinary contribution towards improvement in child welfare and well-being in 1987. In 2017 appointed a Kentucky Colonel by the Commonwealth of Kentucky, the highest honor the governor can bestow to a person. Email: jmerrick@zahav.net.il

About the Department of Pediatric and Adolescent Medicine, Western Michigan University Homer Stryker MD School of Medicine (WMed), Kalamazoo, Michigan, United States of America

The medical school is a collaboration of Western Michigan University (WMU) and Kalamazoo's two teaching health systems—Ascension Borgess and Bronson Healthcare. The inaugural medical student class graduated in 2018 after completing an innovative, patient-centered, four-year curriculum that prepared them to be exceptional clinicians, leaders, educators, advocates, and researchers of tomorrow. WMed also offers three Master of Science degree programs in biomedical sciences, clinical informatics and medical engineering. More than 200 residents and fellows train in ten residencies and five fellowships accredited by the Accreditation Council for Graduate Medical Education. WMed residents and fellows serve patients throughout southwest Michigan in affiliate hospitals and in the WMed Health outpatient clinics. To support its mission to educate and inspire lifelong learners, WMed has Joint Accreditation for interprofessional continuing education, which incorporates accreditation by the Accreditation Council for Continuing Medical Education.

WMed Health is the clinical practice of the medical school with more than 330 providers (including residents and fellows) offering comprehensive primary care and specialty services in several locations throughout Kalamazoo and Portage. The 350,000 square foot educational building on the WE Upjohn MD Campus located in downtown Kalamazoo, that includes research laboratories and a state-of-the-art Simulation Center that is accredited by the Society for Simulation in Healthcare.

WMed is building upon Kalamazoo's century-long foundation of drug discovery and medical device development with a strategic investment in clinical, laboratory, community, and educational research. The Center for Immunobiology, Center for Clinical Research, WMed ForenTox, Research Histology Lab, Innovation Center, Division of Epidemiology and Biostatistics, and Human Research Protection Program contribute to WMed's advancement of knowledge through innovation and discovery.

The WMed Department of Pediatric and Adolescent Medicine, with over 100 faculty members, serves to deliver both undergraduate and graduate medical education, as well as a full range of comprehensive pediatric and adolescent medicine primary and subspecialty clinical care. The department faculty members have a long history of consistent engagement in research and scholarly activities and recognition at national and international levels. The faculty members have edited and authored numerous books and hundreds of peer-reviewed publications and served as invited presenters at national and international venues. The department has developed academic ties with a variety of international medical centers and organizations, including the Queen Elizabeth Hospital in Hong Kong, Indian Academy of

Pediatrics (New Delhi, India), the University of Athens Children's Hospital (First and Second Departments of Paediatrics) in Athens, Greece and the National Institute of Child Health and Human Development in Jerusalem, Israel.

Among the many published books, edited and authored by faculty members, include: Essential adolescent medicine (McGraw-Hill Medical Publishers), The pediatric diagnostic examination (McGraw-Hill), Pediatric and adolescent psychopharmacology (Cambridge University Press), Behavioral pediatrics, through 4th Edition (Nova Science, New York), Pediatric practice: Sports medicine (McGraw-Hill), Handbook of clinical pediatrics (Singapore: World Scientific), Neurodevelopmental disabilities: Clinical care for children and young adults (Dordrecht: Springer), Adolescent medicine: Pharmacotherapeutics in medical disorders (Berlin/Boston: De Gruyter), Adolescent medicine: Pharmacotherapeutics in general, mental, and sexual health (Berlin/Boston: De Gruyter), Pediatric psychodermatology (Berlin/Boston: De Gruyter), Substance abuse in adolescents and young adults: A manual for pediatric and primary care clinicians (Berlin/Boston: De Gruyter), Tropical pediatrics (New York: Nova), and Pediatric and adolescent sexuality and gynecology (New York: Nova Science).

The Department faculty members have served as invited guest editors for a number of peer-reviewed journal special issues. These include, the Pediatric Clinics of North America, Disease a Month, Pediatric Medicine, Annals of Translational Medicine, Translational Pediatrics, Adolescent Medicine State of the Art Reviews, Primary Care Clinics in Office Practice, Current Psychopharmacology, Indian Journal of Pediatrics, and International Journal of Environmental Research and Public Health.

Contact

Professor and Chair, Dilip R Patel, MD, MBA, MPH, Email: dilip.Patel@med.wmich.edu and Professor and Founding Chair Donald E Greydanus, MD, Email: Donald.greydanus@med.wmich.edu

Department of Pediatric and Adolescent Medicine, Western Michigan University Homer Stryker MD School of Medicine, 1000 Oakland Drive, D48G, Kalamazoo, Michigan 49008-1284, United States
Website: http://www.med.wmich.edu

About Sidra Medicine, Doha, Qatar

Sidra Medicine is a 400-bed women's and children's hospital and research center in Doha, Qatar. The hospital's outpatient facility debuted in 2016, and its inpatient hospital opened in January 2018. Sidra Medicine, is part of the Qatar Foundation for Education, Science, and Community Development (QF). Weill Cornell Medicine-Qatar, Georgetown University, Carnegie Mellon University and HEC Paris are among the leading international institutions in Education City, as are newly established national research institutes such as Qatar Biomedical Research Institute and Qatar Environment and Energy Research Institute.

The **Division of Child and Adolescent Mental Health Services (CAMHS)** in the Department of Psychiatry is one of the primary sources to provide child and adolescent mental health services in the State of Qatar. The division remains at the forefront of providing clinical service, professional education as well as research and the work of the division's faculty members covers a broad range of psychiatric illnesses with a focus on providing world-class care. The Division's multi-disciplinary approach to treatment, research, and education means that child and adolescent mental health services at Sidra Medicine has a strong foundation that spans the psychological underpinnings of diseases to the molecular basis of psychiatric disorders.

The mission of the Division is to advance clinical care, research and education by the exploration of psychopathology in children and adolescents and participating in state of the art research studies. The division is also actively involved in increasing community awareness of the pathophysiology of youth mental health concerns including mood, anxiety, ADHD and autism-related disorders by providing excellent care and community educational seminars.

With an expert team of child and adolescent psychiatrists and psychologists, all of whom are trained in excellent programs and universities abroad, the Division of Child and Adolescent Mental Health provides services to children and adolescents from 5 to 18 years of age. The services are provided through an out-patient clinic, inpatient consultation and liaison team and emergency department team. The target group includes young people with a diagnosable psychiatric disorder whose condition is detrimental to their growth or development and /or who have serious difficulties in their social group, school or family.

About the National Institute of Child Health and Human Development in Israel

The National Institute of Child Health and Human Development (NICHD) in Israel was established in 1998 as a virtual institute under the auspices of the Medical Director, Ministry of Social Affairs and Social Services in order to function as the research arm for the Office of the Medical Director. In 1998 the National Council for Child Health and Pediatrics, Ministry of Health and in 1999 the Director General and Deputy Director General of the Ministry of Health endorsed the establishment of the NICHD.

Mission

The mission of a National Institute for Child Health and Human Development in Israel is to provide an academic focal point for the scholarly interdisciplinary study of child life, health, public health, welfare, disability, rehabilitation, intellectual disability and related aspects of human development. This mission includes research, teaching, clinical work, information and public service activities in the field of child health and human development.

Service and academic activities

Over the years many activities became focused in the south of Israel due to collaboration with various professionals at the Faculty of Health Sciences (FOHS) at the Ben Gurion University of the Negev (BGU). Since 2000 an affiliation with the Zusman Child Development Center at the Pediatric Division of Soroka University Medical Center has resulted in collaboration around the establishment of the Down Syndrome Clinic at that center. In 2002 a full course on "Disability" was established at the Recanati School for Allied Professions in the Community, FOHS, BGU and in 2005 collaboration was started with the Primary Care Unit of the faculty and disability became part of the master of public health course on "Children and society". In the academic year 2005-2006 a one semester course on "Aging with disability" was started as part of the master of science program in gerontology in our collaboration with the Center for Multidisciplinary Research in Aging. In 2010 collaborations with the Division of Pediatrics, Hadassah Hebrew University Medical Center, Jerusalem, Israel around the National Down Syndrome Center and teaching students and residents about intellectual and developmental disabilities as part of their training at this campus.

Research activities

The affiliated staff have over the years published work from projects and research activities in this national and international collaboration. In the year 2000 the International Journal of Adolescent Medicine and Health and in 2005 the International Journal on Disability and Human Development of De Gruyter Publishing House (Berlin and New York) were affiliated with the National Institute of Child Health and Human Development. From 2008 also the International Journal of Child Health and Human Development (Nova Science, New York), the International Journal of Child and Adolescent Health (Nova Science) and the Journal of Pain Management (Nova Science) affiliated and from 2009 the International Public Health Journal (Nova Science) and Journal of Alternative Medicine Research (Nova Science). All peer-reviewed international journals.

National collaborations

Nationally the NICHD works in collaboration with the Faculty of Health Sciences, Ben Gurion University of the Negev; Department of Physical Therapy, Sackler School of Medicine, Tel Aviv University; Autism Center, Assaf HaRofeh Medical Center; National Rett and PKU Centers at Chaim Sheba Medical Center, Tel HaShomer; Department of Physiotherapy, Haifa University; Department of Education, Bar Ilan University, Ramat Gan, Faculty of Social Sciences and Health Sciences; College of Judea and Samaria in Ariel and in 2011 affiliation with Center for Pediatric Chronic Diseases and National Center for Down Syndrome, Department of Pediatrics, Hadassah Hebrew University Medical Center, Mount Scopus Campus, Jerusalem.

International collaborations

Internationally with the Department of Disability and Human Development, College of Applied Health Sciences, University of Illinois at Chicago; Strong Center for Developmental Disabilities, Golisano Children's Hospital at Strong, University of Rochester School of Medicine and Dentistry, New York; Centre on Intellectual Disabilities, University of Albany, New York; Centre for Chronic Disease Prevention and Control, Health Canada, Ottawa; Chandler Medical Center and Children's Hospital, Kentucky Children's Hospital, Section of Adolescent Medicine, University of Kentucky, Lexington; Chronic Disease Prevention and Control Research Center, Baylor College of Medicine, Houston, Texas; Division of Neuroscience, Department of Psychiatry, Columbia University, New York; Institute for the Study of Disadvantage and Disability, Atlanta; Center for Autism and Related Disorders, Department Psychiatry, Children's Hospital Boston, Boston; Department of Pediatric and Adolescent Medicine, Western Michigan University Homer Stryker MD School of Medicine, Kalamazoo, Michigan, United States; Department of Paediatrics, Child Health and Adolescent Medicine, Children's Hospital at Westmead, Westmead, Australia; International Centre for the Study of Occupational and Mental Health, Düsseldorf, Germany; Centre for Advanced Studies in Nursing, Department of General Practice and Primary Care, University of Aberdeen,

Aberdeen, United Kingdom; Quality of Life Research Center, Copenhagen, Denmark; Nordic School of Public Health, Gottenburg, Sweden, Scandinavian Institute of Quality of Working Life, Oslo, Norway; The Department of Applied Social Sciences (APSS) of The Hong Kong Polytechnic University Hong Kong.

Targets

Our focus is on research, international collaborations, clinical work, teaching and policy in health, disability and human development and to establish the NICHD as a permanent institute in Israel in order to conduct model research and policy.

Contact

Professor Joav Merrick, MD, MMedSci, DMSc
Director, National Institute of Child Health and Human Development, Jerusalem, Israel.
E-mail: jmerrick@zahav.net.il

Section five: Index

Index

T

U

V

W

X

Z